PUBLIC HEALTH AND MUNICIPAL

T0250917

Historical Urban Studies Series

Series editors: *Jean-Luc Pinol* and *Richard Rodger*

Titles in the series include:

*Testimonies of the City: Identity, Community and Change in a
Contemporary Urban World*
Richard Rodger and Joanna Herbert (eds)

*Medicine, Charity and Mutual Aid: The Consumption of Health and Welfare in
Britain, c.1550–1950*
Anne Borsay and Peter Shapely (eds)

Paris-Edinburgh: Cultural Connections in the Belle Epoque
Siân Reynolds

The City and the Senses: Urban Culture Since 1500
Alexander Cowan and Jill Steward (eds)

*Civil Society, Associations and Urban Places: Class, Nation and Culture in
Nineteenth-Century Europe*
Graeme Morton, Boudien de Vries and R.J. Morris (eds)

*The Transformation of Urban Liberalism: Party Politics and Urban Governance in
Late Nineteenth-Century England*
James R. Moore

Property, Tenancy and Urban Growth in Stockholm and Berlin, 1860–1920
Håkan Forsell

*The European City and Green Space
London, Stockholm, Helsinki and St Petersburg, 1850–2000*
Peter Clark (ed.)

*Resources of the City
Contributions to an Environmental History of Modern Europe*
Dieter Schott, Bill Luckin and Geneviève Massard-Guilbaud (eds)

City Status in the British Isles, 1830–2002
John Beckett

Public Health and Municipal Policy Making
Britain and Sweden, 1900–1940

MARJAANA NIEMI

University of Tampere, Finland

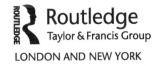

Routledge
Taylor & Francis Group

LONDON AND NEW YORK

First published 2007 by Ashgate Publishing

Published 2016 by Routledge
2 Park Square, Milton Park, Abingdon, Oxfordshire OX14 4RN
711 Third Avenue, New York, NY 10017, USA

First issued in paperback 2016

Routledge is an imprint of the Taylor & Francis Group, an informa business

British Library Cataloguing in Publication Data
Niemi, Marjaana
    Public health and municipal policy making : Britain and Sweden, 1900–1940.
– (Historical urban studies) 1.Urban health – Great Britain – History – 20th century 2.Urban health – Sweden – History – 20th century 3.Medical policy – Great Britain – History – 20th century 4.Medical policy – Sweden – History – 20th century 5.City and town life – Great Britain – History – 20th century 6.City and town life – Sweden – History – 20th century
I.Title
362.1'0941'09041

Library of Congress Cataloging-in-Publication Data
Niemi, Marjaana.
    Public health and municipal policy making : Britain and Sweden, 1900–1940 / Marjaana Niemi.
        p. cm. – (Historical urban studies series)
    ISBN 978-0-7546-0334-4 (alk. paper)
    1. Public health – Political aspects – Great Britain. 2. Medical care – Political aspects – Great Britain. 3. Medical policy – Great Britain. 4. Public health – Political aspects – Sweden. 5. Medical care – Political aspects – Sweden. 6. Medical policy – Sweden. I. Title. II. Series: Historical urban studies.

    RA395.G6N54 2006
    362.10941–dc22

                                                                    2006003896

ISBN 13: 978-1-138-27098-5 (pbk)
ISBN 13: 978-0-7546-0334-4 (hbk)

Contents

List of Figures and Tables   *vii*
General Editors' Preface   *ix*
Acknowledgements   *xi*
List of Abbreviations   *xiii*

1   Knowledge and the City   1
       Scientific Knowledge and Urban Governance   5
       Public Health Officers   7
       Committee Members and City Councillors   13
       Constructed Knowledge and Engineered Ignorance   19

2   Industrial Cities   25
       Social Classes and Urban Space   27
       Housing   32
       Economy and Employment   39
       The Family   44

3   Policy Legacies   47
       Swedish Public Health Strategies   48
       British Public Health Strategies   52
       Public Health Strategies and the New Hygiene   56

4   Regulating Family Life: Campaigns Against
    Infant Mortality, 1900–1940   61
       Introduction   61
       Dysfunctional Families: Two Definitions of One Problem   68
       Infant Welfare Campaigns and Urban Politics   90
       Conclusion   108

5   Shaping Urban Society: Campaigns Against Tuberculosis, 1900–1940   113
       Homes and Habits: Two Definitions of Tuberculosis   118
       Anti-tuberculosis Campaigns and Urban Politics   130
       For or Against the BCG Vaccination?   144
       Conclusion   155

6   Contesting and Negotiating Public Health Policies   159
       Women's Reform Activities   161
       The Working Class and Tuberculosis   173
       Conclusion   178

7   Conclusion   181
    Unruly Urban Life and Neat Scientific Categories   182
    Choosing the 'Right' Results   184
    Rival Interpretations   186
    Science and Urban Society   187

Bibliography   *189*
Index   *219*

List of Figures and Tables

Figures

1.1	Death rate per 1,000 inhabitants in Birmingham and Gothenburg, 1890–1938.	4
2.1	Decennial population growth (%) in Birmingham and Gothenburg, from the 1800s to the 1930s.	30
2.2	Typical working-class flats (*landshövdingehus*) in Albogatan, Gothenburg.	33
2.3	Plan of two typical working-class flats in Gothenburg.	34
2.4	Bagot Street in the centre of Birmingham, *c.* 1905.	37
2.5	Percentage of insured workers unemployed in Liverpool, Manchester and Birmingham, December 1929–July 1934.	42
2.6	Percentage of illegitimate births of all live births in Gothenburg and Birmingham, 1904–1936.	45
4.1	Infant mortality per 1,000 live births in Germany, France, England and Wales, and Sweden, 1875–1905.	66
4.2	Infant mortality per 1,000 live births in Birmingham and Gothenburg, 1875–1905.	67
4.3	Infant mortality in London, Liverpool, Birmingham, Manchester and Sheffield, five-year means, 1876–1900.	69
4.4	Infant mortality in Stockholm, Malmö, Norrköping and Gothenburg, five-year means, 1876–1900.	80
4.5	Milkshop Audumbla in Norrlandsgatan, Stockholm, *c.* 1895.	89
4.6	An infant welfare centre in Birmingham.	95
4.7	Plan of a new infant welfare centre from the 1920s, Warren Farm Estate, Kingstanding, Birmingham.	96
4.8	Milk inspectors at work in Gothenburg in the 1920s.	107
4.9	Infant mortality per 1,000 live births in Birmingham and Gothenburg, 1900–1936.	111
5.1	Tuberculosis mortality per 1,000 population in Gothenburg and Birmingham, 1875–1905.	116
5.2	Tuberculosis map, Birmingham, 1912.	125
5.3	Tuberculosis map, Gothenburg, 1904.	126
5.4	The brand new tuberculosis hospital in Kålltorp, Gothenburg, *c.* 1913.	133
5.5	Summer colony for children from deprived homes in the 1920s.	151
5.6	Cropwood open-air school in Birmingham.	153
5.7	A school day in the Cropwood open-air school.	154
5.8	Tuberculosis mortality per 1,000 population in Gothenburg and Birmingham, 1900–1938.	157

Tables

4.1   Infant mortality and mother's employment in St Stephen's
       and St George's Wards in Birmingham, 1908–1912.   78
5.1   Housebuilding in Gothenburg, 1920–1924.   138

Historical Urban Studies
General Editors' Preface

Density and proximity are two of the defining characteristics of the urban dimension. It is these that identify a place as uniquely urban, though the threshold for such pressure points varies from place to place. What is considered an important cluster in one context – may not be considered as urban elsewhere. A third defining characteristic is functionality – the commercial or strategic position of a town or city which conveys an advantage over other places. Over time, these functional advantages may diminish, or the balance of advantage may change within a hierarchy of towns. To understand how the relative importance of towns shifts over time and space is to grasp a set of relationships which is fundamental to the study of urban history.

Towns and cities are products of history, yet have themselves helped to shape history. As the proportion of urban dwellers has increased, so the urban dimension has proved a legitimate unit of analysis through which to understand the spectrum of human experience and to explore the cumulative memory of past generations. Though obscured by layers of economic, social and political change, the study of the urban milieu provides insights into the functioning of human relationships and, if urban historians themselves are not directly concerned with current policy studies, few contemporary concerns can be understood without reference to the historical development of towns and cities.

This longer historical perspective is essential to an understanding of social processes. Crime, housing conditions and property values, health and education, discrimination and deviance, and the formulation of regulations and social policies to deal with them were, and remain, amongst the perennial preoccupations of towns and cities – no historical period has a monopoly of these concerns. They recur in successive generations, albeit in varying mixtures and strengths; the details may differ

The central forces of class, power and authority in the city remain. If this was the case for different periods, so it was for different geographical entities and cultures. Both scientific knowledge and technical information were available across Europe and showed little respect for frontiers. Yet despite common concerns and access to broadly similar knowledge, different solutions to urban problems were proposed and adopted by towns and cities in different parts of Europe. This comparative dimension informs urban historians as to which were systematic factors and which were of a purely local nature: general and particular forces can be distinguished.

These analytical and comparative frameworks inform this book. Indeed, thematic, comparative and analytical approaches to the historical study of towns and cities is the hallmark of the Historical Urban Studies series which now extends to over 30 titles, either already published or currently in production. European urban historiography has been extended and enriched as a result and this book makes another important addition to an intellectual mission to which we, as General Editors, remain firmly committed.

Richard Rodger   *University of Leicester*
Jean-Luc Pinol   *Université de Lyon II*

Acknowledgements

The list of people who have provided support and encouragement over the last years is long, and includes colleagues, friends and family. A few I would like to single out for special recognition. First of all, I would like to thank my family for all the affection and support they have given to me.

I would also like to express my thanks to Richard Rodger for his constructive criticism and unfailing encouragement, and to Marjatta Hietala for her enthusiasm and invaluable advice. This book would never have materialized without their continual support. My sincere appreciation goes to those who read earlier drafts and offered valuable comments, including Lucy Faire, Sally Horrocks, Robert Lee and the late David Reeder. I also benefited greatly from discussion of my work with Patricia L. Garside, Chris A. Williams, Marie C. Nelson, Lars Nilsson, Tanja Vahtikari, Peter Clark, Pertti Haapala, Lud'a Klusakova and Denise McHugh. I learnt a great deal from those who listened to papers I presented at various seminars and conferences. In particular, I would like to mention conferences on urban environmental history, where I had an opportunity to discuss my work with Dieter Schott, Christoph Bernhardt, Bill Luckin, Helen Meller, Michèle Dagenais, Geneviève Massard-Guilbaud and Harold Platt.

Archivists and librarians have guided me throughout the project. I am especially grateful to the staff of the Birmingham City Archives, the Local Studies and History Department in Birmingham Central Library, the Gothenburg City Archives, the Archives of the Gothenburg City Museum, and the Gothenburg University Library. I am also greatly indebted to JP Lehtonen, Risto Kunnari and Jouni Keskinen for helping me to produce graphs and maps and for sustaining me when my computer abilities failed me. Warm thanks go to Virginia Mattila for checking my English. Her suggestions have often helped me to find the proper articulation of my thoughts.

On the publishing side, I would like to thank Tom Gray and Emily Ebdon at Ashgate for seeing my book through the process.

Finally, I would like to thank Mari Rantasila, Katariina Mustakallio, JP Lehtonen, Mika Hakkarainen, Harri Rinta-aho and Kirsi Ahonen, who have offered the crucial support of friendship.

Funding for this study has come from the Academy of Finland and the Emil Aaltonen Foundation. I am indebted to them for their financial assistance.

List of Abbreviations

BCA	Birmingham City Archives
BIHS	Birmingham Infants' Health Society
CMO	Chief Medical Officer
GSA	Göteborgs Stadsarkiv
GSH	Göteborgs Stadsfullmäktiges Handlingar
GUB	Göteborgs Universitetsbibliotek
HC	Birmingham Health Committee
HVN	Göteborgs Hälsovårdsnämnd
HVN I	Göteborgs Hälsovårdsnämnd, I avdelningen
HVN II	Göteborgs Hälsovårdsnämnd, II avdelningen
KA	Kvinnohistorisk arkiv
LGB	Local Government Board
M&CWC	Birmingham Maternity and Child Welfare Committee
M&SWSC	Birmingham Maternity and Child Welfare Sub-Committee
MOH	Medical Officer of Health
PHC	Birmingham Public Health Committee
PH&HC	Birmingham Public Health and Housing Committee
PH&MCWC	Birmingham Public Health and Maternity and Child Welfare Committee
PRO	Public Record Office, Kew
SOU	Statens Offentliga Utredningar

CHAPTER 1

Knowledge and the City

Public health policies had a profound impact on urban life in the late nineteenth and early twentieth centuries, and yet relatively few people took an active interest in the formulation of these policies. The importance of health campaigns was widely acknowledged, there is no doubt of that, but it was one thing to endorse the health campaigns, quite another to familiarize oneself with the details of sewerage treatment systems and anti-tuberculosis schemes. In Britain, the Local Government Board deplored the state of affairs in its report in the 1880s. The Board commented that most urban policy makers had no interest in public health matters and that there was a rush for the doors as soon as these matters came up on the agenda.[1] The situation was not to change radically over the following decades. In early twentieth-century Britain and Sweden, public health committees were among the few arenas where women participated directly in the official policy making process – a clear sign that the seats on public health committees were not among the most sought-after positions.[2]

Owing to the faltering interest in public health matters, leading public health officials – both elected and administrative – were influential in the formulation of municipal health policies. In many cases, albeit not all, they were largely left to get on with their job and were not required to explain the details of their proposals to the rank and file of the city council, let alone to the general public. This suited leading health officials well. Indeed, they were often working hard to isolate public health practice even better from different political pressures surrounding questions concerning health and environment. They emphasized that if city governments were to succeed in their aim of improving the health of cities, then public health activities had to be planned along scientific lines by scientifically trained experts, and not left to ever-changing political whims. The use of latest scientific knowledge would guarantee, firstly, that health and environmental problems were dealt with as efficiently as possible. Secondly, municipal health policies which were anchored in

---

[1]   A.S. Wohl, *Endangered Lives: Public Health in Victorian Britain* (London 1984), 169.

[2]   For example, the Birmingham Public Health and Housing Committee got its first woman member in 1912, the Gothenburg Public Health Committee in 1921. Moreover, many studies have shown that women were influential in shaping one particular area of health policy – maternal and child welfare – even before they participated in the official policy making process. For discussion, see S. Koven and S. Michel, 'Womanly duties: maternalist politics and the origins of welfare states in France, Germany, Great Britain, and the United States, 1880–1920', *American Historical Review* **95** (4) (1990), 1,076–108; P.M. Thane, 'What difference did the vote make? Women in public and private life in Britain since 1918', *Historical Research* **76** (192) (2003), 268–85.

scientific knowledge would be value-free and therefore would not serve any special interests or political causes.[3] The use of scientific knowledge would enable public health officials, so it was argued, to analyse and organize the life of the city in a way which was above class antagonisms, gender conflicts and ethnic tensions, serving the best interest of the whole community.

However, municipal health authorities[4] had other important functions than just promoting the health of the community. These other functions, which inevitably influenced the way in which authorities understood health problems, were rarely discussed. This was partly because public health officials themselves were not fully aware of them, and partly because they preferred them unstated and undiscussed.[5] Firstly, municipal health authorities had an important role in maintaining social order in cities. They could ease tensions and confine conflicts in urban society by repairing some of the damage – ill health and other forms of social need – which the economic life inevitably left behind it. They could also seek to stabilize urban society by defending its fundamental principles, and in particular by maintaining the

---

[3]   For discussion about the legitimizing authority of science, see for example N.B. King, 'The scale politics of emerging diseases' and C. Sellers, 'The artificial nature of fluoridated water: between nations, knowledge, and material flows', in G. Mitman, M. Murphy and C. Sellers (eds), *Landscapes of Exposure: Knowledge and Illness in Modern Environments/Osiris* **19** (2004), 62–76, 182–200; S. Dierig, J. Lachmund and J.A. Mendelsohn, 'Introduction: toward an urban history of science', in S. Dierig, J. Lachmund and J.A. Mendelsohn (eds), *Science and the City/Osiris* **18** (2003), 1–19; E.A. Hachten, 'In service to science and society: scientists and the public in late-nineteenth-century Russia', in L.K. Nyhart and T. Broman (eds), *Science and Civil Society/Osiris* **17** (2002), 171–209; D. Pestre, 'Science, political power, and the state', in J. Krige and D. Pestre (eds), *Science in the Twentieth Century* (Amsterdam 1997); D.S. Barnes, *The Making of a Social Disease: Tuberculosis in Nineteenth-century France* (Berkeley, CA 1995); R.N. Proctor, *Cancer Wars: How Politics Shapes What We Know and Don't Know About Cancer* (New York 1995); T.M. Porter, *Trust in Numbers: The Pursuit of Objectivity in Science and Public Life* (Princeton, NJ 1995); K. Johannisson, 'Folkhälsa: det svenska projektet från 1900 till 2:ra världskriget', *Lychnos* (1991), 139–95; C. Hamlin, *A Science of Impurity: Water Analysis in Nineteenth-century Britain* (Bristol 1990); B. Luckin, *Questions of Power: Electricity and Environment in Inter-War Britain* (Manchester 1990); J.W. Scott, *Gender and the Politics of History* (New York 1988).

[4]   'Municipal health authorities' and 'public health authorities' will be used throughout this book to refer to elected and professional public health officials who participated in the formulation of health policies. In both British and Swedish cities, the responsibility for health policies was shared among elected governors (city councillors, public health committee members, child welfare committee members and so on) and professional officers working for the public health department and for municipal hospitals.

[5]   For the different roles of local states, see M. Savage and A. Warde, *Urban Sociology, Capitalism and Modernity* (London 1993), 147–87; B.M. Doyle, 'The changing functions of urban government: councillors, officials and pressure groups', in M. Daunton (ed.), *The Cambridge Urban History of Britain, Volume III: 1840–1950* (Cambridge 2000), 287–313; R.J. Morris, 'The state, the elite and the market: the "visible hand" in the British industrial city system', in H. Diederiks, P. Hohenberg and M. Wagenaar (eds), *Economic Policy in Europe Since the Late Middle Ages: The Visible Hand and the Fortune of Cities* (Leicester 1992), 177–99.

work ethic and buttressing the family institution. Children without parents, mothers without husbands and men without jobs were often singled out for attention as problem groups, whose conduct had to be regulated in the name of health.[6]

Secondly, all municipal authorities, health authorities included, played a vital role in regulating the local economy. Economic growth was believed to be in everyone's interests, and therefore health authorities tended to support the local economy and accommodate the demands of the local business community. The local economy could be buttressed by a number of ways, for example, by securing amenable planning decisions or by developing basic urban infrastructure that was vital for the manufacturing and distribution of goods. However, municipal health authorities could also restrict the operation of local industries and trades by imposing regulations that were aimed at curtailing pollution, at improving housing standards or at protecting children and women employed in factories.[7] What is of greatest interest here, however, is that municipal health and housing authorities could intervene (or refrain from intervening) in the medical market or the housing market – a decision that inevitably had implications for the development of the private sector.

Thirdly, municipal authorities were important intermediaries in the formation of collective identity. On the one hand, they could encourage associational life based around workplaces, schools, clubs and societies. These collectivities had an important role in modern urban society, since they provided 'a basis for orderly belonging', diminishing apathy and disaffection. On the other hand, organized groups could also cause problems; their endless claims for rights and resources were difficult to fulfil and their protests could threaten public order. Consequently, municipal authorities might prefer 'to disorganize such people, to fragment and individualize the social body.'[8]

These other functions meant that leading public health officers and the members of public health committees, while not holding the most sought-after positions in municipal government, could be very influential in regulating and re-organizing the life of their city. By sheltering behind the authority of 'value-free' scientific knowledge – behind systematic investigations, impersonal statistics, bare facts and balanced reports – they were able to discuss controversial issues, to offer opinions and answers without having to acknowledge that they themselves were deeply involved in many political and social conflicts.

---

[6]   Many writers have discussed the ways in which health and welfare policies have served to maintain social order but only few of them have used an urban focus to analyse this question. Most writers have concentrated either on state strategies or on encounters between clients and the members of 'helping' professions. See, for example, D. Vincent, *Poor Citizens: The State and the Poor in Twentieth-century Britain* (London 1991), in particular 39–45, 141–7; J. Lewis, *The Politics of Motherhood: Child and Maternal Welfare in England, 1900–1939* (London 1980); S. Pedersen, *Family, Dependence, and the Origins of the Welfare State: Britain and France, 1914–1945* (Cambridge 1995); H. Waitzkin, 'A critical theory of medical discourse: ideology, social control, and the processing of social context in medical encounters', *Journal of Health and Social Behaviour* **30** (1989), 220–39.

[7]   Savage and Warde, *Urban Sociology*, 148–9; Morris, 'The state, the elite and the market'.

[8]   Savage and Warde, *Urban Sociology*, 150–51.

In this book, the impact of different political aims and pressures on 'scientific' health policies is explored by analysing early twentieth-century public health programmes in the second cities of Britain and Sweden: Birmingham and Gothenburg. The ways in which public health campaigns were shaped by political and social concerns is sharply revealed by examining policies pursued by officials who had access to similar scientific findings. The British and Swedish public health experts were part of one public health community, enjoying close links, attending the same international conferences and contributing to the same journals. They had access to the same body of medical knowledge, and they claimed firm scientific grounds for their programmes. The problems they dealt with were also very similar. Both Birmingham and Gothenburg were relatively healthy industrial cities, and the overall health status of the population in these cities was about the same, if the crude death rate is used as a measure (see Figure 1.1). On the basis of these factors, one could assume that the public health policies pursued by the Birmingham and Gothenburg health authorities would have been relatively close to each other. Yet they were often strikingly different, and these differences were not necessarily related to the severity of the specific problem. The Birmingham and Gothenburg authorities clearly gave different emphases to the same medical findings and drew different, yet equally logical, conclusions from the same medical facts.

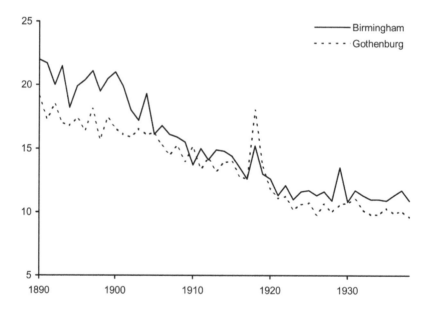

Figure 1.1   Death rate per 1,000 inhabitants in Birmingham and Gothenburg, 1890–1938.

Source: Annual Report of the MOH for Birmingham 1910, 11; 1938, 254; Statistisk årsbok för Göteborg 1949, 21–3.

Scientific Knowledge and Urban Governance

This book explores the political and cultural history of public health, examining in particular how health authorities, wittingly and unwittingly, used 'value-free' scientific knowledge about health and illness to advance political and social aims in early twentieth-century industrial cities. In order words, the aim is to combine the analysis of urban governance with the enhanced understanding of the authority of science in society. The scientific knowledge in which public health policies in Britain and Sweden were anchored was partly 'produced' by professional health officers themselves. By using sanctioned scientific methods, and especially statistical techniques, health officers produced 'value-free' knowledge, for example, about the incidence of diseases among different sections of the population and about the links between particular ways of life and the exposure to disease and death. Alongside this type of statistical knowledge, they made use of the findings of medicine and natural and social sciences to analyse urban health problems and to respond to them.[9]

How did the statistical and the scientific knowledge on which public health programmes were based further political and economic interests and reinforce cultural and moral norms? Debates about the socio-cultural dimensions of medicine and health care have provided useful insights into this theme. Particularly important is the recognition that the basic social implications of capitalist economic arrangements, the family system and the nation state have fundamentally shaped our knowledge about health and illness during the last two centuries. Hence the identification of collective well-being with the market economy, the family system and the major national interests has been implicit in basically all definitions of public health problems and in responses to them. This in turn has meant that the tools of public health medicine, while sharp for some health problems, have often been dull for problems that derive, for example, from economic insecurity, gender inequality or ethnic discrimination.[10] By building on these insights, this book aims to shed light on the ways in which the scientific knowledge that municipal health authorities produced or used reflected and reinforced local economic and social arrangements.

The comparative study brings two points into sharp relief. Firstly, it shows that public health officials in large cities, together with medical civil servants in central government, exerted considerable influence on what was taken as scientific knowledge in society. They themselves 'produced' scientific knowledge about health

---

[9] In this chapter, a distinction is made between the production of knowledge and its deployment in order to clarify the argument. This distinction is artificial; producing and using knowledge cannot be separated from each other.

[10] See, for example, A. Sears, '"To teach them how to live": the politics of public health from tuberculosis to AIDS', *Journal of Historical Sociology* **5** (1) (1992), 61–83; Proctor, *Cancer Wars*; G. Kearns, 'Tuberculosis and the medicalisation of British Society, 1880–1920', in J. Woodward and R. Jütte (eds), *Coping with Sickness: Historical Aspects of Health Care in a European Perspective* (Sheffield 1995), 147–70; Waitzkin, 'A critical theory of medical discourse'; B. Harrison, 'Women and health', in J. Purvis (ed.), *Women's History: Britain, 1850–1945: An Introduction* (London 1995), 157–92. For an overview of research on socio-cultural dimensions of medicine and health care, see D. Lupton, *Medicine as Culture: Illness, Disease and the Body in Western Societies* (London 1995).

and illness, they encouraged scientists to produce a certain type of knowledge, and when they 'consumed' knowledge produced outside public health departments, they used it selectively, reshaping and reconstructing it to suit broader political purposes.[11] In particular, municipal health authorities shaped scientific knowledge about health and illness in a way which enabled them to reconcile their different aims and to mediate conflicts between social classes and between different gender, ethnic and age groups. Reconciling different, often conflicting, aims was a continuous process. For example, there seemed to be irreconcilable divergences between supporting the family institution and facilitating free market mechanisms. Similarly, there were clearly some tensions between the measures which aimed at improving the well-being of women and the measures which supported the male bread-winner family model. Having alleviated one set of problems, municipal authorities often realized that they had made another set worse.[12] However, no matter how unstable and fragmented health policies were, when placed on a firm 'scientific' foundation they appeared relatively coherent and consistent. Irrespective of the fact that they clearly reinforced existing relationships of power and structures of inequality, they could be defended as impartial and value-free.

Secondly, this book shows clearly the large extent to which political decisions were (and are) justified by appeals to the authority of 'value-free' science. Despite the enormous power that scientific knowledge has had as a legitimizing rhetoric in municipal policy making, the role of experts and scientific knowledge in mediating urban conflicts and in regulating the life of city has only recently been studied systematically by urban historians.[13] Even less attention has been paid to the ways in which scientific knowledge has been used by the groups that have had no direct access to the production of scientific knowledge. By comparing health policies in

---

[11]   For the different ways in which science and the city have interacted, see also Dierig, Lachmund and Mendelsohn, 'Introduction'.

[12]   Savage and Warde, *Urban Sociology*, 147–87; A. Oakley, *Man and Wife: Richard and Kay Titmuss: My Parents' Early Years* (London 1997), 6. Jose Harris has argued that the belief in natural unity of social and market concerns began to fragment around the turn of the century. J. Harris, 'Economic knowledge and British social policy', in M.O. Furner and B. Supple (eds), *The State and Economic Knowledge. The American and British Experiences* (Cambridge 1990), 397.

[13]   See for example, H.L. Platt, '"Clever microbes": bacteriology and sanitary technology in Manchester and Chicago during the Progressive Age', in Mitman, Murphy and Sellers, *Landscapes of Exposure*, 149–66; Dierig, Lachmund and Mendelsohn, 'Introduction'; D. Pomfret, 'The city of evil and the great outdoors: the modern health movement and the urban young, 1918–40', *Urban History* **28** (3) (2001), 405–27; R.J. Morris, 'Governance: two centuries of urban growth', in R.J. Morris and R.H. Trainor (eds), *Urban Governance: Britain and Beyond Since 1750* (Aldershot 2000), 1–14; I. Maver, 'Glasgow's civic government', in W.H. Fraser and I. Maver (eds), *Glasgow, Volume II: 1830 to 1912* (Manchester 1996), 441–85; S. Sturdy, 'The political economy of scientific medicine: science, education and the transformation of medical practice in Sheffield, 1890–1922', *Medical History* **36** (1992), 125–59. However, the role of scientific knowledge in municipal policy making and the interaction between science and the city have received relatively scant attention in important collections such as M. Daunton (ed.), *The Cambridge Urban History of Britain, Volume III: 1840–1950* (Cambridge 2000).

two early twentieth-century industrial cities, it is possible to discuss the extent to which the regulation of urban society was legitimized by scientific knowledge about health and illness. Furthermore, this approach also opens an opportunity to discuss how different groups contested authorities' views and how they used scientific knowledge to articulate their demands.

Finally, this study does not argue that municipal health authorities *abused* science to advance political aims or suggest that they could have *used* science in a better, apolitical way. An approach of this type would imply that there were value-free scientific ideas and theories that some right-minded, enlightened health authorities could have used to the 'real' benefit of the whole community. This certainly was not the case: all scientific theories and ideas as well as their applications were affected by political and social concerns.[14] By looking at the policies that the Birmingham and Gothenburg health authorities pursued, this study examines processes whereby power structures were legitimized and challenged in urban societies, and the role which scientific knowledge and 'scientific' public health policy played in these processes. Making moral judgements about what individual public health officers or committee members did or did not do is of no interest here.

Before developing the research questions further, it is important to discuss in more detail why medical power grew in municipal policy making and why science and medicine became so important as a source of authority. In the 1850s and 1860s, science and medicine had not yet been established as sources of authority to which public health officials could automatically resort for the legitimization of their programmes. By the early twentieth century, they had become such ultimate arbiters in many health and social matters, and public health authorities themselves had helped to bring about the change. Both public health officers and elected public health officials actively built up the prestige of science in the late nineteenth and early twentieth centuries.[15] The different reasons why they promoted a new scientific policy making culture, and the negotiations and conflicts through which they managed to build up their own status and that of science will be discussed in the next two sections.

Public Health Officers

The status and power of the whole of the medical profession rose significantly in the late nineteenth and early twentieth centuries. Studies concerned with the professionalization of medical doctors show that the social basis of their authority varied considerably from country to country, but the studies also reveal some close parallels. What was common to all medical doctors across national borders was

---

[14]   For criticism of the use/abuse model, see L. Jordanova, *Sexual Visions: Images of Gender in Science and Medicine between the Eighteenth and Twentieth Centuries* (New York 1989), 15–16; L. Jordanova, 'The social construction of medical knowledge', *Social History of Medicine* **8** (3) (1995), 367; M. Tiles, 'A Science of Mars or of Venus?', *Philosophy* **62** (1987), 293–306; R.N. Proctor, *Value-free Science? Purity and Power in Modern Knowledge* (Cambridge, MA 1991), 1–11.

[15]   Sturdy, 'The political economy'; Jordanova, 'The social construction', 367–8.

that the success of their professional project did not depend on the efficacy of their therapeutic or preventive measures. The assumption that doctors' growing authority was based on their capacity to transform scientific discoveries into effective practical procedures that cured illnesses and alleviated suffering is convenient for many purposes, and not least for doctors themselves, but there is hardly any evidence to support the hypothesis. Efficiency, as many writers have shown, was not an important criterion of occupational status at the turn of the twentieth century any more than it seems to be at the present time. Neurologists are highly respected despite the fact that they are only rarely able to cure serious neurological conditions, whereas venereologists, whose therapeutic measures are usually successful, are not.[16]

Thus, the authority of the medical profession was not based on practitioners' capacity to utilize the content of science. Rather, it was based on their determination to build up the prestige of science and their ability to turn this newly created prestige to their own advantage. Medical doctors increasingly invoked scientific findings to verify the efficiency of their actions and to improve their professional status. This in turn gave science and medicine more credibility and visibility as a source of judgement in society and paved the way for further expansion of these fields.[17] In Britain, because of different traditions, the development of the interconnection between science and professional authority followed somewhat different lines from that in Sweden.

The differences are relevant to this study since they shed light on public health doctors' standing in Britain and Sweden and on their power and prestige in relation to other segments of the medical profession and to the state bureaucracy.[18] Why did the pursuit of scientific 'objectivity' and 'neutrality' in the creation of health policies

---

[16] M.J. Peterson, *The Medical Profession in Mid-Victorian London* (Berkeley, CA 1978); S.E.D. Shortt, 'Physicians, science, and status: issues in the professionalization of Anglo-American medicine in the nineteenth century', *Medical History* **27** (1983), 51–68; T. McKeown, *The Role of Medicine: Dream, Mirage or Nemesis?* (Oxford 1979), xii; K. Johannisson, *Medicinens öga: Sjukdom, medicin och samhälle – historiska erfarenheter* (Stockholm 1990), 30–41; Proctor, *Cancer Wars*, 265–70.

[17] For the growing emphasis on personal medical care in public health policy in the early twentieth century, see for example J. Lewis, *What Price Community Medicine? The Philosophy, Practice and Politics of Public Health since 1919* (Brighton 1986), 1–10; J. Lewis, 'Providers, "consumers", the state and the delivery of health-care services in twentieth-century Britain', in A. Wear (ed.), *Medicine in Society: Historical Essays* (Cambridge 1992), 317–45; S. Cherry, *Medical Services and the Hospitals in Britain, 1860–1939* (Cambridge 1996), 17–20, 48–51; W. Kock (ed.), *Medicinalväsendet i Sverige 1813–1962* (Stockholm 1963); Johannisson, 'Folkhälsa'.

[18] For the discussion about the role and professional status of British medical officers of health and tuberculosis officers, see D. Porter, 'Stratification and its discontents: professionalization and conflict in the British public health service, 1848–1914', in E. Fee and R.M. Acheson (eds), *A History of Education in Public Health: Health that Mocks the Doctors' Rules* (Oxford 1991), 83–113; Lewis, *What Price Community Medicine?*, 8–12; W.S. Walton, 'The history of the Society of Medical Officers of Health 1856–1956', *Public Health* **69** (8) (1956), 160–226; L. Bryder, *Below the Magic Mountain: A Social History of Tuberculosis in Twentieth-century Britain* (Oxford 1988), 72–4. For public health doctors in the Nordic countries, see Johannisson, *Medicinens öga*, 30–41; E. Riska, 'The medical profession in the

become an essential part of public health officers' professional project? Exactly what could health officers expect to gain by convincing elected policy makers and the public that they were able to view health and social problems objectively and impartially? Depending on the country, there are different answers to this question, but Theodore M. Porter's conclusion that '[o]bjectivity lends authority to officials who have very little of their own' can be applied, with modification, to public health officers in both Britain and Sweden.[19]

A New Hierarchy in British Medicine: A New Order in Industrial Cities

Although all British doctors across the wide spectrum of medical careers saw science as a vehicle for enhancing their authority, the profession, as Christopher Lawrence shows, was 'extremely variegated ... in its definition, evaluation and use of science'.[20] The men at the top of the profession were selective in invoking the authority of science, since they considered science both an opportunity and a threat. In the late nineteenth century, the professional authority of the British medical elite was still largely founded on their classical education, on their appointments at voluntary hospitals and medical schools, and on their wealthy clientele, who chose their doctors on the basis of class background, not medical skills and scientific merit. While these pre-eminent physicians often emphasized the scientific basis of medicine, many of them were strongly opposed to reforms which threatened to reduce clinical medicine to a body of technical, scientific knowledge which could be mastered by anyone who had medical training. It was in their interest to draw a distinction between 'ordinary' scientific knowledge and the knowledge that was needed in good clinical practice. The knowledge which the great clinicians possessed, they argued, was 'incommunicable' and private, since it came only with long experience and with the bearing of a gentleman, whereas scientific knowledge was 'communicable', public and, at least in theory, available to everyone.[21]

Despite the determined rearguard action fought by some elite members of the medical profession, scientific research methods and laboratory-based techniques steadily gained ground in the British medical world, from medical research to public health care, and finally to bedside medicine.[22] The great appeal of scientific techniques for public health doctors is not surprising. In late nineteenth-century

Nordic countries', in F.W. Hafferty and J. McKinlay (eds), *The Changing Medical Profession: An International Perspective* (New York 1993), 150–61.

[19]   Porter, *Trust in Numbers*, 8.

[20]   C. Lawrence, 'Incommunicable knowledge: science, technology and the clinical art in Britain, 1850–1914', *Journal of Contemporary History* **20** (4) (1985), 503.

[21]   C. Lawrence, *Medicine in the Making of Modern Britain, 1700–1920* (London 1994), 66–9; Lawrence, 'Incommunicable knowledge', 503–20; W.F. Bynum, *Science and the Practice of Medicine in the Nineteenth Century* (Cambridge 1994).

[22]   For the growing involvement of new scientific knowledge and laboratory-based techniques in British and American medical practice, see Sturdy, 'The political economy'; J.D. Howell, 'Machines and medicine: technology transforms the American hospital', in D.E. Long and J. Golden (eds), *The American General Hospital: Communities and Social Contexts* (Ithaca, NY 1989), 109–34.

and early twentieth-century industrial cities, public health officers – not hospital consultants or general practitioners – were in the front line of mediating class conflict and other social tensions, and of regulating those aspects of urban life which appeared to threaten public health and the prevailing social order. As Steve Sturdy shows, scientific knowledge and techniques contributed significantly to the development of new managerial and administrative responses to these problems and tensions. In the new administrative culture, which reflected the political shift from Tory paternalism to more Liberal views, public health officers surveyed society, identified appropriate sites for intervention and sought to intervene at these sites with maximum efficiency and with minimum cost and criticism. The public health science that located problems and suggested 'value-free' responses to them became indispensable to the running of large industrial cities.[23]

Another reason why many public health doctors were at the forefront of the introduction of scientific techniques was that they saw in this approach a chance of elevating their own status within the medical profession and in society in general. Thus, if the elite doctors who opposed scientific techniques were not completely disinterested, nor were the public health doctors who advocated these reforms. Both groups had their own interests at heart. The push for a scientific approach in both public health medicine and clinical medicine came mainly from aspiring young doctors who were soundly read in basic sciences rather than classics, and whose class background was not likely to smooth their way to the positions of power. For them, the best chance of accumulating professional authority was to build up the prestige of science and of scientifically trained experts.

The challenge to the old order had partial success both in the field of clinical medicine and in that of public health. Full-time medical officers of health in particular succeeded in improving the economic and social status of their office by introducing stricter scientific standards for their work.[24] Yet the changes which the scientific approach brought about within the medical profession were by no means radical. Once the medical elite acknowledged that scientific techniques had come to stay and that further resistance would be futile, they concentrated on controlling the direction of the change. As a result, the new hierarchy of British medicine that took shape in the early twentieth century largely reflected and reinforced the same class divisions as the old one. While the social and economic position of the leading public health officers improved, they were still far from the top of the profession.[25]

---

[23]   Sturdy, 'The political economy'; M. Niemi, 'Public health discourses in Birmingham and Gothenburg 1890–1920', in S. Sheard and H. Power (eds), *Body and City: Histories of Urban Public Health* (Aldershot 2000). See also B. Latour, *The Pasteurization of France* (Cambridge, MA 1988); Barnes, *The Making of a Social Disease*. For the growing role of managerial and administrative strategies, see H. Perkin, *The Rise of Professional Society: England since 1880* (London 1990), 286–358.

[24]   A. Ransome, H.E. Armstrong and J.F.J. Sykes, 'The training and qualification of medical officers of health', *Public Health* (1893–94), 242–8; Porter, 'Stratification and its discontents'.

[25]   Sturdy, 'The political economy'; Porter, 'Stratification and its discontents'. For the ways in which elites have regulated the direction and pace of social and economic change, see for example, R. Rodger, 'Managing the market – regulating the city: urban control in

A New Deal Between Experts and the Swedish State

In Sweden, the adoption of new scientific knowledge and techniques in public health medicine was stimulated by the same factors as in Britain. Public health doctors working in urban areas were interested in reforming their work, since new scientific techniques provided them with means of 'knowing' the population and efficient methods of managing it.[26] Moreover, many public health doctors hoped that by forging a new scientific identity for their speciality they could raise their professional status. However, the locus of the status competition was one feature that clearly distinguished the development of new 'scientific' public health medicine in Britain and in Sweden. In Britain, the leading public health officers, together with university professors and aspiring general practitioners, allied themselves to the development of science to strengthen their status in society in general and in relation to the old medical elite, which consisted almost exclusively of upper-class and upper-middle-class doctors. In Sweden, by contrast, the medical profession invoked the authority of science to enhance their prestige and power in relation to the state bureaucracy. These distinctive characteristics are largely traceable to the extent and nature of state intervention in the medical market in these countries.[27]

The development of the British medical profession shows that state intervention in health care and a high level of professional autonomy and control on the part of medical doctors were not necessarily irreconcilable. The 1858 Medical Act had set the seal on the partnership between the state and orthodox medicine, giving registered medical doctors official recognition and distinguishing them from 'unqualified' practitioners such as homeopaths, bone-setters and medical botanists. In the late nineteenth and early twentieth centuries, the state further supported medical dominance in the arena of health and disease by blocking avenues of advancement for other health workers such as midwives, nurses, radiographers and physiotherapists.[28] At the same time, the medical profession was largely allowed to set its own standards and rules, and the role of the state in regulating and expanding the market for medical services was relatively limited. Local authorities offered medical practitioners full-time careers and part-time posts as medical officers of health, poor

---

the nineteenth-century United Kingdom', in Diederiks, Hohenberg and Wagenaar, *Economic Policy in Europe*, 200–219.

[26] Niemi, 'Public health discourses'; K. Johannisson, 'The people's health: public health policies in Sweden', in D. Porter (ed.), *The History of Public Health and the Modern State* (Amsterdam 1994), 174–8; Johannisson, 'Folkhälsa'.

[27] For comparative accounts, see G. Kearns, W.R. Lee and J. Rogers, 'The interaction of political and economic factors in the management of urban public health', in M.C. Nelson and J. Rogers (eds), *Urbanisation and the Epidemiological Transition* (Uppsala 1989), 22–4; I. Waddington, 'Medicine, the market and professional autonomy: some aspects of the professionalization of medicine', in W. Conze and J. Kocka (eds), *Bildungsbürgertum im 19. Jahrhundert. Teil I: Bildungssystem und Professionalisierung in internationalen Vergleichen* (Stuttgart 1992), 388–416.

[28] G. Larkin, *Occupational Monopoly and Modern Medicine* (London 1983); A. Witz, *Professions and Patriarchy* (London 1992); I. Waddington, *The Medical Profession in the Industrial Revolution* (Dublin 1984), 135–52; Lawrence, *Medicine*, 55–7.

law medical officers, factory inspectors and, in the early twentieth century, as school medical officers. However, these office-holders were in a minority in the medical profession. The National Insurance Act of 1911 increased state involvement in the medical market substantially, but medical doctors' control over their own work was ensured by giving them considerable scope to participate in the administration of the Act.[29]

In Sweden, state intervention placed more constraints on the professional autonomy of medical doctors. On the one hand, the state contributed to the professionalization of medicine, smoothing the way up the social and professional ladders for medical men.[30] On the other hand, the state actively expanded and regulated the market for medical services throughout the nineteenth century, drawing the medical profession into a network of state-bureaucratic relationships and limiting the autonomy and control they had over their work.[31] The development of private health care services was slow in Sweden, mainly because of low population density, low levels of urbanization and late industrialization. The potential as well as the actual size of the private medical market remained small, and the state was instrumental in providing the infrastructure for the expansion of modern medicine and a modern medical profession. The vast majority of medical practitioners, including the medical elite, were in public service, even though many public health doctors also maintained a private practice to supplement their salaries. Not less than 90 per cent of Swedish medical practitioners held a public appointment in 1880, and about 63 per cent in 1900 and 1920.[32]

Thus, the expansion of both preventive and curative medicine in eighteenth- and nineteenth-century Sweden was a case of exchange: the Crown provided medical practitioners with posts and pensions, and medical practitioners did their best to combat epidemics and to improve the nation's health. While state patronage was undoubtedly advantageous to the medical profession, the state emerged as the main beneficiary of this interdependent relationship, the priorities of the government

---

[29] B.N. Armstrong, *The Health Insurance Doctor: His Rôle in Great Britain, Denmark and France* (Princeton, NJ 1939); J.L. Brand, *Doctors and the State: The British Medical Profession and Government Action in Public Health, 1870–1912* (Baltimore, MD 1965); A. Digby, *Making a Medical Living: Doctors and Patients in the English Market for Medicine, 1720–1911* (Cambridge 1994), 16, 120–24, 169, 289–90; A. Digby and N. Bosanquet, 'Doctors and patients in an era of national health insurance and private practice, 1913–1938', *Economic History Review* **41** (1) (1988), 74–94; Lewis, 'Providers'.

[30] Women did not enter the profession until the late nineteenth century.

[31] On the shifting balance of power between the state and the medical profession, see Kearns, Lee and Rogers, 'The interaction of political and economic factors', 19–22; H. Ito, 'Health insurance and medical services in Sweden and Denmark 1850–1950', in A.J. Heidenheimer and N. Elvander (eds), *The Shaping of the Swedish Health System* (London 1980), 44–67.

[32] H. Bergstrand, 'Läkarekåren och provinsialläkareväsendet', in Kock, *Medicinalväsendet*, 120–46; Ito, 'Health insurance'; Riska, 'The medical profession'; M.C. Nelson and J. Rogers, 'Cleaning up the cities: application of the first comprehensive public health law in Sweden', *Scandinavian Journal of History* **19** (1) (1994), 17–20; Kearns, Lee and Rogers, 'The interaction of political and economic factors', 22–5.

weighing more heavily in policy making than the professional interests of medical doctors. However, in the last decades of the nineteenth century the situation began to change. The medical profession still derived great prestige from its connection with the state, but at the same time, together with other professionals such as engineers, they successfully promoted a new culture in which science was an important source of cultural authority.[33] The adoption of new scientific knowledge and scientific techniques in public health and clinical medicine was a central part of the process whereby medical doctors assumed an influential role in shaping health policies at both national and local level. Thus, while in Britain the introduction of new scientific techniques was a vehicle for creating a new social and intellectual hierarchy within the medical profession, for Swedish doctors scientific expertise was primarily a means of making a new deal with the state, of re-negotiating the status of the profession and the state bureaucracy. This deal, which emerged in the late nineteenth and early twentieth centuries, provided a basis for the close co-operation between government and medical authority, or between the state and experts in general, which has been so characteristic of the Nordic countries ever since.[34]

Committee Members and City Councillors

The appearance of impartiality and progressive responsibility which scientific rhetoric could impart was also important for elected city governors. In both Britain and Sweden, city councils and council committees were presumed to place the common good before vested interests, especially in questions such as the health of the population. These bodies sought to appear reasonably disinterested, since failure to do so served to erode their credibility and authority. Individual members of these bodies naturally engaged in party politics and were sometimes openly political, advancing the interests of the groups that had elected them.[35] But even they

---

[33] K. Johannisson, 'Why cure the sick? Population policy and health programs 18th-century Swedish mercantilism', in A. Brändström and L.-G. Tedebrand (eds), *Society, Health and Population During the Demographic Transition* (Stockholm 1988), 323–30; Johannisson, *Medicinens öga*, 30–41; Kearns, Lee and Rogers, 'The interaction of political and economic factors', 22–4. For the professionalization of engineers in Sweden, see R. Torstendahl, 'Engineers in Sweden and Britain 1820–1914: professionalisation and bureaucratisation in a comparative perspective', in Conze and Kocka, *Bildungsbürgertum*, 543–60.

[34] On the important role that experts – medical doctors, economists and engineers – had in policy making in Sweden, see Johannisson, 'The people's health'; M. Weir and T. Skocpol, 'State structures and the possibilities for "Keynesian" responses to the Great Depression in Sweden, Britain, and the United States', in P.B. Evans, D. Rueschemeyer and T. Skocpol (eds), *Bringing the State Back In* (Cambridge 1985), 107–63; Torstendahl, 'Engineers'. For contemporary accounts, see for example B. Thomas, *Monetary Policy and Crises: A Study of Swedish Experience* (London 1936), xix–xxi; D.V. Glass, 'Population policies in Scandinavia', *Eugenics Review* **30** (2) (1938), 89–100. For Britain, see G. Savage, *The Social Construction of Expertise: The English Civil Service and Its Influence, 1919–1939* (Pittsburgh, PA 1996).

[35] See, for example, I. Maver, 'The role and influence of Glasgow's municipal managers, 1890s–1930s', in R.J. Morris and R.H. Trainor (eds), *Urban Governance: Britain and Beyond Since 1750* (Aldershot 2000), 69–85.

often emphasized, with calculation or conviction, that the reforms they tried to push through would serve the best interests of the whole community.

Legitimizing Policy Decisions

Fusing group interests and 'the common good' in public health rhetoric was comparatively easy for the groups that were at the centres of political power and cultural production. They exerted a powerful influence on how 'the best interest of the community' was defined, ensuring that this ideal was never too far away from their own aims and interests. Moreover, many of their policy proposals seemed neutral and value-free simply because they did not usually challenge the status quo in society. Keeping things as they are generally appears less political than changing them.[36] Thus, influential groups did not necessarily need to conceal their aspirations and interests. Yet they often preferred to do so. As long as they were able to achieve important aims by expressing their political interests in a 'value-free', scientific form, there was no point in antagonizing opponents and in being too demonstrative in the use of power. By couching proposals in scientific terms, they could claim that the measures they proposed were the 'right' answers to urban health problems, not a means of promoting narrow party or group interests.

Science was also important for groups that were on the political and cultural margins. These groups had little influence on how 'the best interest of the community' was defined. Consequently, the reforms they called for and the proposals they put forward tended to clash with the prevailing definitions of the common good and to appear very political. By using scientific language and by emphasizing those aspects of their proposals which were broadly in line with the current notions of the common good, these groups were able to tone down the political flavour of their proposals and to make them more palatable to other policy makers.

Legitimizing the Existing Political System

Yet to concentrate exclusively on day-to-day policy making is to risk missing out on what was at least as essential: while new scientific knowledge and techniques were useful in legitimizing specific policy decisions, they could also provide 'up-to-date' explanations and justification for the existing political system as a whole. In the late nineteenth and early twentieth centuries, scientific knowledge about the health of the population generally reinforced the view that existing class and gender arrangements, for example the unequal distribution of political power, were essentially natural. The fact that men wielded more political power than women did indeed follow logically from natural, scientifically proven differences between the sexes. Opening some new opportunities for women in the political arena was possible, and perhaps even desirable, but absolute equality in terms of political power would clearly be

---

[36] S. Tesh, *Hidden Arguments: Political Ideology and Disease Prevention Policy* (New Brunswick, NJ 1988); S. Tesh, 'Disease, causality and politics', *Journal of Health Politics, Policy and Law* **6** (3) (1981), 369–90.

against Nature.[37] Similarly, while the working class was gradually absorbed into local and national political life, it was often considered natural that middle-class people continued to occupy a more exalted place in central and local governments. This arrangement was sanctioned by scientific findings which showed that 'talent' was more thinly spread among the working class than among the middle class.[38]

Those privileged groups and individuals who did not want to explain the current political and social system exclusively in terms of inherited abilities often argued that the initiative, skill and effort of individuals were important determinants of social position. New scientific knowledge also offered powerful support for their views. For example, statistical information about the health, hygiene and habits of different sections of the population, convincingly presented in charts and maps, drew a clear distinction between healthy and unhealthy residential areas, and between rational and irrational townspeople. Statistical and scientific knowledge of this type served to build up the confidence of the middle class and to create the rationale for them to lay claim to political power at local and national level. Similarly, scientific knowledge served to sanction the unequal distribution of political power between the respectable working class and the poor by 'demonstrating' that the poorest segment of the population possessed neither moral character nor economic independence.[39] Health and hygiene were great dividers. In Northern European societies, which embraced the democratic ideal, scientific 'value-free' knowledge about health and illness was one of the mechanisms sanctifying power relationships.

However, drawing upon scientific findings was also an important way in which to challenge and transform existing political and social structures. The groups that were excluded from the centres of political and social power did not have cultural autonomy, they did not have their own 'language' to describe social problems or their own scientific methods to analyse them. They had to make use of the language and scientific methods of the prevailing culture.[40] Their success in transforming

---

[37]   O. Moscucci, *The Science of Woman: Gynaecology and Gender in England, 1800–1929* (Cambridge 1993), 36–41; C. Dyhouse, *Feminism and the Family in England 1880–1939* (Oxford 1989), 74–81.

[38]   P. Bourdieu, *The State Nobility: Elite Schools in the Field of Power* (Cambridge 1998); H. Hendrick, *Children, Childhood and English Society 1880–1990* (Cambridge 1997), 65–73; G.R. Searle, 'Eugenics and class', B. Norton, 'Psychologists and class', and G. Sutherland, 'Measuring intelligence: English local education authorities and mental testing, 1919–1939', in C. Webster (ed.), *Biology, Medicine and Society 1840–1940* (Cambridge 1981), 217–42, 289–314, 315–35.

[39]   For the 'mapping' of cities, see Niemi, 'Public health discourses'; C. Topalov, 'The city as *terra incognita*: Charles Booth's poverty survey and the people of London, 1886–91', *Planning Perspectives* **8** (4) (1993), 395–425. For social structures and people's behaviour, see N. Elias, *The Civilizing Process: The History of Manners & State Formation and Civilization* (Oxford 1994); L. Davidoff and C. Hall, *Family Fortunes: Men and Women of the English Middle Class 1780–1850* (London 1992), 382–3, 445–9; J. Frykman and O. Löfgren, *Den kultiverade människan* (Malmö 1979).

[40]   Some feminist writers argue (or assume) that there is a fundamental, universal difference between feminine and masculine moral reasoning and that women have a degree of cultural autonomy. See for example, C. Gilligan, *In a Different Voice: Psychological Theory*

social structures depended on whether they were able to draw upon these methods and language for their own ends. For example, both feminists calling for a wider role for women and their opponents desirous of limiting women's role in policy making often built their campaigns on the same 'scientifically proven' assumption of women's distinctive characteristics.[41] The opponents argued that since women were fundamentally different from men, they should concentrate on their role as wives and mothers. The feminists, for their part, claimed that society could achieve its full potential only if women were allowed to participate more fully in policy making. Women, the feminists argued, had unique insights into such issues as health and social welfare, and therefore society would benefit from all reforms which opened up new opportunities for them in these policy areas.[42]

Beyond the Reach of Political Argument

While both public health officers and elected city governors regarded science as an important basis for social consensus, they did not necessarily agree on where the boundary between political questions and scientific questions should be drawn in each case. If a specific health problem was perceived as being primarily a technical question to be resolved on the basis of scientific criteria, public health officers had the initiative and they were able to define the problem to politicians.[43] This led health officers to emphasize the technical nature of health problems, and the value of their own expertise in solving these problems. Politicians naturally enough had more ambivalent feelings about the role of technical expertise in policy making. In many cases, placing health issues beyond the reach of political argument was also in their interests. They, too, preferred to operate quietly, to shelter behind the

and Women's Development (Cambridge, MA 1982); B. Smith, *Ladies of the Leisure Class: The Bourgeoisie of Northern France in the Nineteenth Century* (Princeton, NJ 1981); T. Skocpol, *Protecting Soldiers and Mothers: The Political Origins of Social Policy in the United States* (Cambridge, MA 1992); Koven and Michel, 'Womanly duties'. For a critical evaluation of this approach, see for example Scott, *Gender*, 28–50; L. McNay, *Foucault and Feminism: Power, Gender and the Self* (Cambridge 1992), 91–7. See also Chapter 6.

[41]   I use 'feminism', following Pat Thane, to refer to 'any women or group who placed prominently on their agenda the advancement of women's relative position in any respect.' P. Thane, 'Women in the British Labour Party and the construction of state welfare, 1906–1939', in S. Koven and S. Michel (eds), *Mothers of a New World: Maternalist Politics and the Origins of Welfare States* (New York 1993), 345.

[42]   S. Koven and S. Michel, 'Introduction: "mother worlds"', in Koven and Michel, *Mothers of a New World*, 1–42; K. Östberg, 'Män, kvinnor och kommunalpolitik under mellankrigstiden', in M. Taussi Sjöberg and T. Vammen (eds), *På tröskeln till välfärden* (Stockholm 1995), 202–26; Y. Hirdman, 'Särart – likhet: kvinnorörelsens scylla och karybdis? Reflektioner utifrån spröda empiriska iakttagelser rörande svensk kvinnorörelse historia under 1900-talet', in I. Frederiksen and H. Rømer (eds), *Kvinder, mentalitet, arbejde: Kvindehistorisk forskning i Norden* (Århus 1986), 27–40.

[43]   P. Starr and E. Immergut, 'Health care and the boundaries of politics', in C.S. Maier (ed.), *Changing Boundaries of the Political: Essays on the Evolving Balance between the State and Society, Public and Private in Europe* (Cambridge 1987), 221–54; R. Klein, *The New Politics of the National Health Service* (London 1995), 49–53.

authority of science, away from the glare of publicity and overt party political controversies. Yet politicians did not want the balance of power tipping in favour of public health officers. They always identified some health problems or aspects of them as political questions that were open to lay judgement and therefore under the control of political officials rather than scientific or medical experts. In these cases, public health officers usually lost the initiative, and sometimes their role was limited to providing scientific legitimization for the policies which health executives were determined to pursue.

In some policy areas, professional health officers were clearly having difficulty in claiming authority. The question that frequently sparked off fierce political controversy in the early twentieth century was defective housing. In the eyes of some property owners, public health measures that aimed to alleviate housing problems were only 'thinly disguised weapons of a great Socialistic raid upon property'. Left-wing critics, for their part, accused health officers of being cowards who did not dare to touch 'the pockets of the owners of … vile slums.'[44] Similarly, health issues concerning reproduction and sex often inspired heated debates and angry protests. The opponents of birth control insisted that public health officers should adhere to their view and save society from moral collapse, whereas the advocates urged them to provide family planning counselling and save thousands of women from serious health problems.[45] In these cases, health officers could not win. If they did nothing, they laid themselves open to charges of inaction and political bias; if they took action, they were frequently criticized for going too far and, again, serving political ends. Their stance was always contested, no matter how much scientific evidence they produced to support it.

However, most health issues, or important aspects of them, were defined as technical questions and thus removed from the political agenda. Leading public health officers and senior members of health committees may not have theorized about how the boundaries of political and technical spheres changed, but they were aware that they could pull health questions away from politics. What they had to do was to convince other policy makers and the public that there was specialized knowledge about these questions, and that they had privileged access to this knowledge. In a debate which was published in the journal of the Society of Medical Officers of Health in Britain in the early 1890s, it was pointed out several times that a medical officer of health often had to convince both elected policy makers and the public 'as to the propriety

---

[44] Birmingham City Archives (BCA), Birmingham Public Health Committee minutes 28 Feb. 1913, item 1224; A. Gough, *Objections to the Housing and Town-Planning Bill of the Right Honourable John Burns; and to the Housing of the Working Classes Bill Introduced by Mr. Bowerman: With Birmingham's Experience of the Housing Acts* (Birmingham 1908), 2; *Göteborgs Stadsfullmäktiges Handlingar 1913:337*; *1923:328* and minutes 13 Sept. 1923 and discussion; G. Göthlin, 'Några bostadshygieniska reformkrav', Göteborgs Läkaresällskaps förhandlingar 13. 9., *Hygiea* **79** (21) (1917), 1,151–69.

[45] 'Kvinnokongressen i Stockholm', *Ny Tid*, 7 Aug. 1908; 'Sexuell hygien: Dr Alma Sundqvists föredrag å soc.dem. kvinnokongressen', *Ny Tid*, 11 Aug. 1908; 'Det tomma intet', *Ny Tid*, 9 May 1910; 'Mot ofruktsamhets-propagandan: gårdagens stora opinionsmöte', *Göteborgs-Posten*, 9 May 1910; BCA Birmingham Maternity and Child Welfare Committee minutes 5 Mar. 1931, item 585; 13 Mar. 1931, item 590.

of a certain course of action, and he cannot do this without being himself a master of the subject'.[46] In practice, being a master of the subject usually meant that health officers made use of new scientific knowledge, techniques and terminology that put health issues beyond the easy scrutiny of those who were not themselves within the field. Health officers were often able to determine which issues were put on the agenda for action by accentuating some aspects of the problem and by concealing others. From the point of view of health officers, statistics was particularly useful in policy making. Statistical methods gave health officers and the leading members of health committees an opportunity to define health questions, to reveal some aspects of them, and to conceal the others. At the same time, statistics gave the public the impression that they had a means of judging the accomplishments of public health authorities. Statistics was supposed to provide knowledge that anyone could read, thoroughly public knowledge appropriate for new democratic societies.[47]

Clearly, public health officials were actively building up the prestige of science in policy making. Yet this is not to say that invoking the authority of science was always a conscious strategy to exercise power and a calculated enterprise to control the life of the city. Scientific rhetoric would never have been so effective and widely used as it was if public health officers, elected policy makers and the public had not truly believed in the ideal of science as a value-free means of analysing and solving social and health problems. Despite their apparent scepticism about some specific research findings, they all retained their confidence in science in general.[48]

Scientific investigation was supposed to yield objective and unbiased knowledge about the order of society, and in particular about the order of Nature.[49] Medical and public health research, so it was thought, would get at the real causes of diseases and suggest effective and appropriate measures. Most people agreed that, in the case of many health problems, this ultimate aim had not yet been achieved and probably would not be achieved in the near future. Very few studies and reports published in the field of medicine and public health in the early twentieth century made a pretence of providing a complete and totally accurate description of such health problems as infant mortality, tuberculosis or cancer. By contrast, most experts readily acknowledged that they were ill-informed about many aspects of these problems and that more research was needed to fill the gaps in the existing knowledge. Sometimes they even exaggerated their ignorance. Yet it was generally believed, firstly, that a

---

[46]   Ransome, Armstrong and Sykes, 'The training and qualification', the quote on p. 243.

[47]   Porter, *Trust in Numbers*. See also T.M. Porter, 'The management of society by numbers', in Krige and Pestre, *Science in the Twentieth Century*, 97–110.

[48]   For discussion, see R.D. Apple, *Vitamania: Vitamins in American Culture* (New Brunswick, NJ 1996); C. Hamlin, 'Environmental sensibility in Edinburgh, 1839–1840: the 'fetid irrigation' controversy', *Journal of Urban History* **20** (3) (1994), 311–39; Hamlin, *A Science of Impurity*, 1–15, 299–305; B.J. Good, *Medicine, Rationality, and Experience: An Anthropological Perspective* (Cambridge 1994), 1–24.

[49]   L. Jordanova, 'Introduction', in L. Jordanova (ed.), *Languages of Nature: Critical Essays on Science and Literature* (London 1986), 15–47. For the growing interest in social research concerning the nature of urban society and urban life, see Savage and Warde, *Urban Sociology*, 7–22; Topalov, 'The city'.

major part of existing knowledge was accurate, and secondly, that it was possible for medical and public health experts to fill the gaps. Scientists and other experts would gradually advance the frontiers of knowledge, working out the whole truth about health problems and finding the right answers to them.[50]

Constructed Knowledge and Engineered Ignorance

In the course of the twentieth century, the image of science and scientists was to change. The idealized view of the life of science – scientists keeping themselves at a safe distance from politics and dedicating their lives to the relentless pursuit of accurate, value-free knowledge – clashed with what people had seen and experienced. Not only had scientists been politically active outside their laboratories and studies, but they had also, wittingly and unwittingly, 'allowed' political and social concerns to affect the direction and content of their work. Nazi science, Soviet science and late twentieth-century Big Science – military research choreographing the Third World War, medical science promoting expensive high-tech strategies, and tobacco companies spending millions on research in order to buy time – have clearly shown that scientists have been ready to vindicate basically any political rule or commercial interest through scientific legitimization.[51] Similarly, scientific knowledge, and especially its applications, are no longer regarded as innocent, and many writers have raised the question of whether science is just 'other means of politics'.[52] While this question may be open to debate, it is certain that many political and social aims which could not have been achieved through political politics have been achieved through scientific, 'neutral' policies and procedures.

These critical debates, which initially arose out of the social and political upheavals of the 1960s and 1970s, have inspired a wealth of studies on what kind of knowledge science actually provides, and how this knowledge affects societies. The contributions which feminist writers have made to this debate have been particularly important. In seeking to uncover the processes which have ensured the continuance of the economic and social subordination of women, feminist researchers have analysed, for example, the production and deployment of scientific knowledge. They have shown, through theoretical argument and empirical studies, that scientific knowledge and its applications play a major role in maintaining and legitimizing

---

[50] What contemporaries meant by objectivity and truth differed from one occasion to another, see A. Megill, 'Introduction: four senses of objectivity', *Annals of Scholarship* **8** (3) (1991), 301–20.

[51] Proctor, *Value-Free Science?*; Proctor, *Cancer Wars*. See also, D.A. Hollinger, 'Free enterprise and free inquiry: the emergence of laissez-faire communitarianism in the ideology of science in the United States', *New Literary History* **21** (4) (1990), 897–919; Apple, *Vitamania*; D.A. MacKenzie, *Statistics in Britain, 1865–1930: The Social Construction of Scientific Knowledge* (Edinburgh 1981).

[52] Latour, *The Pasteurization*, the quote p. 142. For discussion, see also E. Fox Keller, *Secrets of Life. Secrets of Death: Essays on Language, Gender and Science* (New York 1992), 1–12; E. Fox Keller and H.E. Longino, 'Introduction', in E. Fox Keller and H.E. Longino (eds), *Feminism and Science* (Oxford 1996).

gender hierarchies of power. An important reason why science has been effective in reinforcing the existing structures of inequality is that its *direction, content* and *practice* have all been affected by social and political interests and, in this particular case, by historically specific ideologies of gender. Scientists and other experts have reproduced, at the level of 'universal' scientific knowledge, historically specific assumptions about femininity and masculinity. Social sciences have played a part in legitimizing women's role and position, but natural sciences have had an even more important role, biomedical sciences being the final arbiters in many issues relating to the role of women. Biomedical sciences have been influential in 'defining' the social roles of women and men, since the ultimate authority which they have invoked is Nature.[53] 'And nature [is] a difficult authority to challenge.'[54]

The issue around which this debate has revolved is sexual difference. Most present-day feminists distinguish between biological sexual difference, which is a natural phenomenon, and knowledge about this difference, gender, which is a social and cultural construct. Gender, as Joan Scott argues, is the knowledge which establishes meanings for natural physical differences between women and men. 'These meanings vary across cultures, social groups, and time, since nothing about the body ... determines univocally how social divisions will be shaped.' Thus, unequal distribution of political power between men and women or a sexual division of labour at home are (human) constructs, not a natural state of affairs.[55] Science and its applications, especially in the early twentieth century, but also, to an

---

[53]   L. Bland, *Banishing the Beast: English Feminism and Sexual Morality 1885–1914* (London 1995), esp. ch. 2; K. Johannisson, *Den mörka kontinenten: Kvinnan, medicinen och fin-de-siècle* (Stockholm 1995); Harrison, 'Women and health'; Scott, *Gender*; A. Kessler-Harris, J. Lewis and U. Wikander, 'Introduction', in U. Wikander, A. Kessler-Harris and J. Lewis (eds), *Protecting Women: Labor Legislation in Europe, the Unites States, and Australia, 1880–1920* (Urbana, IL 1995), 15–6. For a feminist analysis of scientific language, see Jordanova, *Sexual Visions*; Jordanova, 'Introduction', and 'Naturalizing the family: literature and the bio-medical sciences in the late eighteenth century', in Jordanova, *Languages of Nature*, 15–47 and 86–116; Keller, *Secrets of Life*. For natural sciences, see L. Schiebinger, *Nature's Body: Sexual Politics and the Making of Modern Science* (London 1993); D.J. Haraway, *Simians, Cyborgs, and Women: The Reinvention of Nature* (London 1991); S. Harding, *Whose Science? Whose Knowledge? Thinking from Women's Lives* (Milton Keynes 1991). For social sciences, see S. Farganis, 'Feminism and the reconstruction of social science', in A.M. Jaggar and S.R. Bordo (eds), *Gender/Body/Knowledge: Feminist Reconstructions of Being and Knowing* (New Brunswick, NJ 1992). See also, Proctor, *Value-free Science*; R. Smith, *Inhibition: History and Meaning in the Sciences of Mind and Brain* (Berkeley, CA 1992).

[54]   J.W. Scott, *Only Paradoxes to Offer: French Feminists and the Rights of Man* (Cambridge, MA 1996), x.

[55]   Scott, *Gender*, 1–11, the quote on p. 2. See also Jordanova, *Sexual Visions*; M. Poovey, *Uneven Developments: The Ideological Work of Gender in Mid-Victorian England* (Chicago, IL 1988), 1–23. Some feminist writers have strongly criticized the theoretical approach chosen by Scott, Jordanova and Poovey. For example, June Purvis attacks, to my mind unsuccessfully, their views and argues that feminists writers should focus on women, not on gender. J. Purvis, 'From "women worthies" to poststructuralism? Debate and controversy in women's history in Britain', in Purvis, *Women's History*, 1–22.

extent, at present, have promoted a very different view. They have established and consolidated sexual difference as a natural phenomenon and a natural fact which cannot be altered, which cannot have different meanings in different cultures and which determines the social roles of women and men.[56] Women who challenged this vision wanted 'biologically unnatural changes that would bring grief to the human race'.[57]

Science has also legitimized other structures of inequality than gender.[58] However, while late nineteenth and early twentieth-century science and scientists were confident that sexual difference belonged to the realm of Nature, they were less certain about whether racial and class differences were natural or social. In medical and public health literature concerned with indigenous peoples in the colonial world or with the urban poor in Europe, the view that race and class hierarchies were due to social and cultural factors was often inextricably interwoven with the view that these hierarchies were natural. Sometimes indigenous peoples and 'slum dwellers' were seen as innately inferior, as biologically different from their superiors. Sometimes they were defined as 'backward people' who lagged behind the 'advanced' races and social groups in the evolutionary process but who could improve themselves if they followed in the footsteps of the leaders. Finally, in some cases, race and class hierarchies were attributed largely to cultural and environmental factors such as poverty and lack of education.[59] Irrespective of where exactly the emphasis was placed, medical science and its applications conceptualized indigenous peoples so that imperialism seemed justified, and defined slum dwellers and slums in such a way as to legitimize municipal intervention.

The 'slum dwellers' apart, class difference was mainly seen as a social rather than a natural phenomenon, a (human) construct rather than a (natural) given. Yet the fact that medical science did not speak of class in the same 'universalizing' and 'naturalizing' utterances it used for gender does not mean that its role in legitimizing and depoliticizing class hierarchies was unimportant. The basic parameters of the existing economic system and institutions influence what is taken as knowledge in society. Thus, the direction, content and practice of Western medicine have been, to an extent, guided by the parameters of a capitalist economy, whereas, for example, Soviet medicine was influenced by the parameters of a socialist economy. In both these systems, medical knowledge and its applications have reinforced people's 'ability *not* to see' the inequality, social distress and economic waste for which their own economic system is responsible. At the same time, medicine has highlighted

---

[56] See, for example, Jordanova, *Sexual Visions*; Moscucci, *The Science of Woman*, 36–41.

[57] A. Fausto-Sterling, *Myths of Gender: Biological Theories about Women and Men* (New York 1992), 4.

[58] For discussion, see D. Arnold, *Colonizing the Body: State Medicine and Epidemic Disease in Nineteenth-century India* (Berkeley, CA 1993); D. Arnold, 'Introduction: disease, medicine and empire', in D. Arnold (ed.), *Imperial Medicine and Indigenous Societies* (Manchester 1988), 1–26; M. Harrison, *Public Health in British India: Anglo-Indian Preventative Medicine* (Cambridge 1994), esp. ch. 2; Good, *Medicine*.

[59] J. Harris, *Private Lives, Public Spirit: Britain 1870–1914* (London 1994), 233–7; Bland, *Banishing the Beast*, 73–6; Arnold, 'Introduction'.

the bedrock principles and values of these economic systems, for example Western medicine has emphasized the value of rationally based entrepreneurship.[60] Medicine, both research and practice, has sought to solve health problems in the existing institutional contexts, and thus it has served to maintain existing structures, including class hierarchies.[61]

This book concentrates on early twentieth-century campaigns against infant mortality and tuberculosis, examining how these campaigns served to depoliticize and 'naturalize' local economic arrangements, social structures and moral norms. The focus is therefore on different, and often conflicting, objectives of municipal health policy and on the complex ways in which scientific knowledge was used to reconcile and depoliticize these goals. By reconstructing scientific knowledge to suit political purposes, health authorities were able to represent themselves as active promoters of health and welfare even when they clearly gave priority to the economic interests of local businesses or to the professional aspirations of medical doctors. By sheltering behind the authority of scientific knowledge, they could claim that they concentrated on improving the health of men, women and children, while their primary focus may have been to maintain the work ethic and to buttress the family institution and its hierarchy of roles.

Processes whereby different political and social concerns became embedded in 'value-free' health policy are examined in Chapters 4 and 5, which occupy a large proportion of the book. Chapter 4 looks at infant welfare campaigns in early twentieth-century Birmingham and Gothenburg, exploring, firstly, how scientific knowledge was used to link the well-being of infants to the efforts to regulate working-class family life and gender roles in particular. Secondly, the chapter discusses the ways in which the promotion of infant welfare was reconciled with the aspirations of the medical profession and with the needs of the local economy. Chapter 5 examines how the Birmingham and Gothenburg authorities defined and responded to the problem of tuberculosis. The main purpose of this chapter is to discuss the extent to which anti-tuberculosis campaigns served to regulate urban life in general and to legitimize municipal intervention or non-intervention in the homes and in the housing market and the medical market. The foci of attention in this chapter are the relations between social classes and between adults and children.

Before examining the role that municipal health policy played in regulating urban life, it is necessary to discuss the economic, social and administrative contexts in which health policies were constructed in early twentieth-century Birmingham and Gothenburg. Chapter 2 examines the diverse socio-economic conditions within these cities, concentrating especially on the aspects which were likely to influence how health problems were understood and defined. The chapter deals with the demographic pressures to which health policy was subject in Birmingham and Gothenburg, examines spatial arrangements in these cities, sheds light on housing conditions and work opportunities, and analyses family patterns and ideals. However, the creation of health policies was affected not only by social relations, but also by administrative structures and policy legacies. In particular, pre-existing administrative arrangements

---

[60]   See, for example, Jordanova, 'Introduction', 25.
[61]   Waitzkin, 'A critical theory of medical discourse'.

and policy legacies served as a catalyst and an impediment to the formulation of new ideas and policies. By analysing government structures and public health traditions in Britain and Sweden and by describing widely held views about the appropriate role of health authorities, Chapter 3 opens up an opportunity to identify and discuss some fundamental patterns and continuities in British and Swedish public health policies.[62]

The comparative international approach chosen in this study provides a fresh perspective on how public health authorities organized and regulated the life of the city and mediated conflicts in urban society. A comparative study provides an opportunity to explore why health authorities knew what they knew, since it shows very clearly that they could have known otherwise. By revealing what happened but also what did not, a comparative approach clarifies the choices British and Swedish health officials made – what they accepted or just assumed, and what they rejected. Furthermore, since this book concentrates on two cities, it is focused enough to do justice to the full complexity of decision-making and to illuminate a wide range of political, social and moral concerns which were threaded through public health campaigns. On the other hand, two important themes have been deliberately left outside the scope of this study.

Firstly, this research concentrates almost exclusively on the 'political' origins and 'political' repercussions of public health policies, and says very little about the life-and-death consequences of these policies. In other words, the aim of this research is not to discuss in detail how efficient the measures taken in Birmingham and Gothenburg were in reducing mortality and morbidity rates and in improving the health and well-being of the city population.[63] The attempt is to explore how these measures served to regulate the life of the city.

Secondly, this research does not discuss in detail the party politics in Birmingham and Gothenburg or the aims and achievements of different political factions in the public health arena. Party politics has been left out partly because this study concentrates on the early twentieth century, when the City Council in both Birmingham and Gothenburg was governed by Liberals and Conservatives and the key positions in municipal policy making were occupied by men of substantial

---

[62]   T. Skocpol, 'Bringing the state back in: strategies of analysis in current research', in Evans, Rueschemeyer and Skocpol, *Bringing the State Back In*, 3–37; Sears, '"To teach them how to live"'.

[63]   Thomas McKeown and many other researchers in his wake have claimed that public health measures were only of secondary importance, and that other factors such as improved nutritional standards should be given most of the credit for the decline in mortality in the late nineteenth and early twentieth centuries. This view has been challenged, for example, by Gerry Kearns, Simon Szreter, Samuel Preston and Etienne van de Walle, who have conceived of sanitary measures as a key determinant of falling death rates. T. McKeown, *The Modern Rise of Population* (London 1976), 110–42, 152–63; G. Kearns, 'The urban penalty and the population history of England', in Brändström and Tedebrand, *Society, Health and Population*, 213–36; S. Szreter, 'The importance of social intervention in Britain's mortality decline c. 1850–1914: a reinterpretation of the role of public health', *Social History of Medicine* **1** (1) (1988), 1–37; S. H. Preston and E. van der Walle, 'Urban French mortality in the nineteenth century', *Population Studies* **32** (2) (1978), 275–97.

wealth and influence. Had the subject been the public health campaigns which were launched in the 1920s and 1930s, it would have been more important also to discuss party politics. In Birmingham, the Conservatives and Liberals continued to dominate the City Council in the 1920s and 1930s, while in Gothenburg these parties had to relinquish their power. From 1919, the Social Democrats were the largest party in Gothenburg.[64]

Another reason for excluding party politics is that an international comparison is a problematic method of analysing the influence of political parties on welfare policies. Theda Skocpol and Susan Pedersen, who have used an approach of this type, have argued that 'working-class strength' does not correlate in any simple way with social policy.[65] However, many writers who have concentrated on a single country have argued that the degree of working-class strength is a key determinant of welfare policies. For example, Martin Powell, who has studied regional variations in health care provision in inter-war Britain, has shown that the political constellation of the City Council influenced the comprehensiveness and the quality of services.[66] Lara Marks has examined the same theme in her study on maternal and infant welfare services in four boroughs in London. She argues that health care provisions were dependent on the political outlook and social relations within each area.[67]

Although this book does not discuss party politics, it explores the ways in which health authorities' views were challenged. The authorities' views mattered in both Birmingham and Gothenburg, but they were by no means unquestioned. Chapter 6 examines how different groups – middle-class women and working-class women and men – challenged the authorities' views or, perhaps more importantly, how these groups seized on contradictions in health policy to change things and to further causes they supported.

---

[64]   A. Attman, S. Boberg and A. Wåhlstrand, *Göteborgs Stadsfullmäktige 1863–1962. III: Stadsfullmäktige, stadens styrelser och förvaltningar* (Göteborg 1971), 70–99; B.-M. Olsson, 'Stadens styrelse – ett upplyst fåvälde?', in *För hundra år sedan – skildringar från Göteborgs 1880-tal* (Göteborg 1984), 227–40; E.S. Griffith, *The Modern Development of City Government in the United Kingdom and the United States*, vol. II (London 1927), 675; A. Briggs, *History of Birmingham, Volume II: Borough and City 1865–1938* (London 1952).

[65]   Pedersen, *The Origins of the Welfare State*; Weir and Skocpol, 'State structures'.

[66]   M. Powell, 'Did politics matter? Municipal public health expenditure in the 1930s', *Urban History* **22** (3) (1995), 360–79; M. Powell, 'Hospital provision before the National Health Service: a geographical study of the 1945 hospital surveys', *Social History of Medicine* **5** (3) (1992), 483–504.

[67]   L. Marks, *Metropolitan Maternity: Maternal and Infant Welfare Services in Early Twentieth Century London* (Amsterdam 1996).

CHAPTER 2

Industrial Cities

Images of cities are important political instruments. Late nineteenth-century Birmingham was often characterized as 'the best-governed city in the world', a reputation which was most agreeable to the Birmingham civic leaders and which says much about their skills in managing the image of their city. Reforms introduced by Joseph Chamberlain, Mayor of Birmingham from 1873 to 1876, and his political heirs did not always achieve their objectives. Nor did these reforms break new ground; Glasgow and Liverpool were several years ahead of Birmingham in widening the sphere of local government action.[1] However, the skilful way in which Chamberlain manipulated the meaning of municipal reforms was not surpassed by any contemporary civic leader. He persuaded policy makers and the public to perceive the Birmingham town improvement schemes as expressions of modernity and progressive responsibility, and as a result, the Birmingham city administration appeared innovative and forward-looking, and the city itself, 'one of the ugliest towns in England', emerged as a respectable metropolis.[2]

Equally important was the city's reputation as 'the workshop of the world'. The message which the Birmingham civic leaders sought to convey in the 1920s and 1930s was that their city, with its Unionist-dominated City Council, diverse and adaptable small businesses, skilled workforce, harmonious industrial relations and good public services, had more to offer modern industrial enterprises than did other provincial cities.[3] Again their message seemed to get across. While many manufacturing towns and cities suffered economic stagnation or decline, Birmingham grew smoothly into

---

[1] H. Fraser, 'Municipal socialism and social policy', in R.J. Morris and R. Rodger (eds), *The Victorian City: A Reader in British Urban History 1820–1914* (London 1993), 258–80; I. Maver, 'Glasgow's civic government', in W.H. Fraser and I. Maver (eds), *Glasgow, Volume II: 1830 to 1912* (Manchester 1996), 441–85; A. Mayne, *The Imagined Slum: Newspaper Representation in Three Cities 1870–1914* (Leicester 1993), 57–62; E.P. Hennock, *Fit and Proper Persons: Ideal and Reality in Nineteenth-century Urban Government* (London 1973), 104–30, 172.

[2] D. Smith, *Conflict and Compromise: Class Formation in English Society 1830–1914: A Comparative Study of Birmingham and Sheffield* (London 1982), 226–7; Hennock, *Fit and Proper Persons*, 170–6. Chamberlain privately regarded Birmingham as 'one of the ugliest towns in England' which could be 'choked in its own growth', see Mayne, *The Imagined Slum*, 59.

[3] See, for example, W.S. Body (ed.), *Birmingham and Its Civic Managers: The Departmental Doings of the City Council* (Birmingham 1928), 146.

a modern industrial city that produced electrical equipment, bicycles and Austin cars.[4]

The Gothenburg civic leaders, for their part, emphasized the cosmopolitan atmosphere of their city. Nineteenth-century Gothenburg was often described as 'the England of Sweden' or 'Little London', since many of the city's wealthy merchants and industrialists had come from Scotland or England.[5] In the early twentieth century, when the British and other foreigners had largely acculturated, close international contacts remained an important feature of Gothenburg's image. The city was 'the gateway to the world' for Swedish pulp and paper and for a million emigrants, and 'the gateway to Sweden' for American cotton, British coal and Brazilian coffee. Gothenburg was also successful in attracting export industries, mainly shipbuilding, metalworking and mechanical engineering. As a bustling centre of commerce and export industries, Gothenburg ranked high in the Swedish urban hierarchy, below the capital city Stockholm, but clearly above the industrial cities of Malmö and Norrköping.[6]

For local elites, the image of Gothenburg as an international city was an invaluable political tool. It facilitated economic, political and intellectual contacts with Western Europe and, in local politics, the image was used to push through substantial public projects such as the extension and improvement of port facilities.[7] While integration into the world market gave Gothenburg wealth and prestige, it also left the city's economy susceptible to sudden fluctuations. The volatility of the local economy and the instability of employment prospects, in turn, may have contributed

---

[4]   A. Briggs, *History of Birmingham, Volume II: Borough and City 1865–1938* (London 1952), Ch. 3 and 9; G.E. Cherry, *Birmingham: A Study in Geography, History and Planning* (Chichester 1994), 125–9. For less successful promotional campaigns, see for example R.J. Marshall, 'Town planning in Sheffield', in C. Binfield et al. (eds), *The History of the City of Sheffield 1843–1993, Volume II: Society* (Sheffield 1993), 17–32.

[5]   M. Åberg, *En fråga om klass? Borgarklass och industriellt företagande i Göteborg 1850–1914* (Göteborg 1991), 67–8; B. Jordansson, 'Women and philanthropy in a liberal context: the case of Gothenburg', in B. Jordansson and T. Vammen (eds), *Charitable Women: Philanthropic Welfare 1780–1930: A Nordic and Interdisciplinary Anthology* (Odense 1998), 65–88; A. Attman, *Göteborgs Stadsfullmäktige 1863–1962*, vol. I.1: *Göteborg 1863–1913* (Göteborg 1963), 11–3. See also autobiographies, A.O. Elliot, *Minnen från det gamla Göteborg* (Stockholm 1930), 65–7, 138; J.G. Richert, *Minnesanteckningar* (Stockholm 1929), 99–106.

[6]   M. Fritz, *Göteborgs historia: Näringsliv och samhällsutveckling: Från handelsstad till industristad 1820–1920* (Stockholm 1996), 112–21, 185–91, 231–76; K. Olsson, *Göteborgs historia: Näringsliv och samhällsutveckling: Från industristad till tjänstestad 1920–1995* (Stockholm 1996), 77–88, 100–129; W.C. McEwen, 'Working-class Politics in Gothenburg, Sweden 1919–1934: A Study of a Social Democratic Party Local in an Industrial and Urban Setting' (unpublished PhD thesis, Case Western Reserve University 1970), 71–87; *Statistisk årsbok för Göteborg 1930*, 142–55; *1935*, 116–29.

[7]   For urban elites and public spending, see for example M. Daunton, 'Taxation and representation in the Victorian city', in R. Colls and R. Rodger (eds), *Cities of Ideas: Civil Society and Urban Governance in Britain, 1800–2000* (Aldershot 2004), 21–45. For the political controversies over plans to enlarge the port in Gothenburg, see A. Attman, *Göteborgs Stadsfullmäktige 1863–1962*, vol. I.2: *Göteborg 1913–1962* (Göteborg 1963), 275–7; Attman, *Göteborg 1863–1913*, 349–52, 364–7.

to some dramatic changes that took place in the party political arena. In 1919, 'the wealthy Gothenburg', the birthplace of the Swedish bourgeoisie and the stronghold of liberalism, became a city governed by the Social Democratic Party, and by the 1950s Gothenburg acquired a reputation as 'Sweden's reddest city'.[8]

These images provide one perspective on Birmingham and Gothenburg. The following sections widen the picture by looking at other aspects of urban development. They deal with the spatial configuration of the cities, discuss demographic trends, analyse economic development and social structures, and trace the development of municipal policies in housing and town planning. The main aim of this chapter is to provide a basis for discussion as to how political and social concerns pervaded 'scientific' public health campaigns and how these campaigns, in turn, served to regulate the life of the cities.

Social Classes and Urban Space

At the beginning of the twentieth century, the city of Birmingham had a population of 522,000 and the suburban areas outside the municipal boundaries were home to a further 238,000 people, a large proportion of whom commuted into Birmingham to work. In 1911, when the surrounding districts were incorporated into the city, Birmingham became England's largest provincial city with a population of 840,000, and around 1930 the population of the city reached one million.[9] The expansion of the municipal boundaries in 1911 was welcomed among others by the Medical Officer of Health (MOH), Dr John Robertson, and the Chairman of the Housing Committee, John Nettlefold. By dramatically increasing the available building land, the reform helped the city accommodate its growing population and expanding industries, but it also opened up opportunities to reorganize the urban space according to the principles of modern town planning. German town extension schemes, which the Birmingham Housing Committee had inspected during their visit to Germany in 1905, and British garden cities had convinced both Robertson and Nettlefold that town planning was the answer to many deep-seated urban problems. They emphasized that building new suburbs *per se* would not solve health and environmental problems in large cities. The mistakes of the past could be avoided only if suburban growth and the redevelopment of the city centre were carefully planned and controlled.[10]

---

8 G. Therborn, *Borgarklass och byråkrati i Sverige: Anteckningar om en solskenshistoria* (Lund 1989), 87–95; Fritz, *Från handelsstad till industristad,* 182; Olsson, *Från industristad till tjänstestad,* 85–6; A. Attman, S. Boberg and A. Wåhlstrand, *Göteborgs Stadsfullmäktige, 1863–1962,* vol. III: *Stadsfullmäktige, stadens styrelser och förvaltningar* (Göteborg 1971), 75–99; McEwen, 'Working-class Politics', 71–87, 180, 289–311, 362–3.

9 B.R. Mitchell, *British Historical Statistics* (Cambridge 1990), 26–7; *Report of the Boundaries Committee for Presentation at the Special Meeting of the Council on the 13th July, 1909* (Boundaries Committee, Birmingham 1909), 17–18; Briggs, *History of Birmingham,* 138–57.

10 J. Nettlefold, *Practical Housing* (Letchworth 1908); *Report of the Medical Officer of Health (MOH) on the Unhealthy Conditions in the Floodgate Street Area and Municipal Wards of St. Mary, St. Stephen and St. Bartholomew* (Health Department, Birmingham 1904), 21–3;

In Birmingham, as in many other British cities, middle-class suburban migration had begun in the early nineteenth century. Suburbs – or more precisely the interdependent relationship between suburbs and slums – were an inalienable part of the growing economic and political power of the British upper middle class. Merchants, manufacturers and professionals celebrated their success by moving from dense central areas to exclusive suburbs. Furthermore, the rise of suburbia went hand in hand with the new form of male domination and the hegemony of the middle-class nuclear family. The separation of home and workplace drastically limited job opportunities for married middle-class women, compelling a division of labour within the family. The lower middle classes and the more prosperous sections of the working class followed in the wake of the manufacturers and merchants in the late nineteenth and early twentieth centuries. New housing estates in the outlying districts of Birmingham, though monotonous and lacking many public amenities, corresponded more closely to their aspirations than the old city centre with its decaying houses and polluting factories.[11]

In the early twentieth century the Birmingham City Council, which until then had remained a passive spectator in the process of suburbanization, changed its mind. At the instigation of reformers such as Nettlefold and Robertson, the Council set about securing the continuation of suburban growth. In the first phase the Council promoted suburbanization by preparing town planning schemes, and in the 1920s it proceeded to build large council estates, where thousands of working-class and lower-middle-class families were to enjoy 'the health-giving opportunities of the country'.[12] While focusing on the new estates in the outlying districts, the Birmingham authorities neglected the central wards. The policy of patching up slums was condemned as unsatisfactory by the early 1920s, but relatively little was done during the inter-war

---

Annual Report of the MOH for Birmingham (hereafter *Annual Report*) *1906*; 'Extract from the Annual Report of the MOH for Birmingham for 1918', in J.E. Lane-Claypon, *The Child Welfare Movement* (London 1920), Appendix VII, 304. See also C. Chinn, *Homes for People: 100 Years of Council Housing in Birmingham* (Exeter 1991), 22–4; Cherry, *Birmingham*, 93–4, 102–9; H.W. Pooler, *My Life in General Practice* (London 1948), 82; Birmingham City Archives (BCA) Birmingham Public Health Committee (PHC) minutes 30 Jan. 1925, item 8825.

[11]   R. Rodger, 'Slums and suburbs: the persistence of residential apartheid', in P. Waller (ed.), *The English Urban Landscape* (Oxford 2000), 233–68; L. Davidoff and C. Hall, *Family Fortunes: Men and Women of the English Middle Class 1780–1850* (London 1992); H.J. Dyos and D.A. Reeder, 'Slums and suburbs', in H.J. Dyos and M. Wolff (eds), *The Victorian City: Images and Realities*, vol. I (London 1973), 359–86; Cherry, *Birmingham*, 89–94; S. Saegert, 'Masculine cities and feminine suburbs: polarized ideas, contradictory realities', *Signs* **5** (3) (1980), Supplement, 96–111. Elizabeth Wilson argues that 'urban life, however fraught with difficulty, has emancipated women more than rural life or suburban domesticity'; see E. Wilson, *The Sphinx in the City: Urban Life, the Control of Disorder, and Women* (London 1991), 10.

[12]   Quote from Nettlefold, *Practical Housing*, 5. See also, Chinn, *Homes for People*, 31–74; Cherry, *Birmingham*, 89–124; H. Meller, *European Cities 1890–1930s: History, Culture and the Built Environment* (Chichester 2001), 221–55.

years to redevelop the central wards.[13] Old factories, workshops and warehouses and the poorest of the poor, who were often represented as a pathological social underclass, remained in the central districts, while new industrial enterprises and 'respectable' working-class people left the urban core for the space and convenience of the fringes.[14]

The authorities were optimistic that suburbanization would indirectly alleviate impoverished living conditions in the slums. Providing the growth of the population was slow, the people who remained in the central wards would benefit from the additional, better quality houses vacated by families who moved to the new estates.[15] In early twentieth-century Birmingham, conditions seemed to be conducive to this kind of 'filtering process'. The city had experienced its most rapid growth as early as the 1820s, when its population had increased by over 40 per cent within a decade (Figure 2.1).[16] After 1830 the growth had gradually levelled off, and between 1910 and 1930 the population increased by only 10 per cent in a decade. However, even in these circumstances, the effect of suburbanization on the living conditions in the slum areas was limited.

Gothenburg was a smaller city than Birmingham. Its population exceeded 100,000 in 1889 and 200,000 in 1919, reaching 280,000 by 1940.[17] The growth rate had been at its highest in the 1850s, 1870s and 1880s, exceeding 35 per cent in each decade, and was still around 25 per cent in the 1890s, although extensive emigration to the United States served to retard urban growth. During the first two decades of the twentieth century, the growth rate was about 20 per cent, being considerably higher than that in Birmingham. The post-war depression between 1920 and 1926, however, halted the flow of immigrants to Gothenburg and the growth rate decreased to 8 per cent, increasing again to 15 per cent in the 1930s.[18]

---

[13]   For a discussion on 'slum patching', BCA PHC minutes 9 Mar. 1923, item 7421; 25 May 1923, item 7561.

[14]   P. Garside, '"Unhealthy areas": town planning, eugenics and the slums, 1890–1945', *Planning Perspectives* 3 (1) (1988), 24–46; Chinn, *Homes for People*, 70–74; Cherry, *Birmingham*, 121–4; A. Sutcliffe and R. Smith, *History of Birmingham, Volume III: Birmingham 1939–1970* (Oxford 1974), 220–32.

[15]   Garside, '"Unhealthy areas"', 27; C.G. Pooley, 'England and Wales', in C.G. Pooley (ed.), *Housing Strategies in Europe, 1880–1930* (Leicester 1992), 93–8; Mayne, *The Imagined Slum*, 85–93.

[16]   C.M. Law, 'The growth of urban population in England and Wales, 1801–1911', *Transactions of the Institute of British Geographers* 41 (1967), 125–43.

[17]   *Statistisk årsbok för Göteborg 1939*, 8–10; *Historisk statistik för Sverige. Del 1* (Stockholm 1969), 63.

[18]   Altogether 1.2 million people emigrated from Sweden to the United States and to some other countries in the years 1850–1914. Despite massive emigration, the rates of urban growth and general population growth were high in Sweden throughout the period. See, for example, L. Nilsson, *Den urbana transitionen: Tätorterna i svensk samhällsomvandling 1800–1980* (Stockholm 1989), 182–93, 248; *Historisk statistik för Sverige. Del 1*, 61–6; Attman, *Göteborg 1913–1962*, 199.

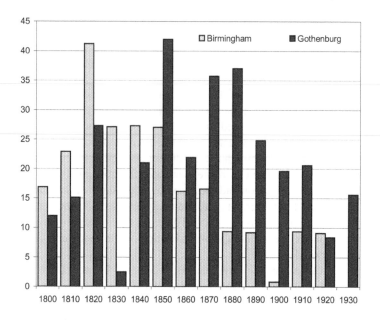

Figure 2.1 **Decennial population growth (%) in Birmingham and Gothenburg, from the 1800s to the 1930s.**

Source: Statistisk årsbok för Göteborg 1939, 8; Historisk statistik för Sverige. Del 1 (Stockholm 1969), 63–5; *Census of England and Wales 1911. Summary Tables. Area. Families and Separate Occupiers and Population,* tables 14 and 15, 64–7; B.R. Mitchell, *British Historical Statistics* (Cambridge 1990), 26–7.

Spatial expressions of urban inequality were noticeable in Gothenburg too, but the relationship between social classes and urban space was different from that in Birmingham. While in Birmingham the economic and political elite regulated the city from their secluded enclaves outside the city centre, the Gothenburg upper middle class, a smaller and more closely knit group, remained in the centre or its vicinity. In Gothenburg, middle-class suburban migration did not begin in earnest until the 1950s and 1960s. Furthermore, various reports published in the late nineteenth and early twentieth centuries suggest that many municipal wards in Gothenburg had a fairly wide mix of social classes.[19] For example, the variation in death rates between different wards was small in comparison to that in Birmingham. The death rates for wards in Gothenburg varied from 13 to 19 per thousand of the population in

[19] H. Wallqvist, *Bostadsförhållandena för de mindre bemedlade i Göteborg: Studie sommaren 1889* (Stockholm 1891), 3–11; C. Lindman, *Sundhets- och befolkningsförhållanden i Sveriges städer 1851–1909,* vol. I: *Text* (Hälsingborg 1911), 66–95. See also, M. Niemi, 'Public health discourses in Birmingham and Gothenburg 1890–1920', in S. Sheard and H. Power (eds), *Body and City: Histories of Urban Public Health* (Aldershot 2000), 123–42; R. Enmark, 'Bo och leva i Annedal – kvarteret Ananasen', in *För hundra år sedan – skildringar från Göteborgs 1880-tal* (Göteborg 1984), 154–7; Fritz, *Från handelsstad till industristad,* 299–308, 317.

the 1890s, whereas in Birmingham they ranged between 14 and 29.[20] Residential segregation appeared to develop slowly in Gothenburg and in consequence the poor and the well-to-do still lived relatively close to each other at the turn of the century. For example, a considerable number of poor people were dispersed throughout some prosperous central areas, occupying cheap flats and houses which were tucked away in courtyards and narrow back streets.[21]

In discussing the spatial arrangements in the two cities, it is important to bear in mind that Gothenburg had not grown 'spontaneously'. It had been founded by the Crown and built according to a town plan produced by a Dutch engineer in the early 1620s. The original town plan was revised and extended in 1808, when the fortifications were removed, and again in the 1860s, in the midst of rapid population growth (Figure 2.1). A new plan for the eastern and southern districts of the city was approved in 1907. However, the Gothenburg planning authorities were not able to keep up with the expansion of the city and therefore a significant proportion of urban growth took place outside the planned areas. Predictably, the districts where building ordinances imposed no restrictions on housebuilding attracted the poorest people. A desire to prevent the development of insanitary shantytowns in outlying areas was one of the driving forces behind Swedish town planning until the early twentieth century.[22]

The City Architect for Gothenburg, Albert Lilienberg, who was the leading advocate of modern town planning in Sweden in the 1910s and 1920s, introduced some ideas from the British garden city movement into Swedish planning. However, the way in which these ideas were implemented in Gothenburg and in Sweden in general was different from that in Britain. Swedish planners and social reformers may have been inspired by the same anti-urbanism that permeated the British town planning movement, but most speculators and municipal authorities in large Swedish cities favoured more efficient exploitation of the building land. Hence many new residential areas were dominated by relatively high and closely grouped buildings.[23]

---

[20] *Göteborgs hälsovårdsnämnds årsberättelse* (hereafter *Årsberättelsen*) *1892*, 46; *1898*, table 18; *Annual Report 1897*, 8–9; *1898*, 8–9; *1899*, 7.

[21] For the patterns of residential segregation, see also Åberg, *En fråga om klass?*, 133–6; Wallqvist, *Bostadsförhållandena*, 7; Olsson, *Från industristad till tjänstestad*, 39–50.

[22] B. Andersson, *Göteborgs historia: Näringsliv och samhällsutveckling*, vol. 1: *Från fästningsstad till handelsstad 1619–1820* (Stockholm 1996), 25–35; T. Hall, 'Urban planning in Sweden', in T. Hall (ed.), *Planning and Urban Growth in the Nordic Countries* (London 1991), 167–206; G. Linden, 'Town planning in Sweden after 1850', in W. Hegemann (ed.), *International Cities and Town Planning Exhibition, Gothenburg, Sweden 1923: English Catalogue* (Gothenburg 1923), 270–71 and 250–61.

[23] T. Hall, 'Planning history: recent developments in the Nordic countries, with special reference to Sweden', *Planning Perspectives* 9 (2) (1994), 153–79; T. Hall, 'Urban planning in Sweden', and 'Concluding remarks: Is there a Nordic planning tradition?', in Hall, *Planning and Urban Growth*, 247–59.

Housing

Wooden three-storey tenements (*landshövdingehus*) divided into small flats, each normally comprising one room and a kitchen, sometimes two rooms and a kitchen, dominated working-class areas in Gothenburg (Figures 2.2 and 2.3). Although the vast majority of working-class people lived in small flats, the housing market in working-class areas was by no means undifferentiated. The standard of housing available for different groups varied greatly according to income. The Annedal district, which was inhabited by lower-middle-class people and 'the elite of the working class', was a model quarter of the city at the turn of the century. In the eyes of many contemporaries, this area was an example of what could be done by careful planning. Tenements and other houses were structurally sound and carefully designed, flower beds were well arranged, and public buildings reflected civic pride. In Masthuggsbergen, Kvarnberget and Otterhällorna, by contrast, most inhabitants lived in badly built houses, and the poorest of them occupied dilapidated cellars and attics.[24]

Overcrowding remained a critical aspect of the housing problem in Gothenburg throughout the period reviewed here. If the contemporary definition of overcrowding, more than two persons per room, is applied, about 38 per cent of Gothenburg's population lived in overcrowded accommodation in 1910.[25] Owing to the lack of space within the home, Swedish working-class families were not able to live up to the same standards of 'decency' and 'propriety' that large sections of the English working class imposed on themselves. The small number of rooms per tenement flat prevented any great specialization in the use of rooms, and it was often difficult, if not impossible, to ensure privacy between parents and children, between sons and daughters, and between daughters and male lodgers.[26]

---

[24] Wallqvist, *Bostadsförhållandena*, 3–11; G. Lönnroth, 'Stadsbilden – praktfulla palats och usla kåkar', and Enmark, 'Bo och leva i Annedal', in *För hundra år sedan*, 22–62 and 141–57; G. Schönbeck, *Victor von Gegerfelt – arkitekt i Göteborg: En yrkesman och hans verksamhetsfält 1841–1896* (Göteborg 1991), 233–40; Attman, *Göteborg 1863–1913*, 265–81; Attman, *Göteborg 1913–1962*, 202–6.

[25] *Statistisk årsbok för Göteborg 1930*, 12, 120; *1935*, 96–100. See also Attman, *Göteborg 1863–1913*, 278–9. Attman argues that 47 per cent of the population lived at a density of more than two persons per room in 1910. However, he has only looked at flats/houses with less than five rooms and the section of the population which lived in these houses. If larger houses are taken into account, 'only' 38 per cent of the population lived in overcrowded accommodation. See also, G. Jansson and R. Sterner, 'Bostadssociala förhållanden inom vissa städer och stadsliknande samhällen', in *Statens Offentliga Utredningar* (hereafter *SOU*) *1935:2*, Bilaga 2, 62–78.

[26] For a discussion on privacy within the home and about specialized use of rooms, see H. Wallqvist, *Om arbetarebostäder* (Stockholm 1890). See also, M. Foucault, *The History of Sexuality, Volume I: An Introduction* (London 1990), 45–6; J. Burnett, *A Social History of Housing 1815–1985* (London 1986), 154.

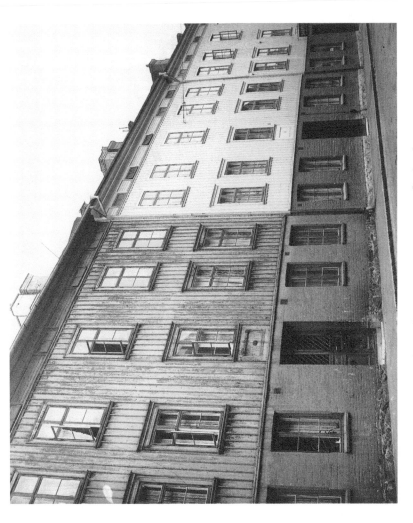

Figure 2.2 Typical working-class flats (*landshövdingehus*) in Albogatan, Gothenburg.
Source: Gothenburg City Museum.

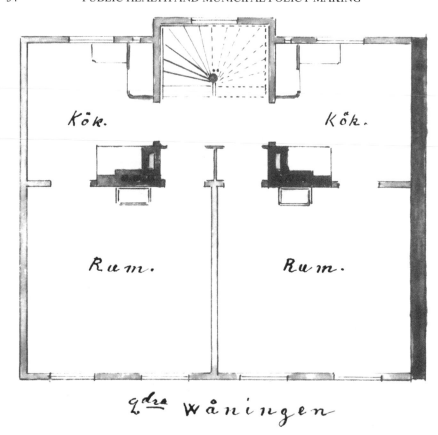

Figure 2.3   Plan of two typical working-class flats in Gothenburg. Most working-class flats consisted of a kitchen (*kök*) and one room (*rum*).
Source: Gothenburg City Museum.

Speculative builders were the most active providers of new housing in Gothenburg in the late nineteenth and early twentieth centuries, but working-class houses were also built on a non-speculative basis. Some employers provided houses for their workers in order to attract skilled labour, while various philanthropic and co-operative associations built houses to improve the health and morals of the working class. The Gothenburg City Council maintained its faith in the philanthropic and private sectors until well into the 1910s, restricting its own activities to the provision of cheap building land for such organizations. In 1915, however, the municipal policy makers decided in favour of building municipal housing, and in the 1920s and 1930s, when the Social Democratic Party had a majority of seats on the City Council, the public efforts to ease the housing shortage and improve housing conditions were further intensified.[27]

---

[27]   B. Nyström, 'Åtgärder till förbättring av de mindre bemedlades bostadsförhållanden i vissa städer', in *SOU 1935:2*, Bilaga 1, 11–4; Fritz, *Från handelsstad till industristad*, 324–31;

Pushing through housing and slum clearance schemes was not easy, since all expensive municipal projects required a two-thirds majority in the Gothenburg City Council. The Social Democrats had to win not only Communist support, but also some Liberal or Conservative backing.[28] During the most difficult housing crises, the Conservatives and Liberals were ready to accept municipal intervention in the housing market, but in general most of them favoured non-interventionist policies. Despite the opposition, the Social Democrats often managed to achieve the necessary two-thirds majority. By 1934 the Gothenburg corporation had built 2,700 flats for the rental sector and 674 houses and flats for owner-occupiers. Furthermore, the corporation had helped finance 2,400 flats and houses built by housing associations. Compared to Stockholm, Gothenburg had a substantial involvement in municipal housing, but at the same time the financial support it provided for housing associations was rather modest.[29] From the point of view of this study, two aspects of Gothenburg's municipal housing policy are particularly important. Firstly, the corporation did not usually provide improved accommodation for those whose housing need was greatest. Although many municipal tenements were initially meant for people evicted from slum quarters, in practice the new houses were usually occupied by relatively affluent working-class families. Secondly, local authority provision only made small inroads into the problem of overcrowding, since a large proportion of the new municipal housing consisted of two-roomed flats. In 1920, about 62 per cent of the housing stock in Gothenburg had only one or two rooms, and 54 per cent of houses still belonged to this category in 1939. However, the standards of amenities in the houses improved considerably. For example, the percentage of flats and houses with central heating rose from 8 to 61 during the period 1920–1939.[30]

In Gothenburg, where many affluent middle-class families lived in flats, people did not observe social barriers between different house types. In Birmingham, by contrast, tenement flats were invariably associated with the poorest of the poor. Nineteenth-century Birmingham had managed to accommodate its working-class population in small, self-contained houses – either in back-to-back court dwellings or, after 1858, in terraced houses built in parallel streets to conform to basic standards of construction and sanitary amenities set out in the building byelaw enacted that year – and early twentieth-century Birmingham was determined to continue the tradition. Proposals to build subsidized multi-storey flats were put forward time and again in municipal politics but, as Anthony Sutcliffe has pointed out, 'a strong middle-class distrust and a working-class dislike of flats' served to postpone extensive flat-building projects

Attman, *Göteborg 1863–1913*, 265–79.

[28]   McEwen, 'Working-class Politics', 99, 185–8.

[29]   *Statistisk Årsbok för Göteborg 1935*, 103–4; Nyström, 'Åtgärder', 1–14; Lönnroth, 'Stadsbilden', 43; Attman, *Göteborg 1863–1913*, 265–81; Attman, *Göteborg 1913–1962*, 202–9. For Stockholm, see also T. Strömberg, 'Sweden', in Pooley, *Housing Strategies*, 11–39.

[30]   For dispossessed tenants and municipal housing, see Nyström, 'Åtgärder', 13. For overcrowding and amenities, see Attman, *Göteborg 1863–1913*, 279; Attman, *Göteborg 1913–1962*, 202–6; K. Olsson, *Hushållsinkomst, inkomstfördelning och försörjningsbörda: En undersökning av vissa yrkesgrupper i Göteborg 1919–1960* (Göteborg 1972), 40–43.

until the mid-1930s.[31] For example, in 1925 the MOH and a number of working-class organizations joined forces to defeat a scheme to erect tenement buildings.[32]

In general, housing provision was better and more plentiful in Birmingham than in Gothenburg. In Birmingham only 2 per cent of housing was of one- and two-roomed houses in 1910, whereas the corresponding figure for Gothenburg was 62. Owing to the predominance of self-contained houses with three or more rooms, only 10 per cent of residents in Birmingham lived more than two persons per room, a degree of overcrowding which was a quarter of that in Gothenburg.[33] Consequently, overcrowding as such was not the most pressing issue in Birmingham in the early years of the twentieth century. Instead, health authorities were preoccupied by the question of how to maintain reasonable housing standards in the city centre, which was growing old (Figure 2.4). The large proportion of houses in the central wards were old, dilapidated back-to-back houses which usually comprised three rooms built one upon another: a living-room, a bedroom and an attic. Each house joined to another house at the back and often also both sides, so that the only door and all the windows were on the front wall. Double rows of these houses were built near each other, and courts were closed at both ends by communal privies or by another row of houses.[34]

Social reformers had made back-to-back houses an object of criticism as early as the 1840s, when these houses had constituted about 65–70 per cent of the total housing stock in Birmingham and in many other cities in the Midlands and South Lancashire. High-density back-to-backs and enclosed courtyards hidden from the general gaze and protected from the regulation of outsiders were criticized for being detrimental to the health and morals of their inhabitants.[35] The MOH for Birmingham, Dr Alfred Hill, argued in 1873 that back-to-back houses were the major culprit in keeping death rates high in the central wards of the city. In his opinion, the principal reason why these houses were so detrimental to health was that through ventilation was impossible.[36] Another great disadvantage lay in the sanitary provision. Bad drainage and sewering, irregularly cleaned communal privies, shared water taps which drew impure water from underground wells, and unpaved yards which were sodden with filth made courtyard houses an ideal breeding ground for diseases.

---

[31] A. Sutcliffe, 'Introduction', and A. Sutcliffe, 'A century of flats in Birmingham 1875–1973', in A. Sutcliffe (ed.), *Multi-storey Living: The British Working-class Experience* (London 1974), 1–18, 181–206, the quote on p. 182; Mayne, *The Imagined Slum*, 84–5, 90; Chinn, *Homes for People*.

[32] BCA PHC minutes 30 Jan. 1925, item 8825; 27 Feb. 1925, item 8901.

[33] *Census of England and Wales 1911, Volume VIII: Tenements in Administrative Counties and Urban and Rural Districts*, 662; *Statistisk årsbok för Göteborg 1930*, 28, 114, 120.

[34] Burnett, *A Social History of Housing*, 166–7; Chinn, *Homes for People*, 1–8. See also K. Dayus, *Her People* (London 1982), 3.

[35] B. Bramwell, 'Public space and local communities: the example of Birmingham, 1840–80', in G. Kearns and C.W.J. Withers (eds), *Urbanising Britain: Essays on Class and Community in the Nineteenth Century* (Cambridge 1991), 36–9; Chinn, *Homes for People*, 1–30; R. Rodger, *Housing in Urban Britain 1780–1814: Class, Capitalism and Construction* (London 1989), 32–4.

[36] *Annual Report 1873*, 19; *1898*, 8–15, 34–9.

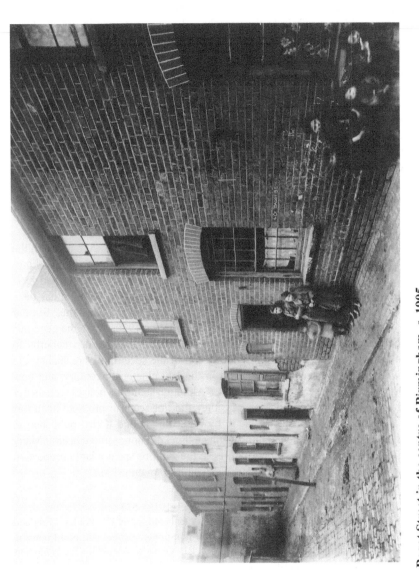

Figure 2.4 Bagot Street in the centre of Birmingham, *c.* **1905.**
Source: Local Studies and History, Birmingham Central Library.

Despite the fierce criticism, there were still 42,000 back-to-backs in Birmingham on the eve of the First World War, and for a long time no serious attempt was made to replace them. In 1919, the *British Medical Journal* stated that the victory over Germany in the war seemed to have made decision-makers blind to enormous domestic problems, one of which was the housing crisis in cities such as Birmingham: 'We, too, may add as a refrain to the speeches of our strong men in praise of our national exertions and prophesying a new heaven and earth, this sentence: In the city of Birmingham 200,000 persons live in back-to-back houses.'[37] The Birmingham decision-makers were not blind to the housing crisis, far from it, but back-to-back houses were no longer regarded as the core of the problem in the aftermath of the First World War. The housing shortage had been exacerbated during the war, so that even many lower middle-class families were having difficulty finding decent housing. In the new situation, addressing the housing problems of the poorest strata became a less pressing need, and attention shifted away from the urban core to the fringe, where new houses were being built for respectable lower-middle-class and working-class families. In the interwar years, Birmingham built about 50,000 council houses, more than any other local authority in England. Nearly 39,000 back-to-backs, which still remained in the central wards in 1936, were occupied by the poorest section of the population, who could not afford to rent a council house.[38]

Housing conditions in working-class suburbs varied enormously. At one end of the housing spectrum was the garden village of Bournville, where respectable working-class families lived in spacious well-built houses with a front and back garden and good facilities. Moreover, the estate as a whole was carefully planned: 'Nothing has been allowed to obstruct the free circulation of air and a maximum of sunshine.' Similar principles were followed in municipal housebuilding in the 1920s. With the generous support of central government, Birmingham built high-quality garden suburbs to house the 'decent' working class. At the other end of the spectrum were shabby old suburbs which private developers had built in the late nineteenth century, and new council estates built for the poor in the 1930s.[39] Although suburban houses were better built and equipped than the back-to-backs, they did not seem to promote health as much as the authorities expected. A study by MacGonigle and Kirby, published in 1937, indicated that environmental improvement alone did not promote health. Many poor families who grasped new opportunities in the suburbs spent a large proportion of their incomes on rent and consequently suffered from malnutrition.[40]

---

[37] 'The Housing Question', *British Medical Journal* (1919), 574.

[38] Chinn, *Homes for People*, 37–74; Garside, '"Unhealthy areas"'; Pooley, 'England and Wales'. For the primacy of local authorities over non-governmental, non-profit housing organizations in providing working-class houses, see P.L. Garside, 'Modelling the behaviour of non-profit housing agencies in Britain and France', in C. Zimmermann (ed.), *Europäische Wohnungspolitik in vergleichender Perspektive 1900–1939/European Housing Policy in Comparative Perpective 1900–1939* (Stuttgart 1997), 42–59.

[39] A.G. Gardiner, *Life of George Cadbury* (London 1923), 131–56, the quote on p. 149; M. Harrison, 'Bournville 1919–1939', *Planning History* **17** (3) (1995), 22–31; Chinn, *Homes for People*.

[40] G.C.M. MacGonigle and J. Kirby, *Poverty and Public Health* (London 1937). For discussion about housing and health, see Garside, '"Unhealthy areas"', 39–40; P. Mein Smith

Economy and Employment

During the late nineteenth and early twentieth centuries, Gothenburg evolved from a city of merchants to one of the nation's leading industrial centres. The growth of industry accelerated in the 1890s. Textile firms, sugar and tobacco factories and breweries, many of which had been established before the 1850s, were the first to seize new opportunities, and the wood processing and paper-making industries soon followed their example. However, the early years of the twentieth century witnessed the expansion of the metal industry and engineering, and in the 1910s these newcomers surpassed textiles and clothing as the most important industries. In 1930 no less than 43 per cent of the workers were employed by metal and engineering firms, the most important of which were two shipyards, Götaverken and Eriksberg, and a ballbearing manufacturer, Svenska Kullagerfabriken (SKF), which became a global concern in the 1920s.[41]

Owing to the dominance of export industries, the local economy was acutely affected by fluctuations in international trade. The problem was especially serious during the world-wide recession in the early 1920s. The reduction in metal employment was such that at one point during the winter of 1921–22 almost 70 per cent of unionized metal workers in Gothenburg were unemployed. A decade later, in 1932, the unemployment rate among metal workers was again high, at 35 per cent. The recessions aside, metal employment in Gothenburg was essentially regular and mainly skilled or semi-skilled. The textile and food processing industries, which served the domestic market, offered a better prospect of job security, and Gothenburg was also able to attract new industries. Vital for the future of the city was the establishment of the Volvo car plant in 1927.[42]

In Gothenburg, the labour market was characterized by a high degree of horizontal gender segregation. The old industries, textiles and food processing, were keen to employ female labour, and at the turn of the century, when these sectors still dominated, women comprised 47 per cent of all industrial workers in Gothenburg.[43] However, their proportion of the total industrial workforce was to decline during the first decades of the twentieth century, when the metal and engineering industries

---

and L. Frost, 'Suburbia and infant death in late nineteenth- and early twentieth-century Adelaide, *Urban History* **21** (2) (1994), 251–72; R.A. Cage, 'Infant mortality rates and housing: twentieth century Glasgow', *Scottish Economic and Social History* **14** (1994), 77–92; N. McFarlane, 'Hospitals, housing, tuberculosis in Glasgow, 1911–51', *Social History of Medicine* **2** (1) (1989), 59–85.

[41]   Fritz, *Från handelsstad till industristad*; Olsson, *Från industristad till tjänstestad;* Attman, *Göteborg 1863–1913*; Attman, *Göteborg 1913–1962.*

[42]   Olsson, *Från industristad till tjänstestad*, 127–35; Attman, *Göteborg 1913–1962*, 11–55, 210–13; McEwen, 'Working-class Politics', 79–80, 85; H. Wallentin, *Arbetslöshet och levnadsförhållanden i Göteborg under 1920-talet* (Göteborg 1978), 40–42, 56–75; I. Elison, *Arbetarrörelse och samhälle i Göteborg 1910–1922* (Göteborg 1970), 6–12; U. Olsson, *Lönepolitik och lönestruktur: Göteborgs verkstadsarbetare 1920–1949* (Göteborg 1970), 16–22.

[43]   *Bidrag till Sveriges Officiela Statistik 1895, D) Fabriker och Manufacturer*, table 7; C. Lindman, *Dödligheten i första lefnadsåret i Sveriges tjugo större städer 1876–95* (Stockholm 1898), 91.

were expanding. With the exception of the ballbearing manufacturer SKF, which had a significant number of women on its payroll, metalworking and engineering firms employed almost exclusively men. Hence by 1929 the proportion of women in the total industrial workforce had declined from 47 per cent to 29 per cent.[44] Outside the industrial sector, domestic service fell into decline, while the expanding service sector generated new employment opportunities for women of all classes.[45]

The wage differentials between women and men were substantial in Gothenburg. For example, in tobacco factories women usually received lower pay although they performed exactly the same tasks as men. Only 15 per cent of skilled female cigar makers earned more than 800 crowns a year in the late nineteenth century, whereas the corresponding figure for men was 50 per cent. However, compared to other female workers, and even to some male workers, skilled female cigar makers earned high wages and had good terms of employment. This small group of women was also exceptionally active in the trade union, and a large proportion of them continued to work in the factory after marriage. Women employed in the metal industry also had relatively high wages. The ballbearing firm SKF paid women about 60–65 per cent of the average wage of male employees in the 1920s, and 80–85 per cent in the 1930s. In many other industries, women's wages were low. For example, a survey of 3,000 female factory workers conducted in Stockholm in the 1890s showed that 38 per cent of them earned less than 365 crowns a year and therefore were below the basic level of subsistence.[46]

The male-breadwinner ideology was relatively weak in Sweden, and women, both unmarried and married, were often seen as a permanent part of the workforce, not just as a labour reserve. The weakness of the male-breadwinner family model, as Lena Sommestad has pointed out, had its historical roots in emigration and financial stringency. Owing to the shortage of labour, Swedish society needed women's labour power, and many Swedish working-class families would not have survived without women's earnings, since per capita income was low.[47] Therefore Swedish legislators were rather reluctant to introduce restrictions inhibiting women's right to work. Sweden followed the example set by other European countries, prohibiting women's night work in industry in 1909, but attempts to introduce more drastic measures such as the marriage bar were not successful. On the contrary, the Swedish parliament in

---

[44] Olsson, *Lönepolitik och lönestruktur*, 113–19; *Statistisk årsbok för Göteborg 1921*, 174–84, table 159; *1930*, 135–40, table 148.

[45] For women's employment in Gothenburg, see Wallentin, *Arbetslöshet*, 30–40; Attman, *Göteborg 1913–1962*, 210–11; Fritz, *Från handelsstad till industristad*, 141–9; Olsson, *Från industristad till tjänstestad*, 135–50.

[46] B. Skarin Frykman, *Arbetarkultur – Göteborg 1890* (Göteborg 1990), 119–29, 251–61; Olsson, *Lönepolitik och lönestruktur*, 133–5; E. Broomé, 'Kvinnofrågor och kvinnoarbete', in G.H. von Koch (ed.), *Social handbok* (Stockholm 1908), 199–201; K.A. Edin, 'Antalet barnaföderskor bland gifta industriarbeterskor', in *SOU 1929:28*, 105–6.

[47] L. Sommestad, 'Welfare state attitudes to the male breadwinning system: the United States and Sweden in comparative perspective', in A. Janssens (ed.), *The Rise and Decline of the Male Breadwinner Family?/International Review of Social History* **42** (1997), Supplement, 153–74; J. Lewis, 'Gender and the development of welfare regimes', *Journal of European Social Policy* **2** (3) (1992), 159–73.

1939 passed a law which prohibited employees from being dismissed on account of marriage, pregnancy or childbearing.[48]

Despite the relatively tolerant attitude to women's work, the majority of working-class women in Gothenburg gave up formal paid employment on marriage, or at least after the first child was born, and only rarely did they re-enter labour force at a later stage. As a result of rising real wages, a growing number of working-class men were able to provide for their families and therefore their wives devoted more of their time to housewifery.[49] This trend was reflected in the pages of the local Social Democratic newspaper *Ny Tid* in the 1920s. The paper, which had concentrated almost exclusively on local and national politics or on trade union issues, introduced women's pages, where articles and stories centred around household management, childrearing, gardening and fashion. While the majority of mothers in Gothenburg stayed at home, there was a sizeable minority who combined motherhood with paid work. Almost 10 per cent of married women with young children were 'gainfully employed' in the 1920s, and in addition to them there were a significant number of unmarried women with dependent children who had to work for a living.[50]

While Gothenburg's economy was affected by fluctuations in the world market, Birmingham's economic life was less sensitive to trends in the international trade and more capable of adapting to changing circumstances. Birmingham's economy had been built upon industrial production since the late eighteenth century, and in this respect the late nineteenth and early twentieth centuries did not bring any fundamental changes. Industry was undergoing structural transformations, but even these processes were marked by continuities. While some old industries such as jewellery were clearly on the decline, others continued to play a major role in the economic life of the city. For example, the metalworking and engineering sectors managed to retain their position among the key industries by modernizing their production. Alongside the old industries, there were new sectors such as cycle manufacture, electrical trades and the car industry. Owing to the broad base of industrial production, Birmingham avoided the worst effects of the recessions and recovered more rapidly than industrial cities in Northern England (Figure 2.5), Scotland and Wales.[51]

---

[48]   L. Karlsson, 'The beginning of a "masculine renaissance": the debate on the 1909 prohibition against women's night work in Sweden', in U. Wikander, A. Kessler-Harris and J. Lewis (eds), *Protecting Women: Labor Legislation in Europe, the United States, and Australia, 1880–1920* (Urbana, IL 1995), 235–66; B. Hobson, 'Feminist strategies and gendered discourses in welfare states: married women's right to work in the United States and Sweden', in S. Koven and S. Michel (eds), *Mothers of a New World: Maternalist Politics and the Origins of Welfare State* (London 1993), 396–429.

[49]   Attman, *Göteborg 1863–1913*, 289; Attman, *Göteborg 1913–1962*, 218–19.

[50]   Skarin Frykman, *Arbetarkultur*, 183–97; Wallentin, *Arbetslöshet*, 30–33; Olsson, *Hushållsinkomst*, 122–31.

[51]   *Census of England and Wales 1911, Volume X: Occupations and Industries. Part II*, table 13, 593–5; *Census of England and Wales 1951, Industry Tables*, table 2, 92–4; Sutcliffe and Smith, *Birmingham 1939–1970*, 6–9, 154–64; Briggs, *History of Birmingham*, 28–31, 43–66, 278–301; B.M.D. Smith, 'Industry and trade 1880–1960', in W.B. Stephens (ed.),

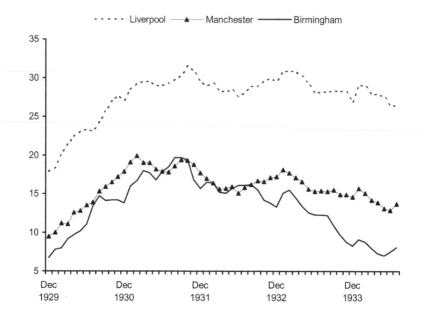

Figure 2.5   Percentage of insured workers unemployed in Liverpool, Manchester and Birmingham, December 1929–July 1934.

Note: The Birmingham figures include men from depressed areas who were attending government training or instructional centres.

Source: Local Unemployment Index, Unemployment Statistics, prepared by the Ministry of Labour (London: HMSO, 1929–34), nos 48–91.

The decades from 1870 to 1910 were a period of increasing gender segregation in Birmingham occupations. By 1911 the horizontal and vertical dividing lines between men's and women's occupations were very clear. Workers employed in the building and transport sectors or in gas and electricity plants were almost exclusively men, whereas laundry workers, dress and shirt makers and seamstresses were women. Jewellery, car and cycle manufacture and the metal industry employed both men and women, but in these sectors women almost invariably found themselves working in lower-grade jobs than men.[52] Irrespective of whether they worked in a female dominated sector or not, women workers usually earned less than half the average weekly earnings of men. In Birmingham factories, the average earnings of married women workers, most of whom had to partially maintain their families, were only 9s. 1d. per week at the beginning of the twentieth century, while unskilled male labourers received between 17s. and 21s. Only women who were 'really first-class workers' or 'exceptionally good machine rulers' could earn as much as unskilled

---

A History of the County of Warwick, vol. VII (London 1964), 171–8, 190–208; Cherry, *Birmingham*, 60–66.

[52]   *Census of England and Wales 1911, Volume X: Occupations and Industries. Part II,* table 13, 593–5; See also *Census of England and Wales 1931, Occupation Tables*, table 16, 362–76; Smith, 'Industry and trade', 176–8.

male workers. In Britain in general, women's pay was about 38–46 per cent of men's pay in the metal industry, and 55 per cent in the textile industry.[53]

In Birmingham, the census of 1911 categorized 18 per cent of married women as 'gainfully employed', but does not provide any information about how many of them had young children.[54] In addition to married women who worked outside the home, a significant number of women were employed as homeworkers or outworkers in the early years of the twentieth century. The commonest tasks which female homeworkers undertook were the carding of hooks and eyes, sewing of buttons onto cards and wrapping up hair pins in paper, but a large number of women also worked in the jewellery and metal trades like metal burnishing and plating. While metal burnishing was relatively well paid, much of the other work which women homeworkers did amounted to sweated labour. The jobs were tiring and repetitive, and the wages were below the subsistence level. To what extent women engaged in this type of work is difficult to estimate, since Census enumerators systematically failed to record married women's part-time work.[55]

Attitudes to married women's work were generally negative in Britain during the first half of the twentieth century. Central and local government, the press, employers and trade unions were all committed to reinforcing the male-breadwinner family model.[56] These attitudes manifested themselves, for example, in legislative restrictions such as the marriage bar, which inhibited women's activity rates and ensured that men had priority in the labour market. Women pursuing professional careers were almost invariably forced to give up their work upon marriage, but a marriage bar was also applied to many other women workers. The Birmingham Public Health Department demanded not only women doctors but also health visitors and nurses renounce their work once they married. Moreover, many British companies employing working-class women, for example Boots and Unilever, operated

---

[53]   *Birmingham Trades for Women and Girls* (Education Committee, Birmingham 1914); G.J. Barnsby, *Birmingham Working People: A History of the Labour Movement in Birmingham 1650–1914* (Wolverhampton 1989), 466–7; C. Chinn, *They Worked All Their Lives: Women of the Urban Poor in England, 1880–1939* (Manchester 1988), 86–8; J. Lewis, *Women in England 1870–1950: Sexual Divisions and Social Change* (London 1984), 162–93. See also B. Drake, *Women in Trade Unions* (London 1984, first pub. 1920), 44; C. Black (ed.), *Married Women's Work: Being the Report of an Enquiry Undertaken by Women's Industrial Council* (London 1983, first pub. 1915).

[54]   *Census of England and Wales 1911, Volume X: Occupations and Industries. Part II*, table 13, 593–5.

[55]   Chinn, *Homes for People*, 19; Smith, 'Industry and trade'; Lewis, *Women in England*, 58–62. See also G.M. Tuckwell, 'The regulation of women's work', in G.M. Tuckwell et al., *Woman in Industry: From Seven Points of View* (London 1908), 1–23.

[56]   Lewis, 'Gender and the development of welfare regimes'; S. Horrell and J. Humphries, 'The origins and expansion of the male bread-winner family: the case of nineteenth-century Britain', in Janssens, *The Rise and Decline of the Male Breadwinner Family?*, 25–64; M. Savage, 'Trade unionism, sex segregation, and the state: women's employment in "new industries" in inter-war Britain', *Social History* **13** (2) (1988), 209–30.

marriage bars in the interwar years.[57] Unsurprisingly, women had mixed feelings about measures which served to curtail their job opportunities. For example, the Labour women, who generally endorsed the male-breadwinner family model, often joined middle-class feminists in defending women's right to work and in opposing measures such as the marriage bar, which circumscribed this right.[58]

The Family

In Gothenburg and in Sweden in general, marriage and family patterns varied widely depending on the social group. Among the urban middle class, family formation and pre-marital relationships were strictly controlled, and in consequence the percentage of illegitimate children was very low. Working-class people in towns and unlanded people in the rural areas, by contrast, had relatively tolerant attitudes to pre-marital sex, non-marital childbearing and co-habitation. Despite public efforts to encourage more orthodox marriage and family patterns, the illegitimate birth rate remained high in Sweden throughout the period covered here. In Stockholm the proportion of illegitimate children had traditionally been very high – almost 50 per cent in the mid-nineteenth century – and in the early twentieth century it was still considerably higher than in other Swedish cities. In Gothenburg, the percentage of illegitimate children among all newborn babies hovered between 16 and 22 per cent from the turn of the century until the 1930s, when it started to decline.[59] However, many illegitimate children were born into relationships similar to marriage, and their parents often got married after the child was born, legalizing their long-standing relationship. Furthermore, a large proportion of unmarried mothers married someone other than the father of their child. Yet in Swedish cities there were a considerable number of women, single mothers, widows and deserted wives who maintained their children entirely by themselves. At the turn of the century, a survey conducted in Stockholm showed that a third of women who had children were solely responsible for them.[60]

---

[57] See, for example, BCA Birmingham Maternity and Child Welfare Committee (M&CWC) minutes 23 Jan. 1931, item 514, document 122. See also Lewis, *Women in England*, 75–9, 97–106, 173, 187; J. Humphries, 'Women and paid work', in J. Purvis (ed.), *Women's History: Britain, 1850–1945: An Introduction* (London 1995), 98–100; Savage, 'Trade unionism'.

[58] For a Birmingham campaign against the marriage bar, see BCA M&CWC 26 Sep. 1930, item 365, 9 Jan. 1931, item 499, 23 Jan. 1931, item 514. See also P. Thane, 'Visions of gender in the making of the British welfare state: the case of women in the British Labour Party and social policy, 1906–1945', in G. Bock and P. Thane (eds), *Maternity and Gender Policies: Women and the Rise of the European Welfare States 1880s–1950s* (London 1991), 98–9; J. Lewis and S.O. Rose, '"Let England blush": protective labor legislation, 1820–1914', in Wikander, Kessler-Harris and Lewis, *Protecting Women*, 91–124, esp. 109–110. See also J. Bourke, *Working-class Cultures in Britain 1890–1960: Gender, Class and Ethnicity* (London 1994), 104.

[59] *Statistisk årsbok för Göteborg 1924*, 52, table 33; *1930*, 36, table 29; *1934*, 28, table 26; *1939*, 28, table 26.

[60] A-S. Ohlander, 'The invisible child? The struggle for a Social Democratic family policy in Sweden, 1900–1960s', in Bock and Thane, *Maternity and Gender Policies*, 63;

In early twentieth-century Britain, marriage and family patterns were much more uniform and attitudes to pre-marital relationships, and in particular to unmarried motherhood, less tolerant than in Sweden.[61] The view that the family consisted of a married couple and children was clearly accepted not only throughout the middle classes but also to a large extent among the working class. Illegitimacy rates were between 4 and 5 per cent until the First World War, when they rose sharply, and then immediately after the war they fell back again. In Birmingham, as in many other large British cities, the rates were even lower, around 3 per cent (Figure 2.6), and unmarried mothers were a small minority. One reason why illegitimacy rates remained so low was that a large proportion, about 70 per cent, of premarital conceptions were legitimized by marriage before the birth.[62] How these structures, attitudes and aims influenced the way in which health authorities approached the problems of infant mortality and tuberculosis is examined in Chapters 4 and 5, but before that, in Chapter 3, there is discussion of policy legacies.

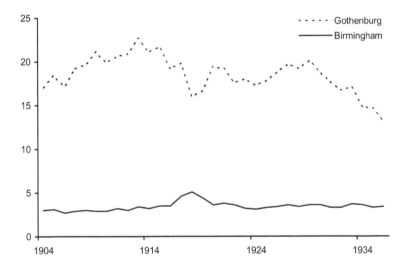

Figure 2.6   Percentage of illegitimate births of all live births in Gothenburg and Birmingham, 1904–1936.
Source: Bidrag till Sveriges Officiella Statistik, A) Befolkningsstatistik 1904–1910; Statistiska årsböcker för Göteborg 1910–1936; Annual Reports of the Registrar General of Births, Deaths and Marriages in England and Wales 1904–1920; Registrar General, Statistical Reviews 1910–1936.

A. Kälvemark, 'Att vänta barn när man gifter sig: föräktenskapliga förbindelser och giftermålsmönster i 1800-talets Sverige', *Historisk Tidskrift* **97** (2) (1977), 181–99.

[61]   Bourke, *Working-class Cultures*, 27–41; E. Roberts, *A Woman's Place: An Oral History of Working-class Women 1890–1940* (Oxford 1984), 72–80.

[62]   J. Lewis, *Women in Britain Since 1945: Women, Family, Work and the State in the Post-War Years* (Oxford 1992), 44; J. Lewis and J. Welshman, 'The issue of never-married motherhood in Britain, 1920–70', *Social History of Medicine* **10** (3) (1997), 401–18; Lewis, *Women in England*, 5–6.

CHAPTER 3

Policy Legacies

Policy making is inherently a historical process. Previously established policies influence present-day decision-making, which in turn shapes future policy options. In mounting campaigns against infant mortality and tuberculosis in the early twentieth century, both British and Swedish health authorities tended to introduce reforms which were broadly in line with local government traditions and which could be incorporated into the existing health services. Instead of formulating entirely new strategies, they usually built on old policies or reacted against them. Similarly, the decisions taken in the early twentieth century inevitably curtailed the number of policy options open to the future decision-makers and, in consequence, the legacy of the early twentieth-century choices remains with us today.

By looking at public health policies and local government structures in nineteenth-century Britain and Sweden, this chapter provides a basis for discussion as to how the policy legacies and pre-existing administrative structures influenced early twentieth-century infant welfare and anti-tuberculosis campaigns. The chapter identifies some important continuities in Swedish and British health policies that partly explain the variation in national responses to the problems of infant mortality and tuberculosis.[1] Firstly, the chapter develops further the themes briefly discussed in Chapter 1: the strength of the public sector and the social status of public health officers. In Sweden, the role of the public sector in health care was very important in the nineteenth and early twentieth centuries. The public sector catered – at least in principle – for all social groups, not only the poor, and the majority of medical doctors, including influential hospital consultants, worked for the public sector. Most hospitals were publicly owned. Furthermore, the leading public health officers held a relatively powerful position in society, especially from the late nineteenth century, and they were influential in the formulation of health policies. In Britain, by contrast, public provision for sickness was of secondary importance, as general practitioners and voluntary hospitals formed the core of the health care system, and British public health officers were less influential than their Swedish counterparts in determining policies.

---

[1] For similar approaches, see S. Pedersen, *Family, Dependence, and the Origins of the Welfare State: Britain and France, 1914–1945* (Cambridge 1995); T. Skocpol, 'Bringing the state back in: strategies of analysis in current research', and M. Weir and T. Skocpol, 'State structures and the possibilities for "Keynesian" responses to the Great Depression in Sweden, Britain, and the United States', in P.B. Evans, D. Rueschemeyer and T. Skocpol (eds), *Bringing the State Back In* (Cambridge 1985), 3–37, 107–63. Skocpol argues that public policies are jointly conditioned by social relations and the pre-existing institutional arrangements of the state.

Secondly, the chapter discusses two other aspects that influenced the way in which Swedish and British officials defined health problems in the early twentieth century: the primary object of intervention in the field of public health in the nineteenth century and the respective powers and jurisdictions of central government and local authorities. Until the end of the nineteenth century, the British public health authorities concentrated on improving physical environment, and the expansion of central government control over local health and sanitary policies was slow. In Sweden, by contrast, the primary focus of the public health policies was the individual, and many aspects of health policies were under central government control.

Swedish Public Health Strategies

In Sweden, central government regulated both public and private health care provision from an early date. At the instigation of influential Stockholm-based physicians and with the support of the Crown, the first regulatory body, the *Collegium Medicum*, was established as early as 1663. The initial purpose of the organization was to restore order in Stockholm's medical market, where physicians had to compete against other healers, but within a few decades the Collegium Medicum developed into a governmental body that supervised health care provision in the entire country. In the eighteenth century, the organization recognized and regulated not only physicians but also barber-surgeons, midwives and pharmacists, distinguishing them from quacks. Moreover, provincial doctors and city physicians, numbering altogether forty or fifty doctors, worked under the control of the Collegium Medicum. They attended patients, but also supervised hospitals and other local health facilities and reported regularly the central government on the conditions in their respective districts.[2]

Mercantilist thinking was the main motivating force for increasing government involvement in the medical market in eighteenth-century Sweden. Convinced that a large and healthy population was a cornerstone of the nation's power, the Swedish government founded the Statistical Bureau (*Tabelverket*) in 1749 to ascertain the number of inhabitants in the country and to compile vital statistics which would help authorities devise strategies to increase the population. The report based on the first national registration of the population was not, however, gratifying to the authorities. The population of Sweden (including Finland) was only two million, a figure so embarrassingly low that it was immediately declared top secret. One solution proposed by decision-makers was to improve the health care system and, above all, to combat epidemics.[3]

---

[2]   E. Björkquist and I. Flygare, 'Den centrala medicinalförvaltningen', and H. Bergstrand, 'Läkarekåren och provinsialläkareväsendet', in W. Kock (ed.), *Medicinalväsendet i Sverige 1813–1962* (Stockholm 1963), 7–40, 120–31; M.C. Nelson and J. Rogers, 'Cleaning up the cities: application of the first comprehensive public health law in Sweden', *Scandinavian Journal of History* **19** (1) (1994), 18–20; J. Rogers and M.C. Nelson, 'Controlling infectious diseases in ports: the importance of the military in central–local relations', in M.C. Nelson and J. Rogers (eds), *Urbanisation and the Epidemiologic Transition* (Uppsala 1989), 88–9.

[3]   K. Johannisson, 'The people's health: public health policies in Sweden', in D. Porter (ed.), *The History of Public Health and the Modern State* (Amsterdam 1994), 166–9.

The following decades saw a steady increase in the number of ordinances regulating health care provision in general and the containment of epidemics in particular. From 1813, local parish priests were obliged to report outbreaks of diseases in their parishes to provincial doctors. If the reported disease proved contagious and serious, free medicine was made available and a temporary hospital was set up in order to isolate patients. In 1816, almost four decades earlier than in Britain, smallpox vaccination was made compulsory.[4] All aspects of health care, with the exception of hospital administration, were under the control of the *Sundhetskollegium,* the new central government department that had replaced the Collegium Medicum in 1813.[5]

During the cholera epidemic of 1834, temporary sanitary committees were established in many Swedish towns to supervise measures taken to attend to the victims and to stop the disease from spreading. Despite these efforts, the epidemic killed 8 per cent of the population in Gothenburg (1,700 people) and 5 per cent in Stockholm, levels significantly above those, for example, in Liverpool.[6] The Epidemic Act of 1857 (*epidemistadgan*) was concerned specifically with cholera and other contagious diseases. It required urban authorities to set up a permanent sanitary committee (*sundhetsnämnden*), whose main task was to ensure that necessary precautionary measures were taken against epidemics and that people who became infected were isolated and treated.[7] Strategies focusing on the individual – vaccination, isolation hospitals and quarantine, and medical treatment – were clearly given priority in the Swedish public health policy of the mid-nineteenth century.

The emphasis on the individual manifested itself not only in the campaigns against epidemics, but also in measures taken to contain venereal diseases (VD). Throughout the nineteenth century, Swedish health authorities devoted a considerable proportion of their resources to hospital treatment for VD and, in particular, syphilis. In 1820, about half of all hospital beds in Sweden were allotted to patients with VD, and in 1881 still 15 per cent. Moreover, during the second half of the nineteenth century, 13 Swedish towns, including Gothenburg, began to regulate prostitution. Women 'identified' as prostitutes by the police were subjected to regular medical inspection and, if found to be suffering from a venereal disease, were interned in a hospital. The regulation of prostitution was not abolished in Sweden until 1918.[8]

---

[4]   S. Edvinsson, *Den osunda staden: Sociala skillnader i dödlighet i 1800-talets Sundsvall* (Umeå 1992), 63–6; H. Nilsson, *Mot bättre hälsa: Dödlighet och hälsoarbete i Linköping 1860–1894* (Linköping 1994), 56.

[5]   The supervision of hospitals was entrusted to the Sundhetskollegium in 1859. The present-day Medicinalstyrelsen (The National Board of Health) replaced the Sundhetskollegium in 1877–78.

[6]   B. Zacke, *Koleraepidemien i Stockholm, 1834: En socialhistorisk studie* (Stockholm 1971); for Gothenburg, see pp. 62–3.

[7]   R. Bergman, 'De epidemiska sjukdomarna och deras bekämpande', in Kock, *Medicinalväsendet*, 364–6; Nelson and Rogers, 'Cleaning up the cities', 20–24.

[8]   S. Hellerström and M. Tottie, 'De veneriska sjukdomarna', in Kock, *Medicinalväsendet*, 405–15; A. Brändström, 'The silent sick: the life-histories of 19th century Swedish hospital patients', in A. Brändström and L.-G. Tedebrand (eds), *Society, Health and Population During the Demographic Transition* (Stockholm 1988), 343–68, 23; T. Lundquist, *Den disciplinerade dubbelmoralen: Studier i den reglementerade prostitutionens historia i Sverige 1859–1918*

The second half of the nineteenth century saw the proliferation of health care services in Swedish towns. The rapid growth of services was possible, firstly, because local authorities assumed wide responsibilities regarding personal health care, and secondly, because they did not develop health care within the confines of the poor law system. Owing to active government involvement, health care provision in Sweden was soon comparable to services available in more affluent societies such as Britain and Germany. Swedish hospital provision in particular stood comparison with that of Britain, a considerable achievement given the wide discrepancy in levels of wealth.[9] In late nineteenth-century Gothenburg, the municipal authorities ran a workhouse infirmary, but also general and special hospitals. While the infirmary provided hospital treatment for the destitute, the general and special hospitals catered mainly for working-class and lower-middle-class people, who usually contributed something towards their treatment and upkeep.[10]

As the public provision for sickness was not subordinate to the poor law in Sweden, the 'respectable' working class and lower middle class did not view this provision with the same profound distrust as did the corresponding social groups in Britain. However, some publicly funded health measures gave rise to criticism even in Sweden. The most vehement objections were raised to reforms such as the smallpox vaccination programme that gave compulsory powers to health authorities and therefore clearly impinged on the individuals' right to make their own decisions in matters concerning their health. Protests against the vaccination legislation, however, were staged rather sporadically and they did not develop into an organized anti-vaccination movement. The campaign against the compulsory screening and treatment of prostitutes did not fare any better, although it was better organized than the anti-vaccination activity.[11]

Awareness of environmental problems increased in Sweden in the 1850s and 1860s. Firstly, the 1857 Epidemic Act required, though in rather vague terms, local sanitary committees to examine the sanitary conditions of their towns and,

---

(Göteborg 1982); A. Lundberg, *Care and Coercion: Medical Knowledge, Social Policy and Patients with Venereal Disease in Sweden 1785–1903* (Umeå 1999). As late as 1914, the Gothenburg health police examined 235 women, 86 of whom were hospitalized. *Göteborgs hälsovårdsnämnds årsberättelse 1914*, 20–21.

[9]   For a comparative analysis of British, German and Swedish public health policies, see G. Kearns, W.R. Lee and J. Rogers, 'The interaction of political and economic factors in the management of urban public health', in Nelson and Rogers, *Urbanisation*. For the development of health care services in Sweden, see also S. Edvinsson and J. Rogers, 'Hälsa och hälsoreformer i svenska städer kring sekelskiftet 1900', *Historisk tidskrift* **121** (4) (2001), 541–64; Nelson and Rogers, 'Cleaning up the cities', 17–20; Edvinsson, *Den osunda staden*; Nilsson, *Mot bättre hälsa*. For the social background of hospital patients in Sweden, see Brändström, 'The silent sick', 346–50.

[10]   A. Attman, *Göteborgs Stadsfullmäktige 1863–1962*, vol. I.1: *Göteborg 1863–1913* (Göteborg 1963), 333–6; G. Carlson et al., *Sjukvården i Göteborg 200 år* (Göteborg 1982), 43–51, 69–102.

[11]   M.C. Nelson and J. Rogers, 'The right to die? Anti-vaccination activity and the 1874 smallpox epidemic in Stockholm', *Social History of Medicine* **5** (3) (1992), 369–88; Lundquist, *Den disciplinerade dubbelmoralen*, 408–21; Lundberg, *Care and Coercion*, 198–214.

if necessary, to take measures and to give advice to townspeople as to how to deal with problems. Secondly, the local government reform in 1862–63 paved the way for more ambitious public intervention. Former governing bodies dominated by the traditional middling class, shopkeepers and artisans, were replaced by a town council representative of all ratepayers. The system where the number of votes was in proportion to the property owned favoured those with large incomes, and in consequence, in Gothenburg and in many other Swedish cities, leading businessmen and manufacturers were influential in the formation of municipal policies in the late nineteenth and early twentieth centuries. In general, this group advocated more liberal public spending than shopkeepers and artisans had done.[12]

Despite these reforms, progress in urban environmental management was uneven and slow. In the 1860s and 1870s several towns supplied piped water to the central districts where middle-class families lived, but did not provide other residential areas with the same service until much later.[13] Attempts to mitigate the problem of insanitary housing were even less enthusiastic, although local building ordinances gave authorities some means of dealing with the question. Many medical doctors and social reformers were in favour of stricter regulation, but Parliament was reluctant to circumscribe the rights of property owners.[14] In Gothenburg, a member of the sanitary committee, Dr Elias Heyman, studied local health conditions and demanded more extensive sanitary measures. His demands fuelled a dispute over sanitary policy which culminated in Heyman leaving Gothenburg for Stockholm in the early 1870s.[15]

The first comprehensive Public Health Act, influenced by both British and German public health legislation, was passed in 1874. The Act required each municipality to set up a public health committee consisting of the city physician, the police chief, a representative of the magistracy, and four other members who were to be appointed

---

[12] O. Wetterberg and G. Axelsson, *Smutsguld och dödligt hot: Renhållning och återvinning i Göteborg 1864–1930* (Göteborg 1995), 97. For the role of businessmen and industrialists in municipal policy making, see H. Nilsson, 'Hälsa och stadsrenhållning under 1800-talet', *Nordisk Arkitekturforskning* **8** (1) (1995), 24; B.-M. Olsson, 'Stadens styrelse – ett upplyst fåvälde', in *För hundra år sedan – skildringar från Göteborgs 1880-tal* (Göteborg 1984), 227–40; Nelson and Rogers, 'Cleaning up the cities', 28–38.

[13] C. Lindman, *Dödligheten i första lefnadsåret i Sveriges tjugo större städer 1876–95* (Stockholm 1898), 126–7; J. Hallström, *Constructing a Pipe-bound City: A History of Water Supply, Sewerage, and Excreta Removal in Norrköping and Linköping, Sweden, 1860–1910* (Linköping 2002), 170–228; R. Castensson, M. Löwgren and J. Sundin, 'Urban water supply and improvement of health conditions', in Brändström and Tedebrand, *Society, Health and Population*, 273–98; Wetterberg and Axelsson, *Smutsguld*, 97–120; Nilsson, 'Hälsa och stadsrenhållning', 24; Kearns, Lee and Rogers, 'The interaction of political and economic factors', 72, table 46.

[14] Edvinsson, *Den osunda staden*, 70–74; Nelson and Rogers, 'Cleaning up the cities', 21–5; Bergman, 'De epidemiska sjukdomarna', 364–6. For the local building ordinances, see T. Hall, 'Urban planning in Sweden', in T. Hall (ed.), *Planning and Urban Growth in the Nordic Countries* (London 1991), 174–8.

[15] K. Linroth, 'Minnesteckning öfver Elias Heyman', *Hygiea* **52** (1890), 59. For Heyman's studies, see for example E. Heyman, 'Några statistiska uppgifter om sunda arbetarebostäders inflytande på dödligheten', *Hygiea* **41** (1879), 73–85.

by the town council. The responsibilities of the committee included the management of sewers, drains and water supply, the control of the sanitary condition of rented houses and flats, and the regulation of the sale of foodstuffs. Moreover, the Public Health Act broadened the responsibilities of medical doctors. They were required to notify the public health authorities of all cases of cholera, smallpox, typhus, typhoid fever, scarlet fever, diphtheria and dysentery. In Britain, the Infectious Disease (Notification) Act was passed somewhat later, in 1889.[16] Despite the important reforms, Sweden clearly lagged behind Britain in sanitary engineering in the late nineteenth century. The acute-care model, which concentrated on the individual and gave priority to medical care, was the tradition that early twentieth-century health authorities in Gothenburg and other Swedish cities inherited from their predecessors.[17]

British Public Health Strategies

Unlike the Swedish government, the British government showed little interest in guiding local communities in questions concerning health care and environmental cleanliness in the seventeenth and eighteenth centuries. Central control, as Christopher Hamlin has pointed out, was almost non-existent: 'to a large degree counties, boroughs, and parishes were responsible for their own affairs, each conducting these with its own traditions, institutions, and ineptitude'.[18] Hence Britain had virtually no national public health legislation when cholera broke out in the country in 1831. Political pressures to guide local policy making and to enforce some degree of uniformity had been increasing over the preceding decades, but it needed a serious crisis such as cholera to actually put public health issues on the national agenda. A temporary central government body, the Board of Health, was established specifically to deal with the cholera epidemic, and another response to the pressures to create centralized bureaucracies was the Poor Law Amendment Act of 1834. The Poor Law Commission, the new central authority, and local poor law unions provided the first administrative network with national coverage of both urban and rural areas. This network was used, for example, to provide a vaccination service for the entire population.[19]

While the British authorities expressly asserted the non-pauperizing nature of the vaccination service, all other poor law medical services were tainted by the stigma of pauperism. The subordination of public provision for sickness to the poor law administration caused some problems. Firstly, a system which actively discouraged

---

[16]   Nelson and Rogers, 'Cleaning up the cities', 21–6, Edvinsson, *Den osunda staden*, 75–7; Nilsson, *Mot bättre hälsa*, 60–67.

[17]   See also Edvinsson and Rogers, 'Hälsa och hälsoreformer'.

[18]   C. Hamlin, 'State medicine in Great Britain', in Porter, *The History of Public Health*, 134.

[19]   M.W. Flinn, 'Medical services under the New Poor Law', in D. Fraser (ed.), *The New Poor Law in the Nineteenth Century* (London 1976), 51–2; E.P. Hennock, 'Vaccination policy against smallpox, 1835–1914: a comparison of England with Prussia and Imperial Germany', *Social History of Medicine* **11** (1) (1998), 49–71; F.B. Smith, *The People's Health 1830–1910* (London 1990), 158–68.

people from applying for medical relief even when they urgently needed it could not be effective in alleviating health problems. Secondly, the development of poor law medical care was seriously hampered by the principle that all services which provided for the destitute ought to be inferior to the medical treatment which 'independent labourers' obtained through sick clubs, friendly societies and voluntary hospitals. In the late nineteenth century, after a number of well-publicized scandals had drawn the public's attention to the state of the ailing poor, efforts were made to remove some of the ambivalence pervading the service. Poor law infirmaries eased the requirement of destitution, also admitting non-pauper patients, and the standard of care and the level of amenities were raised. Despite these changes, poor law infirmaries did not compete on equal terms with voluntary hospitals. In many cities poor law infirmaries provided more than half of all hospital beds at the turn of the century, but they were mainly catering for chronic and long-term patients excluded from voluntary hospitals.[20]

The public health authorities, for their part, were reluctant to assume any responsibilities regarding personal health care. The last decades of the nineteenth century saw a piecemeal expansion of the number of municipal hospitals, but these institutions were almost exclusively designed to isolate and treat patients suffering from infectious diseases. Any wider vision of municipal commitments was repudiated by most decision-makers, who regarded personal health care services either as private and voluntary ventures or, in the case of indigent patients, as the responsibility of the poor law authorities. For example, most local authorities, the Birmingham authorities included, did not start to run general hospitals until the poor law infirmaries were transferred to them in 1929.[21]

The focus of British public health policy was pre-eminently environmental throughout the nineteenth century. In the first half of the century, the initiative lay entirely with local authorities and the pace of reform varied enormously from place to place. Large and wealthy towns, with a few notable exceptions, were the driving force behind attempts to tackle urban environmental problems. In drafting local improvement Acts which would empower them to control the rapidly changing urban environment, they played a dominant role in identifying and defining new statutory needs. Other towns followed in their wake, preparing more limited Acts or taking over clauses from the local Acts of the pioneering towns. In the mid-nineteenth century, central government finally assumed a more active role in the field of public health. One of the first general acts was the Public Health Act of 1848, which empowered local authorities to establish a local board of health and to appoint

---

[20] Flinn, 'Medical services'; M.A. Crowther, *The Workhouse System 1834–1929: The History of an English Social Institution* (London 1983); R. Pinker, *English Hospital Statistics 1861–1938* (London 1966), 60–68; Kearns, Lee and Rogers, 'The interaction of political and economic factors', 18, 56.

[21] Pinker, *English Hospital Statistics*, 72–9; A.S. Wohl, *Endangered Lives: Public Health in Victorian Britain* (London 1984), 129–41; J.V. Pickstone, *Medicine and Industrial Society: A History of Hospital Development in Manchester and Its Region, 1752–1946* (Manchester 1985), 165–9, L. Granshaw, 'The rise of the modern hospital in Britain', in A. Wear (ed.), *Medicine in Society: Historical Essays* (Cambridge 1992), 202–18. For Birmingham, see J. Jones, *History of the Corporation of Birmingham*, vol. V, Part II (Birmingham 1940), 543–5.

a Medical Officer of Health (MOH) to identify houses unfit for human habitation, to manage sewers, drains, wells and water supplies, to remove nuisances and to regulate offensive trades. Local authorities were also given the right to levy local rates and purchase land, which were essential prerequisites of effective implementation of the new legislation. However, in the 1850s and 1860s local authorities could either adopt the powers conferred by general Acts or continue to draft local Acts. The Birmingham authorities, suspicious of any interference from central government, refused to adopt, for example, the 1848 Public Health Act, and drafted a local improvement Act instead.[22]

The 1848 Act also established a new central government department, the General Board of Health, to deal with public health problems and to supervise local authorities in sanitary questions. Its responsibilities were transferred to the Privy Council in 1854 and to the Local Government Board in 1871.[23] Despite the fact that most of the public health legislation was optional until the late nineteenth century, central government nevertheless had a considerable influence on the public health strategies pursued in British cities. Central government was, to an extent, able to define urban health problems by directing local authorities' attention to some questions and by allowing them to ignore others. For example, Edwin Chadwick and other 'ultra-sanitarians' in central government mounted a sustained and successful campaign to convince local policy makers that epidemic diseases were a product of dirt and decomposing matter, and that environmental measures were the answer to these problems.[24]

Moreover, by categorizing towns and districts as healthy or unhealthy on the basis of mortality league tables, central government managed to shame some cities with high death rates into activity. The drawback of the strategy was that comparative tables provided cities with low overall death rates, like Birmingham, with an excuse for not taking decisive action to alleviate environmental problems in their slum areas.[25] Birmingham had been spared the worst ravages of cholera in both 1832 (21 deaths in Birmingham, 1,523 in Liverpool) and 1849 (29 deaths in Birmingham, 5,308 in Liverpool), and it stood favourably in the league tables. Yet the death rates for the central wards of the city were high, and in 1849 the Inspector of the General Board of Health, Robert Rawlinson, reported many serious problems in the city, such as the 'indescribable filthiness' of streets, canals and rivers. Central government's one-sided attention to overall death rates and local decision-makers' determination

---

[22]   E.P. Hennock, *Fit and Proper Persons: Ideal and Reality in Nineteenth-century Urban Government* (London 1973), 4–6; Wohl, *Endangered Lives*, 149–59, 166–74; G. Kearns, 'Zivilis or Hygaeia: urban public health and the epidemiologic transition', in R. Lawton (ed.), *The Rise and Fall of Great Cities: Aspects of Urbanization in the Western World* (London 1989), 112–22.

[23]   Wohl, *Endangered Lives*, 118, 149–58; S.E. Finer, *The Life and Times of Edwin Chadwick* (London 1952), 431–8.

[24]   Not everyone was happy with this narrow definition. See, for example, J.V. Pickstone, 'Dearth, dirt and fever epidemics: rewriting the history of British "public health", 1780–1850', in T. Ranger and P. Slack (eds), *Epidemics and Ideas: Essays on the Historical Perception of Pestilence* (Cambridge 1992), 126–48.

[25]   Wohl, *Endangered Lives*, 149–58.

to keep expenses low made Birmingham one of the most backward boroughs in the country in the 1850s and 1860s. Health and sanitary problems received systematic attention only after the appointment of the first MOH, Dr Alfred Hill, in 1873.[26]

The public health legislation of the 1870s contained a significant number of compulsory clauses, leaving local authorities less room to manoeuvre. However, this was not the only reason why attitudes to public health questions were changing in Birmingham. The economic elite of the city, leading businessmen and manufacturers, gained control over local decision-making by the early 1870s. They were well aware of the significant benefits which more liberal public spending would bring to them personally and to the city in general, and in consequence they started to steer municipal politics in a new direction.[27]

When municipal intervention in the management of private property grew more ambitious, small property owners voiced their grave concern that, while they were made to pay for environmental and sanitary reforms, other groups reaped the benefits. Their concern was not entirely groundless. New environmental regulations left some marginal landlords and workshop owners in desperate financial straits. However, environmental regulations did not seriously erode property rights, and this was the message which Chadwick and other leading sanitary reformers sought to get across. They sold national and local policy makers on the notion that public health reform was a means of ensuring that capitalist market relationships operated effectively and that imperfect competition and other abuses were minimized.[28]

Although the British authorities pinned their hopes on sanitary engineering, they adopted some individualistic public health strategies in order to prevent and contain epidemics. The launching of these strategies often met with protests. For example, during the cholera epidemic of 1831–32 some working-class people

---

[26]   R. Woods, 'Mortality and sanitary conditions in the "Best governed city in the world" – Birmingham 1870–1910', *Journal of Historical Geography* **4** (1) (1978), 36–7; Hennock, *Fit and Proper Persons*, 104–16; D.R. Green and A.G. Parton, 'Slums and slum life in Victorian England: London and Birmingham at mid-century', in S.M. Gaskell (ed.), *Slums* (Leicester 1990), 37–53; D.G. Watts, 'Public health', in *A History of the County of Warwick, Volume VII: The City of Birmingham* (London 1964), 340–42; A. Briggs, *History of Birmingham, Volume II: Borough and City 1865–1938* (London 1952); J.L. MacMorran, *Municipal Public Works and Planning in Birmingham: A Record of the Administration and Achievements of the Public Works Committee and Department of the Borough and City of Birmingham* (Birmingham 1973), 5–10. Alfred Hill was also influential at the national level. He was the first president of the Society of Medical Officers of Health, which came to being in 1889 as a result of the amalgamation of the Metropolitan association and various regional associations. D. Porter, 'Stratification and its discontents: prefessionalization and conflict in the British public health service, 1848–1914', in E. Fee and R.M. Acheson (eds), *A History of Education in Public Health: Health that Mocks the Doctors' Rules* (Oxford 1991), 105–12.

[27]   *Annual Reports of the Medical Officer of Health for Birmingham for 1872–1900*, and in particular *1874*, 15–17; *1882*, 3–4; *1885*, 57–67; *1888*, 46–53; *1897*, 6–10, 20–33; *1898*, 8–15, 34–40. See also A. Mayne, *The Imagined Slum: Newspaper Representation in Three Cities 1870–1914* (Leicester 1993), 57–97.

[28]   G. Kearns, 'Private property and public health reform in England 1830–70', *Social Science and Medicine* **26** (1) (1988), 187, 190–93. See also Kearns, Lee and Rogers, 'The interaction of political and economic factors', 25–9, 35.

perceived emergency measures as an unnecessary disruption to their everyday lives and as a threat to their established rights, and in consequence they responded to the measures either with passive disobedience or with violent resistance. Similarly, protests against the regulation of prostitution and against the poor law authorities' vaccination programme attracted support, and both these protest movements were eventually able to claim success. The campaign against the regulation of prostitution achieved its aim in 1886, when the Contagious Diseases Acts were repealed. The movement protesting against compulsory vaccination won a compromise. The conscience clause which enabled parents to refuse permission for health authorities to vaccinate their children was introduced by the Vaccination Act of 1898.[29] Compared to their Swedish counterparts, the British public health authorities had relatively little experience with individualistic public health strategies in the late nineteenth century, and the strategies they had pursued had met with protests from various quarters.

Public Health Strategies and the New Hygiene

In the late nineteenth century, British and Swedish public health policies were converging. The British health policy shifted away from environmental concerns to a more individualistic focus. However, the new individualistic strategies that the British and Swedish public health authorities devised at the turn of the century differed from the traditional Swedish strategies in one major way. The new techniques were not primarily fixed to identify disease in individual bodies but, as David Armstrong has pointed out, 'in the spaces between people, in the interstices of relationships, in the social body itself'. Disease became increasingly constituted in the social body rather than the individual body, and it was monitored by various agents in the community.[30]

The appointment of the First City Physician for Gothenburg in 1901 clearly illustrates the new attitude. According to the regulations governing the appointment, the minimum qualification for the post was three years' experience as a provincial doctor or a city physician. However, in 1900 the Gothenburg Health Committee managed to convince the City Council that it was a matter of the utmost importance to appeal to central government to change the regulations. What is of interest here is

---

[29]   R.J. Morris, *Cholera 1832: The Social Response to an Epidemic* (New York 1976), 95–128; R. Richardson, *Death, Dissection and the Destitute* (London 1988), 223–9; D. Porter and R. Porter, 'The politics of prevention: anti-vaccinationism and public health in nineteenth-century England', *Medical History* **32** (1988), 231–52; Wohl, *Endangered Lives*, 132–5; Smith, *People's Health*, 158–70; J.R. Walkowitz, *Prostitution and Victorian Society: Women, Class, and the State* (Cambridge 1980).

[30]   D. Armstrong, *Political Anatomy of the Body: Medical Knowledge in Britain in the Twentieth Century* (Cambridge 1983), 8. See also D. Lupton, *Medicine as Culture: Illness, Disease and the Body in Western Societies* (London 1995), 30–32; G. Kearns, 'Tuberculosis and the medicalisation of British society, 1880–1920', in J. Woodward and R. Jütte (eds), *Coping with Sickness: Historical Aspects of Health Care in a European Perspective* (Sheffield 1995), 147–70; K. Johannisson, *Medicinens öga: Sjukdom, medicin och samhälle – historiska erfarenheter* (Stockholm 1990).

the way in which the Gothenburg Health Committee justified their appeal to central government.

The Health Committee claimed that much of the great sacrifices the city had made to improve the health of its population would be wasted if the health policy was directed by a medical doctor whose main qualification was long and loyal service to local authorities or to the Crown. Practical knowledge of administrative systems and procedures was, they argued, an overrated merit, which did not alone render a medical doctor equal to the demands of this important post. Ratepayers would get value for their money only if the Public Health Department was led by a health officer capable of finding scientific solutions to pressing medical and social problems. In other words, the Health Committee was looking for a young aspiring scientist with a first-rate medical education and an interest in research and familiarity with the new 'hygiene movement'. Although the National Board of Health (*Medicinalstyrelsen*) disagreed with the Gothenburg Health Committee, stressing the importance of administrative experience, the regulations were eventually amended.[31] Dr Karl Gezelius, who had worked in a pathological institute and in general hospitals and had made several study trips both to Central Europe and Britain, was appointed as the First City Physician. The Gothenburg Public Health Department was under his leadership until 1931.[32]

This case, even though it ended with the Gothenburg Health Committee getting its way, shows that Swedish central government continued to closely monitor some aspects of health care provision in the twentieth century. In general, however, central government allowed urban authorities considerable leeway when formulating their health policies, since it was heavily involved in providing health care services for the sparsely populated rural areas. Public health care services in towns and cities were, to a very large extent, financed locally and in consequence municipal health committees and leading health officers were able to exercise discretion in exactly how to develop these services in 1900–1940. However, the anti-tuberculosis scheme was an exception. From 1909–10 onwards, Swedish local authorities were eligible for central government grants to establish and maintain tuberculosis sanatoria and hospitals. This meant that local authorities had to bring their anti-tuberculosis schemes broadly into line with government recommendations.[33]

Gezelius, like many other leading health officers in Swedish cities, participated in the formulation of municipal health policies in various roles. He was a member of the Gothenburg City Council from 1903 to 1910, a member of the Public Health Committee from 1900 to 1932 and the chairman of the Public Health Committee's second department, which was responsible for running municipal hospitals, from

---

[31]   *Göteborgs Stadsfullmäktiges Handlingar 1900:13, 1900:78* and *1900:156*, and minutes 1 Mar. 1900, item 2; 31 May 1900, item 11.

[32]   Karl-Johan Gezelius (1866–1947) was the acting First City Physician for Gothenburg from 1900 to 1901 and the First City Physician from 1901 to 1931. For biographical details, see N.J. Wellinder, *Biografisk matrikel över svenska läkarkåren 1924* (Stockholm 1924); M. Fahl, *Göteborgs Stadsfullmäktige 1863–1962*, vol. II: *Biografisk matrikel* (Göteborg 1963).

[33]   G. Neander, 'Anti-tuberkulosarbetets finansiering i Sverige. Återblick. Översikt. Önskemål', in *Det Fjärde Nordiska Tuberkulosläkarmötet i Stockholm 25–27 augusti 1925* (Stockholm 1926), 104–13.

1920 to 1929. Hence he had a key role in the planning of health policies, but he also participated in the actual decision-making in the Public Health Committee and the City Council. Moreover, he was active in voluntary and professional associations. For example, from 1903 to 1908 he was the chairman of the voluntary association operating milk depots in Gothenburg, and in 1920 he was the chairman of the local Medical Association (*Göteborgs läkaresällskap*).[34]

In the early years of the twentieth century, Birmingham was also looking for an innovative Medical Officer of Health. The Health Committee, which had come in for a great deal of criticism, was keen to appoint an MOH who could steer a new course in public health and give credibility to the health policy. Dr John Robertson, who was appointed, had previously held the post of MOH for St Helens and for Sheffield.[35] In both these places he had introduced bacteriological research into the field of municipal health care. In St Helens he had undertaken extensive investigations into combating diphtheria, and had been 'responsible for probably the first bacteriological work done under municipal auspices in this country (Britain).' In Sheffield Robertson had been the MOH, Professor of Public Health and a lecturer in bacteriology in the then newly established university. He had shown his initiative, for example, in the promotion of the first local Act of Parliament for making the notification of tuberculosis compulsory.[36]

To enable Robertson to co-ordinate public health work efficiently, the Birmingham Health Committee reorganized the Public Health Department immediately after his appointment. More power was concentrated in the hands of the MOH, who was to supervise, directly or indirectly, all public health officers in Birmingham.[37] Robertson was also active in many voluntary societies and professional associations and published two books on housing and health.[38] Yet he was less influential in shaping the municipal health policy than his counterpart in Gothenburg. Unlike Gezelius, Robertson was not a member of the City Council or the Health Committee, and in the 1920s he was no longer allowed even to attend the meetings of the Committee.

In Britain, central government became more involved in the infant welfare and anti-tuberculosis campaigns from the second decade of the twentieth century.

---

[34]   *Göteborgs hälsovårdsnämnds årsberättelser 1900–1931*; Fahl, *Göteborgs Stadsfullmäktige 1863–1962*.

[35]   Birmingham City Archives (BCA) Birmingham Health Committee (HC) minutes 6 Apr. 1903, item 8009; 13 May 1903, item 8058; 24 Jun. 1903, items 8111–2; 14 Jul. 1903, item 8146.

[36]   'Obituary: Sir John Robertson', *British Medical Journal* **II** (1936), 1,337–8. See also, 'Obituary: Sir John Robertson', *Lancet* **II** (1936), 1,548–9; S. Sturdy, 'The political economy of scientific medicine: science, education and the transformation of medical practice in Sheffield, 1890–1922', *Medical History* **36** (1992), 125–59; C. Shaw, 'Aspects of public health', in C. Binfield et al. (eds), *The History of the City of Sheffield, 1843–1993, Volume II: Society* (Sheffield 1993), 100–117.

[37]   BCA HC minutes 12 Jan. 1904, item 8402; 8 Mar. 1904, item 8517.

[38]   J. Robertson, *Housing and Public Health* (London 1919); J. Robertson, *The House of Health: What the Modern Dwelling Needs to Be* (London 1925). For the voluntary associations, see for example *Annual Report of the Society for the Study of the Heredity in Its Bearings on the Human Race* (Birmingham 1910–11), 3.

The National Insurance Act of 1911, the introduction of compulsory notification of tuberculosis in 1913, and the Public Health (Tuberculosis) Act of 1921 gave municipal authorities wide responsibilities for the prevention and treatment of tuberculosis. Government grants were available on condition that the sanatoria and hospitals built by local authorities met the standards required by central government and that the medical doctors and nurses appointed had the necessary qualifications. This was also the case with the infant welfare work after the Maternity and Child Welfare Act was passed in 1918.[39] In the 1920s, central government grants covered up to 50 per cent of the approved expenditure on both tuberculosis and child welfare services in Britain. However, even though the role of central government became increasingly important in Britain during the interwar years, local authorities were still 'the major source of initiative and of increased expenditure.'[40] Local policy makers had a say in how much was spent on health care services and consequently there were considerable geographical variations in municipal health care provision.[41] As Hilary Marland argues, and as the following chapter shows, '[e]ven after the passing of the Maternity and Child Welfare Act in 1918, its implementation remained largely a question of local interpretation and policy making'.[42]

---

[39] L. Bryder, *Below the Magic Mountain: A Social History of Tuberculosis in Twentieth-century Britain* (Oxford 1988). J. Lewis, *The Politics of Motherhood: Child and Maternal Welfare in England, 1900–1939* (London 1980); D. Dwork, *War is Good for Babies and Other Young Children: A History of the Infant and Child Welfare Movement in England 1898–1918* (London 1987).

[40] P. Thane, *The Foundations of the Welfare State* (London 1990), 196. See also R. Lee, 'Uneven zenith: towards a geography of the high period of municipal medicine in England and Wales', *Journal of Historical Geography* **14** (3) (1988), 260–80.

[41] M. Powell, 'Did politics matter? Municipal public health expenditure in the 1930s', *Urban History* **22** (3) (1995), 360–79; Lee, 'Uneven zenith', A. Crowther, *Social Policy in Britain 1914–1939* (London 1988), 16–17.

[42] H. Marland, 'A pioneer in infant welfare: the Huddersfield scheme 1903–1925', *Social History of Medicine* **6** (1) (1993), 25–50.

CHAPTER 4

Regulating Family Life: Campaigns Against Infant Mortality, 1900–1940

Introduction

The early twentieth-century infant welfare campaigns began amid uncertainty. Public health authorities in both Britain and Sweden were acutely aware that science provided few immediate answers as to how to fight the diseases and disorders responsible for the high infant mortality. Firstly, in Britain and Sweden, the most common causes of deaths occurring within the first month of life (neonatal mortality) were prematurity, congenital defects and birth injuries. These causes of death had inspired some research that had linked neonatal mortality to the quality of maternity care, hereditary characteristics of the parents, general health of the mother, and her economic and social circumstances. However, experts were incapable of explaining how the different factors operated and helpless to save babies born prematurely or with serious congenital defects.[1]

Secondly, most deaths within months two to twelve (post-neonatal mortality) were attributable to infantile diarrhoea and respiratory diseases. Despite the intense scrutiny to which the problem of infantile diarrhoea had been subjected, investigators had failed to identify the precise micro-organism responsible for the disease. Consequently, the transmission and course of infantile diarrhoea remained a source of confusion and argument in the early twentieth century. Most public health officials, general practitioners, epidemiologists and bacteriologists agreed that bottle-feeding was a major risk factor, but the question of what other factors contributed to the prevalence of the disease and what measures would be appropriate to eradicate the problem yielded no such consensus. Respiratory diseases such as bronchitis and pneumonia proved to be even more perplexing. Much of their aetiology was unclear,

---

[1]   C. Lindman, *Dödligheten i första lefnadsåret i Sveriges tjugo större städer, 1876–95* (Stockholm 1898), 31–42; G. Newman, *Infant Mortality: A Social Problem* (London 1906), 46–89, 281–3; *Special Report of the Medical Officer of Health on Infant Mortality in the City of Birmingham* (hereafter *Special Report on Infant Mortality*) (Health Department, Birmingham 1904), 12–13. See also A. Wallgren, 'The neonatal mortality in Sweden, from a pediatric point of view', *Acta Pædiatrica* **29** (1942), 372–86; L. Marks, *Metropolitan Maternity: Maternal and Infant Welfare Services in Early Twentieth Century London* (Amsterdam 1996), 111–14.

and experts usually confined themselves to stating that exposure to cold and damp made infants susceptible to these diseases.[2]

Although the health authorities clearly did not know what was to be done, when and where, and for whom, they were determined to launch new campaigns to save infant lives. What helped them get started was that they were able to build on old policies. Public concern over high infant mortality had surfaced several times in the course of the nineteenth century, and some measures had already been taken in both Britain and Sweden. How effective these measures had been in saving babies is open to debate, but they had certainly served to accustom the public to state intervention in family relations and to the growing authority of the medical profession.

Policy Legacies

In Britain, infant mortality and infanticide emerged as an acute public problem in the 1860s. Medical practitioners, the police and the press, who all stood to gain something from the crisis, defined the problem. They pointed an accusing finger at 'baby-farmers', working-class women who offered to take care of babies for a small weekly payment or a larger lump sum. It was assumed that in large British cities, 70–90 per cent of the infants placed in the care of baby-farmers died. Referring to these estimates, the opinion-forming groups argued that baby-farmers were at best ignorant and at worst downright dangerous, and that in either case they needed to be watched. The debate developed into moral panic, culminating in the trial and execution of a baby-farmer, Margaret Waters, in 1870, and in the passing of the first Infant Life Protection Act in 1872. The Act, which introduced some level of state regulation for child-carers, was inconsistently enforced and therefore it was to have relatively little effect on infant mortality. However, it was an important change in gender politics, a step towards the 'biologicalization' of motherhood. Any children cared for by someone other than the natural mother were seen as problem children.[3]

---

[2] A. Newsholme, 'Infantile mortality: a statistical study from the public health standpoint', *Practitioner* (1905), 489–500; Newman, *Infant Mortality*, 48–60, 139–76; *Special Report on Infant Mortality*; Lindman, *Dödligheten*, 50–65; E. Almquist, *Allmän hälsovårdslära med särskildt afseende på svenska förhållanden för läkare, medicine studerande, hälsovårdsmyndigheter, tekniker m. fl.* (Stockholm 1897), 792–3; R.I. Woods, P.A. Watterson and J.H. Woodward, 'The causes of rapid infant mortality decline in England and Wales, 1861–1921, Part I', *Population Studies* **42** (3) (1988), 343–66, and 'Part II', *Population Studies* **43** (1) (1989), 113–32; D. Dwork, *War is Good for Babies and Other Young Children: A History of the Infant and Child Welfare Movement in England 1898–1918* (London 1987); A. Hardy, 'Rickets and the rest: child care, diet and the infectious children's diseases, 1850–1914', *Social History of Medicine* **5** (3) (1992), 394.

[3] M.L. Arnot, 'Infant death, child care and the state: the baby-farming scandal and the first infant life protection legislation of 1872', *Continuity and Change* **9** (2) (1994), 271–311; C. Smart, 'Disruptive bodies and unruly sex: the regulation of reproduction and sexuality in the nineteenth century', in C. Smart (ed.), *Regulating Womanhood: Historical Essays on Marriage, Motherhood and Sexuality* (London 1992), 7–32; H. Hendrick, *Child Welfare: England 1872–1989* (London 1994), 43–9.

The Swedish authorities, for their part, awakened to the problem of infant mortality as early as the 1760s, when the Statistical Bureau started to provide information about mortality according to age. The new statistics revealed, or rather confirmed the fears, that one-fifth of infants died in their first year, and that in many northern parishes infant mortality was between 400 and 500 – meaning that out of every 1,000 children born, 400–500 died before reaching their first birthday. These figures, together with the mercantilist principles equating power with population size, prompted the Swedish authorities to carry out some reforms, the most important of which was the campaign to train midwives.[4] The campaign had good chances of success, since Swedish doctors, unlike their British counterparts, were in favour of midwifery training. Most Swedish doctors practised in towns, and therefore they needed staunch allies who would work in the sparsely populated rural areas and campaign against folk healers, upon whom the rural population largely relied. Midwives were well suited to bridge the distance between medical science and popular culture both in the rural areas and among the urban working class, since the majority of them came from social milieus similar to those of their clients. Historians who have examined the midwifery reform in eighteenth- and nineteenth-century Sweden have found some evidence that trained midwives lowered maternal mortality, and convincing evidence that they reduced infant mortality. In particular, the campaign to promote breast-feeding appears to have reduced mortality from infantile diarrhoea.[5]

At the turn of the twentieth century, these previous efforts to reduce infant mortality were deemed insufficient. Both British and Swedish authorities sought to find fresh approaches to the problem and, since science had few immediate answers to offer, they also looked to other countries for ideas. In 1902, British legislators followed the example set by Sweden and the Netherlands, taking the first tentative step towards the regulation of midwives. In the same year, the Swedish Parliament passed a law requiring local authorities to supervise foster families, a reform that was partly modelled on the British legislation.[6] Moreover, both British and Swedish authorities took an active interest in French reforms. The child welfare clinics

---

[4] K. Johannisson, 'Why cure the sick? Population policy and health programs within 18th-century Swedish mercantilism', in A. Brändström and L.-G. Tedebrand (eds), *Society, Health and Population During the Demographic Transition* (Stockholm 1988), 323–30; A. Løkke, 'No difference without a cause: infant mortality rates as a world view generator', *Scandinavian Journal of History* **20** (2) (1995), 75–96; A. Brändström, 'The impact of female labour conditions on infant mortality: a case study of the parishes of Nedertorneå and Jokkmokk, 1800–96', *Social History of Medicine* **1** (3) (1988), 329–58; A. Brändström, S. Edvinsson and J. Rogers, 'Illegitimacy, infant feeding practices and infant survival in Sweden 1750–1950: a regional analysis', *Hygiea Internationalis* **3** (3) (2002), 13–52.

[5] C. Romlid, *Makt, motstånd och förändring: Vårdens historia speglad genom det svenska barnmorskeväsendet 1663–1908* (Stockholm 1998); A. Brändström, *'De kärlekslösa mödrarna': Spädbarnsdödligheten i Sverige under 1800-talet med särskild hänsyn till Nedertorneå* (Umeå 1984), 56–65, 111–25; I. Loudon, *Death in Childbirth: An International Study of Maternal Care and Maternal Mortality 1800–1950* (Oxford 1992), 406–15, 516–17.

[6] Loudon, *Death in Childbirth*, 402–21; H. Isberg, 'Barnavård', in G.H. von Koch (ed.), *Social Handbok* (Stockholm 1908), 72–3.

established by Drs Pierre Budin and Gaston Variot emerged as the most innovative measures against infant mortality in the early twentieth century. The ideas were imported into Britain and Sweden, and the names of Budin and Variot figured prominently in the reports of British and Swedish local authorities and voluntary associations.[7] The early twentieth-century infant welfare movement was clearly an international venture.

Two Legitimizing Strategies

What also distinguished the early twentieth-century infant welfare campaigns from their forerunners was the role of medicine. Medical practitioners had not stood on the sidelines in the nineteenth century, nor had they had a monopoly of the questions of infant welfare. In Britain, for example, the police had claimed relevant expertise to deal with infanticide and infant mortality. In the early twentieth century, despite the considerable confusion about the causes and prevention of infant deaths, the medical profession succeeded in making the strongest claim for authority in the matter. Measures taken to improve infant welfare were increasingly justified by reference to scientific and medical findings.[8]

Public health officials in both Birmingham and Gothenburg emphasized their faith in the capacity of science and medicine to determine the real causes of infant mortality and to specify the measures to be taken. Not all the answers were yet available, it was admitted, but science and medicine provided the best route to reach the answers. In particular in Birmingham, where the status of public health officers was not secure and the problem of infant mortality assumed unprecedented political proportions, meticulous care was taken to ensure that the basic tenets of the campaign could be defended as scientific and rational. Health officers clearly sensed that they could do their work without constant surveillance only if they convinced other policy makers and the public that the campaign was based on a firm factual foundation. In Gothenburg, where the status of health officers was higher and where infant mortality was not an acute political problem in the early twentieth century,

---

[7]   *Report of the Birmingham Infants' Health Society* (hereafter BIHS) *1908*; A. Höjer, 'Mjölkdroppar och barnavårdscentraler', in *Statens Offentliga Utredningar* (hereafter *SOU*) *1929:28*, 44–5. See also G.F. McCleary, *The Maternity and Child Welfare Movement* (London 1935), 8–9; Dwork, *War is Good for Babies*, 93–123; A.-M. Stenhammar et al., *Mjölkdroppen – Filantropi, förmynderi eller samhällsansvar?* (Stockholm 2001), 27–38; G. Weiner, 'De "olydiga" mödrarna: konflikter om spädbarnsvård på en Mjölkdroppe', *Historisk Tidskrift* **112** (4) (1992), 490.

[8]   R.D. Apple, 'Constructing mothers: scientific motherhood in the nineteenth and twentieth centuries', *Social History of Medicine* **8** (1) (1995), 161–78; J. Lewis, *The Politics of Motherhood: Child and Maternal Welfare in England, 1900–1939* (London 1980); K. Johannisson, 'Folkhälsa: Det svenska projektet från 1900 till 2:a världskriget', *Lychnos: Årsbok för idehistoria och vetenskapshistoria* (1991), 154–68; L. Bryder, 'Two models of infant welfare in the first half of the twentieth century: New Zealand and the USA', *Women's History Review* **12** (4) (2003), 547–58. For medical technology and infant welfare, see J.P. Baker, *The Machine in the Nursery: Incubator Technology and the Origins of Newborn Intensive Care* (Baltimore, MD 1996).

the push for scientific rigour in the health debate was somewhat weaker. Health officers did not always need to justify their decisions by scientific evidence, but were allowed to exercise their expert judgement. However, the importance of science as legitimizing rhetoric increased even in Gothenburg, when different views about infant welfare emerged.

By comparing the Birmingham and Gothenburg campaigns, it is possible to examine the wider political and social objectives which municipal health authorities furthered by reshaping and reconstructing scientific knowledge about infant health and illness. Although the Birmingham and Gothenburg authorities had access to the same body of medical knowledge, the Gothenburg authorities clearly 'knew' something which the Birmingham authorities did not know, and vice versa. Some research findings that the Gothenburg authorities presented as hard facts were deemed highly inconclusive in Birmingham, and the scientific results on which the Birmingham authorities based their policies were often completely ignored by their Gothenburg counterparts.

Even many contemporary commentators admitted that, besides scientific progress, there were other factors adding colour and urgency to the infant welfare campaign in the early twentieth century. In particular, they stressed that the high infant mortality deserved 'the most serious consideration by all true patriots', since it posed a threat to national security and prosperity (Figure 4.1).[9] The same insistence on the importance of national interests in explaining the proliferation of infant welfare services can also be found in the works of many present-day scholars. Anxiety about foreign competition and fear of racial deterioration, so it has often been argued, were the most important factors stimulating the interest in infant welfare.[10] However, in order to understand the form and direction the infant welfare campaigns took in different countries, it is necessary to examine not only the national efficiency movements in a narrow sense, but also the wider political and social causes this movement was deployed to advance. Improving national efficiency and pursuing national interests were seen as perfectly legitimate aims, thus they became convenient labels under which many other political and social objectives could be grouped. By looking at the infant welfare campaigns in Birmingham and Gothenburg, it is possible to reveal how the health authorities equated the enhancement of the national well-being with the promotion of what they saw as the core values of the British or the Swedish. In so doing, they legitimized health measures which discriminated against mothers and children who did not embody the 'national virtues.'[11]

---

[9] McCleary, *The Maternity and Child Welfare Movement*, 1–9; Newsholme, 'Infantile mortality', 489–95; J.E. Lane-Claypon, *The Child Welfare Movement* (London 1920), 1–7; F. Carlberg, 'Frivilligt arbete för späda barn i Göteborg', *Social Tidskrift* (1908), 536–40; Isberg, 'Barnavård'; *Göteborgs Stadfullmäktiges Handlingar* (hereafter *GSH*) *1911:27*, 3–9. The quotes are from McCleary and Newsholme.

[10] Dwork, *War is Good for Babies*, 208–20, 228. See also G.R. Searle, *The Quest for National Efficiency: A Study in British Politics and Political Thought, 1899–1914* (Oxford 1971); C. Dyhouse, 'Working-class mothers and infant mortality in England, 1895–1914', in C. Webster (ed.), *Biology, Medicine and Society 1840–1940* (Cambridge 1981), 73.

[11] See also G. Bock, 'Anti-natalism, maternity and paternity in National Socialist racism', in G. Bock and P. Thane (eds), *Maternity and Gender Policies: Women and the Rise*

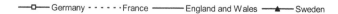

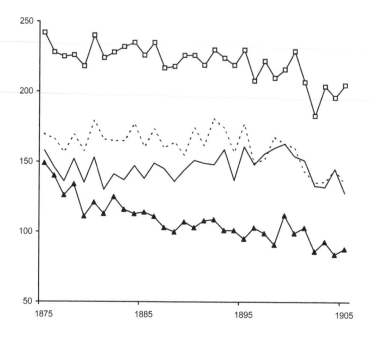

Figure 4.1 **Infant mortality per 1,000 live births in Germany, France, England and Wales, and Sweden, 1875–1905.**

Source: B.R. Mitchell, *International Historical Statistics: Europe 1750–1988* (New York 1992).

The two legitimizing strategies – the discourse of science and discourse of nationalism – diverted attention away from political controversies. When policy makers defined health problems as medical, technical questions, they removed them from the political scene and were able to argue that the policies they pursued were above class antagonisms and gender conflicts. When authorities emphasized the importance of the national interests, they encouraged people to embrace the 'nation' as the most important context for self-definition and to relegate other categories, such as class and gender, which could also have provided a sense of identity.

Infant Welfare and Politics

The first aim of this chapter is to discuss the role which early twentieth-century infant welfare campaigns played in regulating the relationship between the state and the family on the one hand and in controlling urban family life and family relations

---

of the European Welfare States, 1880s–1950s (London 1994), 233–55; M. Poovey, 'Curing the "social body" in 1832: James Philip Kay and the Irish in Manchester', *Gender and History* **5** (2) (1993), 196–211.

on the other. The chapter examines the process whereby two political ideals – the family's responsibility to be self-supporting and the male-breadwinner family model – became embedded in the 'apolitical' campaigns, whose explicit aim was to promote the well-being of infants. The Birmingham authorities managed to reconcile the three objectives. They proved 'scientifically' that the well-being of infants *could be ensured* without direct economic assistance to the poorest families, but that *it could not be ensured* without the 'normal' family form. Because of different economic circumstances and cultural norms, the Gothenburg authorities were unable to reconcile the three aims, and they had to choose between them. Hence the Gothenburg infant welfare campaign offers an interesting contrast to the Birmingham campaign.

Secondly, the chapter discusses how the infant welfare campaigns regulated the relationship between social classes and urban space in early twentieth-century industrial cities. Health policies reflected the spatial arrangements of the city and, perhaps more importantly, health authorities' views about the appropriate relationship between social classes and urban space. Political considerations of this type, and not, for example, the severity of the problem of infant mortality (Figure 4.2), explain the differences between the Birmingham and Gothenburg campaigns. Thirdly, the chapter explores how public health legacies and the interests of the medical profession affected the form taken by the campaigns. In Gothenburg, the majority of medical practitioners worked in the public sector, and the expansion of publicly funded medical care was in their interests. In Birmingham, by contrast, general practitioners often organized themselves against plans to develop public health services.

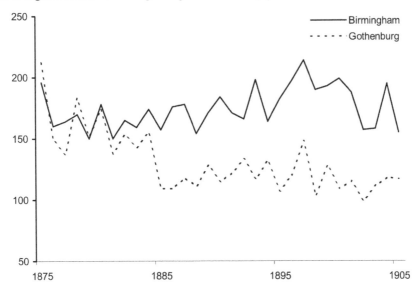

Figure 4.2   Infant mortality per 1,000 live births in Birmingham and Gothenburg, 1875–1905.
Source: Annual Report of the MOH for Birmingham 1910, 15; Statistisk årsbok för Göteborg 1900, 50; 1901–05.

Dysfunctional Families: Two Definitions of One Problem

Birmingham

For most of the nineteenth century, mortality league tables had served to sustain Birmingham's reputation as a healthy manufacturing town and had given local policy makers an excuse to ignore certain important health issues. In the late 1890s, the same tables were instrumental in shattering Birmingham's positive image.[12] Firstly, the general death rate for Birmingham had not improved since the dramatic advances of the 1870s and early 1880s, and in consequence the city had gradually lost the good position it had held among the major British cities. Secondly, an increase in infant deaths in the late 1890s put Birmingham at the top of the infant mortality league.[13] The Birmingham authorities, in defence, argued that the death rates for the city were high mainly because a large proportion of the middle-class families lived outside the municipal boundaries.[14] However, at the turn of the century, when considerable agitation was afoot to improve 'national efficiency' and to promote the health of the working class, excuses of this type were unfavourably received.

Admittedly, the Birmingham authorities were not alone in puzzling over the growing infant mortality. In many British cities infant mortality, and in particular mortality from diarrhoea, showed a slight increase at the turn of the twentieth century. In Birmingham, however, the upturn was sharp (Figure 4.3). Naomi Williams and Graham Mooney argue that the hot dry summers in the late 1890s represented a 'sanitary test' that exposed the cities 'which had failed to secure safe public health through sound methods of environmental management' and in particular the cities 'reliant on conservancy methods of excrement removal, such as privies and ash-closets'.[15] Birmingham seemed to be among the first identified by this test. The Medical Officer of Health (MOH) for Birmingham, Dr Alfred Hill, drew the same conclusion in the late 1890s. He conceived the dramatic increase in diarrhoeal mortality as being an index of environmental degradation and urged the Health Committee to press ahead with sanitary reform in the poorest wards of the city.[16]

---

[12]   J.A. Fallows, *The Housing of the Poor* (Birmingham 1899); Birmingham City Archives (BCA) Birmingham Health Committee (HC) minutes 11 Apr. 1899, item 5687; 23 Apr. 1901, item 6766. For the relative healthiness of Birmingham in the mid-nineteenth century, see S. Szreter and G. Mooney, 'Urbanization, mortality, and the standard of living debate: new estimates of the expectation of life at birth in nineteenth-century British cities', *Economic History Review* **51** (1) (1998), 84–112.

[13]   *Annual Report of the Medical Officer of Health for Birmingham* (hereafter *Annual Report*) *1897*, 3–10, 20–29; *1899*, 10–11; *Special Report on Infant Mortality*, 6. For adverse publicity, see for example Newsholme, 'Infantile mortality', 495–6.

[14]   C.A. Vince, *History of the Corporation of Birmingham, Volume III: 1885–1899* (Birmingham 1902), 125; *Annual Report 1906*, 11–14; *1907*, 12–14.

[15]   N. Williams and G. Mooney, 'Infant mortality in an "Age of Great Cities": London and the English provincial cities compared, c.1840–1910', *Continuity and Change* **9** (2) (1994), 206–8.

[16]   *Annual Report 1897*, 3–10, 20–34; *1898*, 26–8.

Even more critical were local church leaders, reporters and political opponents, who bombarded the Committee with questions and complaints.[17]

The Committee responded by cleaning courtyards, by converting privies into water closets and by experimenting with municipal housebuilding. However, they were not ready to accept full responsibility for 'the enormous death-rate from diarrhoea'. They insisted that some of the blame be attributed to the townspeople themselves.[18] Scientific legitimization for their stance was provided by Dr John Robertson, who became the MOH for Birmingham in 1903. Unlike Hill, a strong advocate of sanitary engineering, Robertson had won his spurs as a bacteriologist and had learnt to think that sanitary reform alone was a relatively ineffective means of dealing with urban health problems.[19]

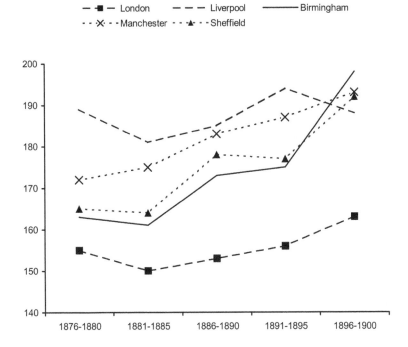

Figure 4.3   Infant mortality in London, Liverpool, Birmingham, Manchester and Sheffield, five-year means, 1876–1900.

Source: Annual Report of the MOH for Birmingham for 1882, 13; *1890,* 15; *1895,* 10; *Special Report of the MOH on Infant Mortality in the City of Birmingham* (Health Department, Birmingham 1904), 6.

---

[17]   BCA HC minutes 11 Apr. 1899, item 5687; 23 Apr. 1901, item 6766; 9 Jul. 1901, items 6901–2; 23 Jul. 1901, items 6933 and 6935; 24 Sept. 1901, item 6979; 22 Apr. 1902, items 7383–4; *Annual Report 1897,* 30; A. Mayne, *The Imagined Slum: Newspaper Representation in Three Cities 1870–1914* (Leicester 1993), 78–93.

[18]   BCA HC minutes 23 Jul. 1901, item 6933; 9 Dec. 1902, item 7774; *Annual Report 1899,* 34–9.

[19]   See Chapter 3.

At the request of the Health Committee, Robertson set out to investigate the problem of infant mortality during the first year of his tenure. His analysis of the problem and recommendations for reform were published in 1904 and distributed to the city councillors and the press.[20] The plan outlined by Robertson and developed in further reports together with Drs Jessie Duncan and Alexandra MacCallum formed a basis for the Birmingham infant welfare campaign. Robertson exerted considerable influence on decision-makers' thinking on the question, and even in cases where the Health Committee did not to follow his advice, the MOH often played an important part: he provided the Committee's decisions with scientific legitimization. To maintain his credibility, the MOH categorically denied having yielded to political pressure and sought to give the impression that he himself had amended the proposals after considering them in the light of new evidence. If a U-turn had to be made, the MOH sought to ensure it undermined his authority as an impartial expert as little as possible.

The impact of Robertson's reports was not confined to Birmingham. Some of them were referred to by Drs George Newman, Arthur Newsholme and Janet Lane-Claypon, who were prime movers in constructing the national infant welfare campaign. They brought Robertson into the national debate and valued his expertise, particularly when discussing the question of how to improve infant welfare in the most deprived urban areas. The central wards of Birmingham, on which Robertson initially concentrated his attention, were considered to be among the worst slums in Britain.[21]

'Important' and 'Unimportant' Causes of Death   While Robertson acknowledged many possible causes of infant death, in practice, like most British MOHs, he equated infant mortality with the problem of infantile enteritis and diarrhoea. The discussion in Birmingham concentrated almost exclusively on these diseases, which caused 15–33 per cent of infant deaths, and was not extended to include other causes until the late 1910s. Robertson justified the narrow scope of the campaign, firstly by contending that 'almost all the other causes of infant deaths are comparatively unimportant when compared with the enormous wastage of human life due to … diarrhoea and enteritis'. Secondly, he argued that deaths from diarrhoea were more easily preventable than deaths from other causes.[22]

---

[20]   *Special Report on Infant Mortality*; BCA HC minutes 27 Oct. 1903, item 8297; 28 Jun. 1904, item 8732; 29 Nov. 1904; 10 Jan. 1905, item 9058.

[21]   Newman, *Infant Mortality*, 189–96; A. Newsholme, 'Report on infant and child mortality', in *39th Annual Report of the Local Government Board* (London 1909–10), Supplement, 57; Lane-Claypon, *The Child Welfare Movement*, Appendix VII. Newman was the MOH for the Metropolitan Borough of Finsbury 1901–7, the CMO at the Board of Education 1907–19 and the CMO at the Ministry of Health 1919–35. Newsholm was the MOH for Brighton until 1908, and the CMO at the Local Government Board from 1908 to 1918. Lane-Claypon was a lecturer at King's College for Women, University of London.

[22]   *Special Report on Infant Mortality*, 12–18; *Report of the MOH on Child Welfare in 1913* (Public Health and Housing Department, Birmingham 1914), 7–10; 'Report of the MOH on maternity and child welfare during 1916', in *Annual Report 1916*, appendix, 11; *Annual*

The MOH was reluctant to suggest any special measures against bronchitis and pneumonia, together accounting for 15 per cent of deaths. The main reasons for his reluctance were apparently that doctors knew little about respiratory diseases, and that even careful mothers had difficulty in warding off attacks of bronchitis. A significant proportion of deaths from bronchitis occurred in respectable artisan or middle-class homes where children were presumably well cared for, hence the MOH addressed the subject in discreet terms.[23] Dealing with prematurity and congenital malformations proved even more difficult. These disorders, together with other 'wasting diseases', accounted for 28–35 per cent of infant deaths, and they caused many deaths in both slums and suburbs. As the MOH discussed the question in the early twentieth century, his lack of enthusiasm was noticeable. Had he attributed the deaths, for example, to the quality of maternal care, he would have cast aspersions not only on the standard of practice of untrained midwives, but also that of the general practitioners who delivered middle-class women. In treading warily through this minefield, the MOH considered it wise to state that the deaths from prematurity and congenital anomalies 'may not be preventable'.[24] The flexibility of these categories is revealed by comparison between the Birmingham and Gothenburg campaigns. It was not uncommon for the Gothenburg authorities to place high on their agenda some causes of death which the Birmingham authorities defined as 'comparatively unimportant'. Furthermore, while the Birmingham authorities argued that a large proportion of deaths might be 'non-preventable', their Gothenburg counterparts sought to convey the message that most diseases would be preventable or curable if only ratepayers were willing to invest more money in medical care.

A Filth Disease The Birmingham MOH was clearly convinced that a pound spent in combating 'easily preventable' diarrhoeal diseases would go much further towards saving infant lives than a pound laid out in campaigning against other diseases. However, had poverty been allowed to emerge as the central issue, even the campaign against diarrhoeal diseases would have been costly. The MOH was acutely aware of this. He often mentioned the problem of poverty, even analysed a possible impact of poverty on infant welfare, but at the same time he was careful not to talk himself into a corner. If need be, he went to great lengths to show that there was no *direct* connection between poverty and mortality. For example, he argued that 'mere size or even cheapness of the house can in itself have little or no effect on the mortality', and reminded his readers that many rural areas where people lived in simple two-roomed cottages had remarkably low infant mortality rates. Likewise, low wages in themselves could not explain the high rates of infant mortality, since

---

Report 1905, 20–23, 48–51; *1906*, 12–20; *1910*, 15–21, 40–46; *1912*, 18–26. See also, Dwork, *War is Good for Babies*, 23–6.

[23] *Special Report on Infant Mortality*, 9, 18; 'Report of the MOH on maternity and child welfare during 1916', 11.

[24] *Special Report on Infant Mortality*, 9, 12; *Annual Report 1906*, 16; 'Report of the MOH on maternity and child welfare during 1916', 11.

in many poor communities the infant mortality was low.[25] The MOH was clearly determined not to raise false hopes that the municipality would offer direct financial assistance to the poorest families.

Another way in which Robertson circumvented the poverty problem was to reduce diarrhoea to 'a filth disease' and to define the concept of filth carefully.[26] In his first reports in 1904 and 1905, the concept was still relatively broad and the blame for the existence of dirt and squalor was placed on the whole community. Courtyards were littered with filth mainly because the tenants did not clean them, but the landlords were not blameless either. They did not keep the yards in good repair. Homes in slum areas were dirty chiefly because the residents 'were dirty in any conceivable way', but at the same time most houses were old and badly constructed. It was difficult to keep them clean. People's bodies and clothes were dirty because people were negligent, but given the lack of washing facilities, little more in the way of personal hygiene could be expected of them. The accumulated dirt in houses and their immediate surroundings, the MOH argued, was the most important cause of diarrhoea, and a concerted effort was to be made to deal with the problem. The municipal authorities, voluntary societies and private landlords were to give people a better chance of being clean and keeping their houses clean, but ultimately the success of the campaign depended on whether the individuals improved their personal and domestic hygiene.[27]

While Robertson was convinced that raising the standard of hygiene would bring down diarrhoeal mortality rates permanently, he expected the change to take time. In the hope of more immediate results, he insisted that special attention should be paid to infant feeding. The simplest way to protect infants from diarrhoea and other potentially food-borne diseases seemed to be to persuade working-class mothers to breast-feed, and where exclusive breast-feeding was not possible, meticulous care was to be taken that cow's milk, the best substitute for mother's milk, was stored and prepared properly.[28] Again, while the MOH criticized slum-dwellers for unsatisfactory infant feeding practices, he admitted that the blame could not be laid at their door alone. Firstly, a study of infant feeding in the poorest areas of Birmingham in 1903 showed that 22 per cent of the mothers who weaned early did so on the advice of their family doctor, and that a further 62 per cent had an insufficient

---

[25]   The quote is from the *Special Report on Infant Mortality*, 10. See also *Report of the MOH on the Unhealthy Conditions in the Floodgate Street Area and the Municipal Wards of St. Mary, St. Stephen, and St. Bartholomew* (Health Department, Birmingham 1904), 14–18; *Annual Report 1906*, 54. An exception to the rule was the report based on the research done by Dr Jessie Duncan. In this report, the MOH argued that poverty *per se* was an important cause of infant death. See J. Robertson, *Report on Industrial Employment of Married Women and Infantile Mortality* (Health Department, Birmingham 1910); *Annual Report 1910*, 21.

[26]   *Special Report on Infant Mortality*, 17.

[27]   *Special Report on Infant Mortality*, 11, 18–21; BCA HC minutes 29 Nov. 1904, items 8994–9008; 10 Jan. 1905, item 9050; 24 Jan. 1905, item 9087; 14 Feb. 1905, items 9115; *Annual Report 1907*, 16–17.

[28]   *Special Report on Infant Mortality*, 15–17, 21–2; *Annual Report 1905*, 49–50.

amount of breast-milk.[29] Secondly, as ignorant as working-class mothers were of proper storage and preparation of food, they were by no means solely responsible for the contamination of cow's milk. The MOH acknowledged that cow's milk was often contaminated before it even reached the customer because of the insanitary conditions under which it was produced, stored and sold.[30] Robertson concluded that the solution to the infant feeding problem lay partly in the hands of midwives and the Health Committee. Midwives were to assist mothers in the initiation of breast-feeding, and the Health Committee was to instruct farmers, inspect milk shops and establish milk depots in order to ensure that uncontaminated cow's milk was available to the remaining bottle-fed babies. However, the MOH stressed that all these efforts would be in vain if the mothers did not do their utmost to save their babies.[31]

Reconciling Divergent Interests   The first reaction to Robertson's analysis in 1904 and 1905 was one of approval. Voluntary agencies welcomed his views, and the local press complimented him on the important recommendations he had made.[32] The Health Committee members and the city councillors, a large proportion of whom were businessmen, were also satisfied with the general tone of the report. The endorsement of the report was hardly unexpected. In defining the problem of infant mortality, Robertson had been careful to accommodate the demands of special interests. Firstly, by putting the question of poverty low on the priority list, he had secured the backing of the Health Committee and the City Council. Most of the Health Committee members and councillors, regardless of party affiliation, continued to cling to the view that the local authority should not intervene in the economy of individual families.[33] Secondly, the MOH had been careful not to provoke general practitioners, who were suspicious of any expansion of local authority health services.[34] In the

---

[29]   *Annual Report 1905*, 21–3. See also P.J. Atkins, 'Mother's milk and infant death in Britain, circa 1900–1940', *Anthropology of Food* 2 (2003); V. Fildes, 'Infant feeding practices and infant mortality in England, 1900–1919', *Continuity and Change* 13 (2) (1998), 251–80.

[30]   *Special Report on Infant Mortality*, 21–5.

[31]   *Annual Report 1905*, 21–3; *Special Report on Infant Mortality*, 11, 17, 21–9; BCA HC minutes 29 Nov. 1904, items 9001–5; 10 Jan. 1905, items 9050–52.

[32]   'Medical Officer's report – important recommendations', *Birmingham Daily Mail*, 12 Dec. 1904; 'Infantile mortality in Birmingham', and 'The Floodgate street area ...', *Birmingham Daily Mail*, 13 Feb. 1904; 'Crusade against dirt', *Birmingham Daily Mail*, 15 Feb. 1904; 'Infantile mortality in Birmingham', *Birmingham Daily Post*, 14 Dec. 1904. For voluntary agencies, see for example *Royal Commission on the Poor Laws and Relief of Distress, 1909*, appendix, vol. IV, Question 44 618 (22).

[33]   BCA HC minutes 29 Nov. 1904, items 8994–9008; 10 Jan. 1905, items 9050–52; 24 Jan. 1905, item 9087; 14 Feb. 1905, items 9115, 9120 and 9134 (HC's report to the CC, 32–8); 11 Apr. 1905, item 9223. See also the discussion about subsidized meals in the 1910s, BCA Birmingham Maternity and Child Welfare Sub-Committee (M&CWSC) minutes 2 Mar. 1917, item 236; 4 May 1917, items 281–2; *Annual Report 1914*, 20–21. For discussion, see Lewis, *The Politics of Motherhood*, 13–21, 165–90; S. Pedersen, *Family, Dependence, and the Origins of the Welfare State: Britain and France, 1914–1945* (Cambridge 1993), 32–59.

[34]   See, for example, BCA HC minutes 26 Jan. 1904, item 8449; 'Medical fees in midwives' cases', *Midland Medical Journal* 3 (2) (1904), 25–6; A.G. Bateman, 'Doctors in Parliament', *Midland Medical Journal* 3 (3) (1904), 38–9.

early years of the twentieth century, it was difficult for poor women and children to gain access to medical and hospital care even in life-threatening situations. For example, there were no hospital beds in Birmingham specially set part for obstetric complications, and the Children's Hospital, run by a charity, suffered for a chronic want of funds.[35] In his reports in 1904 and 1905, the MOH did not touch on these or any other problems concerning the provision of medical care, let alone suggest that the local authority should provide medical services.

Thirdly, Robertson's analysis of infant mortality was in line with other municipal policies and provided legitimization for them, especially for housing policy. In considering solutions to the inner-city housing problems in the early twentieth century, the Birmingham Housing Committee had decided to embark on a programme of piecemeal repairs instead of a large-scale slum clearance. The Committee sought to keep slum houses in a habitable condition by ordering owners to repair them and by opening up courtyards to light. When the MOH discussed the impact of defective housing on infant welfare, he concentrated on these factors: the structural defects of houses and the lack of air and sunshine. Hence he was able to conclude that, though living conditions left much to be desired, the most pressing problems were already being addressed. The Housing Committee was dealing with slum properties 'in an energetic manner', and the progress was 'satisfactory both as regards the houses themselves and as regards the amount of light and fresh air'. The prevention of infant deaths in these 'unhealthy areas', instead of requiring entirely new housing initiatives, primarily demanded changes in people's behaviour.[36]

Finally, the MOH had carefully grounded his analysis in contemporary scientific findings. A large amount of statistical information on infant mortality and numerous clinical observations of different diseases were presented in the reports to convince the readers that the main factors producing high infant mortality had been identified and thoroughly investigated. Surveys of feeding practices, theories about energy requirements and bacteriological analyses of milk were discussed at length to convey the message that the recommendations for reform were based on a firm factual foundation. Moreover, the MOH referred to the social surveys conducted by Charles Booth and Seebohm Rowntree to enhance the credibility of his analysis of poverty and infant mortality.[37]

The 1910s: More Emphasis on Individual Responsibility   After the initial enthusiasm, the Health Committee started to sift through the MOH's proposals, assessing their feasibility. The Committee praised the MOH for giving new insights into the role of ignorance and negligence. The Committee members were now 'strongly convinced

---

[35]   J.E. Jones, *History of the Hospitals and Other Charities of Birmingham* (Birmingham 1909), 55–8, 74–81; R. Waterhouse, *Children in Hospital: A Hundred Years of Child Care in Birmingham* (London 1962), 58–63.

[36]   Quotes from *Special Report on Infant Mortality*, 18, see also 11–12, 19–21; *Report on the Unhealthy Conditions*, 23–9; Mayne, *The Imagined Slum*, 85–93.

[37]   *Special Report on Infant Mortality*. See also Newman, *Infant Mortality*; A. Newsholme, 'Domestic infection in relation to epidemic diarrhoea', *Journal of Hygiene* **6** (1906), 139–48.

that the best method of combating infant mortality is by educational means'. A much more cautious attitude was taken, for example, towards the MOH's recommendations concerning the improvement of the milk supply.[38] In the following five years, when some of the MOH's initial ideas were turned into new municipal services and some others were rejected, the definition of the problem of infant mortality changed. By the 1910s, the emphasis on individual responsibility had become much stronger. Infantile diarrhoea was still defined as a filth disease, but the concept of filth had narrowed considerably. Although the MOH was acutely aware that slum houses were getting beyond repair, defective housing was now almost entirely absent from the discussion on infant mortality, likewise unpaved yards and poor sanitation. The focus of the debate in Birmingham was now on home environment, and the blame for the dirt and squalor was placed entirely on the slum-dwellers.[39]

As to infant feeding, the change in the tone of Robertson's reports was even clearer. While in his earlier writing in 1904 and 1905 the MOH emphasized that farmers, wholesale dealers and retailers were partly to blame for the contamination of milk, in the 1910s he argued that the problem was entirely due to uncleanliness in the home. Even though Birmingham had been relatively active in improving the quality of milk, the measures taken in Birmingham and other British cities before the First World War were far from adequate. For example, Peter Atkins shows that even in the 1920s, '[t]he conditions of milk production were still disgracefully filthy and ill-regulated, with those of transport and sale only marginally better'.[40] Despite the problems concerning the milk supply, the MOH argued in 1911 that 'milk does not carry the disease into the home, although it may be contaminated at the home'. The bottle-fed babies were exposed to death only because their mothers did not 'understand the need for regularity and extreme cleanliness in artificial feeding of babies.'[41]

With the increasing emphasis on individual responsibility, the cohesion of families also came to be seen as a key explanatory variable in determining the level of infant mortality. An assistant MOH, Dr Jessie Duncan, pointed out in 1912 that many mothers were malnourished and therefore unable to feed their children properly. Malnutrition, in turn, was often ascribed to the lack of solidarity in problem families. Husbands spent a large proportion of their income on drink, while their

---

[38]   BCA HC minutes 29 Nov. 1904, and in particular items 9002–5; 10 Jan. 1905, items 9050–52; 24 Jan. 1905, item 9091; 14 Feb. 1905, items 9120 and 9134; 14 Mar. 1905, item 9173; 11 Jul. 1905, item 9390; 12 Mar. 1907, item 424; 25 Jun. 1907, item 628.

[39]   See, for example, *Report of the MOH on Child Welfare in 1913*.

[40]   P.J. Atkins, 'White poison? The social consequences of milk consumption, 1850–1930', *Social History of Medicine* **5** (2) (1992), 207–27; Atkins, 'Mother's milk and infant death in Britain'. For the plans to improve the quality of milk in Birmingham, see for example J. Robertson, 'Prevention of tuberculosis among cattle', *Public Health* **22** (1909), 324–8; J. Robertson, *The Milk Supply: Report on a Visit to American Cities in Regard to Milk Supply* (Public Health Department, Birmingham 1922).

[41]   The quotes are from the *Quarterly Report of the MOH 1911/III*, 12, and from the 'Report of the MOH on maternity and child welfare during 1916', 11. See also Newsholme, 'Domestic infection'.

wives and children suffered acute deprivation.[42] What exacerbated the situation was poor household management. The MOH criticized working-class mothers for their lack of cookery skills: 'the catering and the cookery for the household' was often 'as bad as it well can be'. Furthermore, any improvement in the standards of housekeeping seemed remote, since working-class girls 'employ[ed] themselves in low grade factory labour' instead of preparing themselves for their future role as mothers.[43]

Many writers have shown that the British welfare state, compared with that of France and Sweden, developed along deeply gendered lines.[44] The infant welfare movement was no exception. The Birmingham campaign reflected and reinforced a normative model of the family in which men were assumed to be breadwinners and women were presumed to spend their time caring for their children and home. Securing as great compliance as possible with this ideal was one of the main aims of the Birmingham campaign. The early twentieth-century discussion about infant mortality and married women's industrial employment illustrates this point further. The determination to buttress the conventional family and its hierarchy of roles could override other important considerations, including the well-being of children.

Factory Mothers   The view that female employment predisposed society to high levels of infant mortality was by no means new. The debate on the question had been rumbling along in the pages of medical journals and governmental reports ever since Edwin Chadwick had published his classic *Report on the Sanitary Condition of the Labouring Population* in 1842.[45] At the turn of the twentieth century, the debate regained momentum. Many public health experts, and especially Drs George Newman and George Reid (the MOH for Staffordshire), managed to make a name for themselves with studies 'showing' a clear causal link between infant mortality and the occupation of mothers outside the home.[46] Even though the studies failed to provide conclusive proof of the relationship between infant mortality and women's

---

[42]   J. Duncan, *Report on the Prevention of Infantile Mortality* (Public Health Department, Birmingham 1912); *Report of the MOH on Child Welfare in 1913*, 9–10, 15–16; 'Report of the MOH on maternity and child welfare during 1916', 1; BCA Birmingham Public Health and Housing Committee (PH&HC) minutes 26 Sept. 1913, item 1695; 24 Oct. 1913, item 1785.

[43]   *Annual Report 1914*, 14.

[44]   Pedersen, *The Origins of the Welfare State*; J. Lewis, 'Gender and the development of welfare regimes', *Journal of European Social Policy* 2 (3) (1992), 159–73; L. Sommestad, 'Welfare state attitudes to the male breadwinning system: the United States and Sweden in comparative perspective', in A. Janssens (ed.), *The Rise and Decline of the Male Breadwinner Family?/International Review of Social History* 42 (1997), Supplement, 153–74.

[45]   M. Tennant, 'Infantile mortality', in G.M. Tuckwell et al., *Woman in Industry: From Seven Points of View* (London 1908), 87–119; Newman, *Infant Mortality*, 90–138; E. Chadwick, *Report on the Sanitary Condition of the Labouring Population of Great Britain* (Edinburgh 1842/1965), 205–6.

[46]   Newman, *Infant Mortality*, 90–138; G. Reid, 'Report of proceedings of public medicine section of annual general meeting of British Medical Association', *British Medical Journal* (1892), 275–8; G. Reid, 'Infant mortality and the employment of married women in factory labour before and after confinement', *Lancet* (1906), Part II, 423–4.

employment, they went a long way towards convincing health officials that factory mothers were to blame for the high infant mortality rates.[47] Firstly, it was pointed out that only a small proportion of factory mothers were able to combine their work with intensive breast-feeding. Secondly, working mothers rarely made proper provision for their children's care during the day, and those who did exposed their children to bronchitis by carrying them out to a childminder in the early morning. Thirdly, it was argued that instructing the factory mother in infant care was difficult. During the day she was at work, and 'when the evening comes she is too tired and too busy to welcome the teaching of the Health Visitor'. On the basis of these studies, some social reformers and health experts insisted that mothers of young children should be barred from working in industry.[48]

In Birmingham, much confusion arose when the health officers started investigating the issue after the National Conference on Infant Mortality in 1906. The conference, where local authorities were strongly represented, recommended that central government extend compulsory (unpaid) maternity leave to three months.[49] The Home Office responded by asking local authorities to acquire further information as to the industrial employment of married women and infant mortality. The Birmingham Health Department embarked on a series of investigations, producing several reports on the question during the years 1908–12.[50] Contrary to all expectations, the study conducted in 1908 revealed that in the poorest areas, mortality among babies whose mothers worked in factories or were engaged in charring or washing was lower than among babies whose mothers were not employed. In 1909 the results pointed in the other direction, but again in 1910 and 1911 mortality was lower among the children of working mothers (Table 4.1). This type of result could have been dismissed once as a statistical anomaly, but not three times. The Birmingham health officers were divided over how to interpret the results of their studies.

[47] For present-day analysis of the studies, see R. Millward and F. Bell, 'Infant mortality in Victorian Britain: the mother as medium', *Economic History Review* **54** (4) (2001), 699–733; A.S. Wohl, *Endangered Lives: Public Health in Victorian Britain* (London 1984), 25–32; D. Graham, 'Female employment and infant mortality: some evidence from British towns, 1911, 1931 and 1951', *Continuity and Change* **9** (2) (1994), 313–17; Dyhouse, 'Working-class mothers'.

[48] Tennant, 'Infantile mortality', 89–90, 117–19, the quote is from p. 90; Newman, *Infant Mortality*, 90–138. For Birmingham, see *Annual Report 1906*, 17–20; Robertson, *Report on Industrial Employment*, 16–17, 20–22; BCA M&CWSC minutes 7 Jul. 1916, item 112.

[49] *Annual Report 1906*, 19–20. The 1891 British Factory Act included a clause which obliged women to take a month off after childbirth. Enforcing the clause had proved difficult.

[50] BCA HC minutes 28 May 1907, item 575; Robertson, *Report on Industrial Employment*; J. Duncan, *Report on Infant Mortality in St. George's and St. Stephen's Wards* (Health Department, Birmingham 1911); Duncan, *Report on the Prevention of Infantile Mortality*; *Annual Reports 1908–1912*.

	1908	1909	1910	1911	1912
Mother employed	190	179	153	191	191
Mother not employed	207	169	161	192	174

Table 4.1   Infant mortality and mother's employment in St Stephen's and St George's Wards in Birmingham, 1908–1912.

Source: *Annual Report of the MOH for Birmingham 1913*, 20.

Jessie Duncan, an assistant MOH, drew the conclusion that the influence of industrial employment on infant mortality in the inner-city areas was 'quite small when compared with the influence of acute poverty'. In her reports, she not only provided evidence for this conclusion, but also pointed out fallacies and inconsistencies in other studies. On the basis of her reports, she recommended that central and local governments concentrate on dealing with the problem of poverty before even considering any restrictions on married women's work. She stated:

> [f]rom my own observations amongst these women, I have come to the conclusion that it is not the child of the working mother who has the worst chance. The woman who is thrifty and energetic, and wishes to supplement her husband's earnings, goes to work, and the additional money has an important influence on the prevention of poverty which is one of the greatest causes of infantile mortality.[51]

Central government favoured a different interpretation. Arthur Newsholme, the Chief Medical Officer on the Local Government Board, stated that it would be sheer folly to infer from such studies 'that the industrial occupation of mothers is not a most injurious element in our social life'.[52] The official view in Birmingham was brought into line with his view. Although the MOH admitted his perplexity over the results, he always concluded his reports by drawing readers' attention to the detrimental effects that women's employment had on infant welfare and domestic hygiene.[53] Dr Alexandra MacCallum, the successor of Dr Duncan, supported the MOH's view, emphasizing the findings that illuminated the great disadvantage at which the children of working mothers were placed.[54] Moreover, when the Birmingham delegates, including Robertson and MacCallum, returned from the Fourth English-speaking Conference on Infant Mortality in 1913, they stressed that maternal ignorance and factory work were among the greatest obstacles to improving infant welfare. Poverty

---

[51]   Duncan, *Report on the Prevention of Infantile Mortality*, 9.
[52]   Newsholme, 'Report on infant and child mortality', 57.
[53]   See in particular Robertson, *Report on Industrial Employment*.
[54]   *Annual Report 1912*, 22–6. Dr Duncan resigned from her job in 1912 and accepted an appointment as a School Medical Officer in London. BCA PH&HC minutes 27 Sept. 1912.

and lack of medical care were not mentioned.[55] If the infant welfare campaign was to succeed, women had to be encouraged to concentrate on their role as mothers.

What makes the case interesting is that the Birmingham authorities knew all along – before conducting any investigations – that working mothers were not to blame for the high rates of infant mortality in Birmingham. For example, in the summer 1906 almost 700 infants died in the central wards, and in only 39 of these cases (6 per cent) did the mother work outside the home.[56] No one in the Birmingham Health Department could expect that the campaign against women's work as such would dramatically improve infant welfare. Indeed, they expected the campaign to bring other benefits. By linking infant mortality with working mothers, the authorities conveyed the message that the conventional middle-class family with its breadwinning husband and dependent wife was the 'natural' and, by definition, the best family model. This approach was approved of not only by most middle-class people, but also, for example, by male trade unionists, who feared that cheap female labour would serve to undercut wages.[57] Yet there was one aim which was more important than buttressing the conventional gender roles. If the authorities had to decide whether to provide financial assistance for desperately poor mothers or to allow these mothers to work, they chose the lesser of two evils: they allowed the mothers to work. In the early twentieth century, the principle that families should be economically independent overrode even the wishes to encourage 'normal' domestic relations.[58] In most cases, however, the Birmingham authorities did not have to choose, but were able to construct policies which reflected and reinforced both of these ideals. In Gothenburg, by contrast, combining the ideals proved difficult.

Gothenburg

Like Birmingham, Gothenburg failed the 'sanitary test' in the 1890s. Compared to the other Swedish cities, Gothenburg had responded promptly to perceived community needs for a safe water supply and an effective sewer system, but the technologies the city had employed in addressing these needs failed to adapt to the changing standards of hygiene and to the long-term pressures of growth. For instance, in the early 1890s it was realized that conversion to water closets was not possible until the sewerage system had been modernized. The Gothenburg policy makers, reluctant to allocate money for improving the sewerage infrastructure, shelved plans to introduce water closets, and only began to deal properly with the matter in the early twentieth century. A price for relying on traditional methods was paid in the late 1890s, when the hot and dry summers brought significant increases in infant mortality (Figure 4.4).[59]

---

[55]   BCA PH&HC minutes 26 Sept. 1913, item 1695; 24 Oct. 1913, item 1785. See also minutes 22 Mar. 1912, item 352.

[56]   *Annual Report 1906*, 17. For bottle-feeding and women's employment, see *Annual Report 1905*, 23.

[57]   B. Drake, *Women in Trade Unions* (London 1920/1984); J. Lewis, *Women in England 1870–1950: Sexual Divisions and Social Change* (London 1984), 173–84.

[58]   *Annual Report 1905*, 23; *1906*, 16–20; Robertson, *Report on Industrial Employment*.

[59]   Lindman, *Dödligheten*, 126–7; *Göteborgs hälsovårdsnämnds årsberättelse* (hereafter *Årsberättelsen*) *1906*, 38; O. Wetterberg and G. Axelsson, *Smutsguld och dödligt hot:*

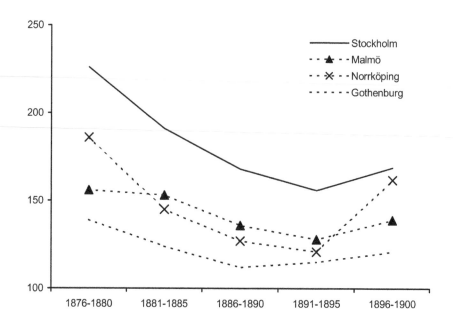

Figure 4.4   Infant mortality in Stockholm, Malmö, Norrköping and Gothenburg, five-year means, 1876–1900.

Source: C. Lindman, *Dödligheten i första lefnadsåret i Sveriges tjugo större städer 1876–95* (Stockholm 1898), 103; *Bidrag till Sveriges Officiella Statistik* (BiSOS), *A) Befolkningsstatistik 1895–1900.*

However, even in the 1890s, the infant mortality rate in Gothenburg was relatively low. Both international and national studies comparing infant mortality in various cities showed Gothenburg in a favourable light. For example, Dr Carl Lindman's study on infant mortality in Sweden, published in 1898, showed that Gothenburg was well ahead of Stockholm, Malmö and Norrköping in tackling the problem.[60] The setback in the 1890s served as a valuable reminder that there was still room for improvement in environmental management, but on the whole the late nineteenth-century sanitary reforms seemed to make Gothenburg a healthier place to live. The general mortality rate decreased considerably, and infants appeared to benefit from

---

Renhållning och återvinning i Göteborg 1864–1930 (Göteborg 1995), 123–69, 210; A. Attman, *Göteborgs Stadsfullmäktige 1863–1962*, vol. I.1: *Göteborg 1863–1913* (Göteborg 1963), 343–7, and vol. I.2: *Göteborg 1913–1962* (Göteborg 1963), 274–5. For the infant death rate in the late 1890s, see *Årsberättelser 1895–1900*.

[60]   Lindman, *Dödligheten*, 17–27, 50–51, 103, 106–31, and in particular 126–7 and appendix, figures 5, 6, 7 and 8. See also Silbergleit, 'Ueber den gegenwärtigen Stand der Kindersterblichkeit, ihre Erscheinungen und ihre Entwickelung in europäischen Großstädten', *Beilage zur Hygienischen Rundschau* 5 (1895), 216–41; Newman, *Infant Mortality*, 6–19 and Appendix I. For a present-day analysis, see M. Poulain and D. Tabutin, 'La mortalité aux jeunes âges en Europe et en Amérique du Nord du XIXe à nos jours', in P. Boulanger and D. Tabutin (eds), *La mortalité des enfants le monde et dans l'histoire* (Liège 1980), 119–24.

the reforms, too. In particular, the reorganization of the waste collection system in 1885 apparently reduced infant mortality dramatically (see Figure 4.2).[61]

Given the relatively low mortality rates, the Gothenburg authorities did not come under pressure from the general public to improve infant welfare. Indeed, the main reason why they took up the matter was not so much criticism from within as influences from outside Sweden. As the infant welfare movement spread across the Western world, health authorities and philanthropic dignitaries in Gothenburg and in other Swedish cities felt that they too should intensify their efforts to safeguard the next generation. Two groups in particular seized on the issue in order to further causes they considered important. Firstly, medical practitioners urged government to take measures to improve child welfare, hoping that these measures would also serve to enhance their professional status. Unlike British doctors, who were divided over state intervention, the Swedish medical profession was often united in campaigning for the expansion of publicly funded medical care. The majority of Swedish medical practitioners worked in the public sector and benefited directly from public investments in health care, but even doctors not holding a public post were acutely aware of the importance of governmental involvement. Central and local governments were the only agencies in Sweden capable of providing the infrastructure for the expansion of modern medicine and for the development of medical specialities such as paediatrics and obstetrics.[62] The second group actively participating in the discussion about child welfare consisted of social reformers. They were concerned about widespread social deprivation in Sweden, and seized on the international infant welfare movement to shame governmental and voluntary agencies into activity. They were convinced that the problem of poverty could be resolved only if the public and voluntary sectors took more responsibility for the physical well-being and moral socialization of children.[63]

'Important' and 'Unimportant' Causes of Death   If the origins of the Gothenburg and Birmingham campaigns were different, so were their main foci. While the Birmingham authorities concentrated almost exclusively on dealing with the problem of infantile diarrhoea, the Gothenburg authorities chose an approach that provided more scope for flexibility. They addressed the prevention of infantile diarrhoea, but the disease never dominated the discussion as it did in Birmingham. Other causes of infant death such as congenital defects, bronchitis and pneumonia also figured in the Gothenburg campaign from an early date.

---

[61]   *Årsberättelsen 1888*, 72–3 and appendix; E. Almquist, 'Dödorsakerna i Göteborg 1861–85'; Almquist, *Allmän hälsovårdslära*, 154, 789–90; Lindman, *Dödligheten*, 124–31; Wetterberg and Axelsson, *Smutsguld och dödligt hot*, 123–57.

[62]   For the state intervention in the medical market, see G. Kearns, W.R. Lee and J. Rogers, 'The interaction of political and economic factors in the management of urban public health', in M.C. Nelson and J. Rogers (eds), *Urbanisation and the Epidemiological Transition* (Uppsala 1989), 9–81.

[63]   K. Ohrlander, *I barnens och nationens intresse: Socialliberal reformpolitik 1903–1930* (Stockholm 1992).

The cause-of-death tables do not help to explain the different approaches.[64] At the turn of the century, diarrhoea was a major cause of infant mortality in both cities. In Gothenburg, the proportion of diarrhoeal deaths of all infant deaths varied from 18 to 33 per cent; in Birmingham, from 15 to 33 per cent. When it came to other causes of infant death, the differences between the cities were somewhat clearer. Firstly, respiratory diseases such as bronchitis and pneumonia were responsible for 18–25 per cent of all infant deaths in Gothenburg, compared with only 12–15 per cent in Birmingham. Secondly, prematurity, congenital defects and other 'wasting diseases' accounted for 23–28 per cent of infant deaths in Gothenburg and for 28–35 per cent in Birmingham.[65] However, these differences do not explain why the Birmingham authorities concentrated on preventing infantile diarrhoea and why the Gothenburg authorities launched a broader campaign. The following sections analyse the way in which the Gothenburg authorities defined the problem of infant mortality, and explain the reasons why they defined it differently from the Birmingham authorities. As the analysis shows, the Gothenburg authorities' decision to launch a broader campaign was as logical (or illogical) as the Birmingham authorities' decision to concentrate on infantile diarrhoea. Both campaigns could be defended as scientific and rational, even though they were shaped by political and social concerns.

A Medical Problem Many commentators expressing their concern about the physical health of children in Gothenburg in the late nineteenth and early twentieth centuries called for the extension and modernization of hospital facilities. The scarcity of medical resources, they contended, was an important contributing factor to the high infant mortality and to the prevalence of poor health among mothers and children. Firstly, the lives of many mothers and their newborn babies were in danger because of overcrowding in the Municipal Maternity Hospital.[66] Secondly, a large number of infants and small children whose illnesses might have been curable were condemned to death or disability due to the lack of access to effective treatment. Citing various investigations, the campaigners argued that the well-being of mothers and children could be vastly improved if only there were enough specialists and hospital facilities in the city. Mothers could be better protected from the perils of childbirth, infants could have a better chance of surviving pneumonia and diarrhoea, and many children suffering from congenital defects or non-pulmonary tuberculosis could be rehabilitated.[67] These campaigns attracted influential support from the First City Physician and the Health Committee, but the main agitators were the doctors

---

[64]   Comparing the cause-of-death tables in Birmingham and Gothenburg is problematic, since infant deaths were often poorly diagnosed and some descriptions such as prematurity were ambiguous.

[65]   *Årsberättelser 1899–1903*; Lindman, *Dödligheten*, 120–24; *Special Report on Infant Mortality*, 5.

[66]   *GSH 1886:71*; *1894:14*; *1896:29*; *1896:55*.

[67]   For the discussion about children's access to medical care, see *GSH 1903:122A*, no. 7; *1903:122B*, no. 14; *1903:196*, 15–19 and 50–56 (the table demonstrates clearly the increasing importance attached to children's health care); *1908:102*, 156 and minutes 17 Sept. 1908, item 11; *1910:269* and minutes 8 Dec. 1910, item 11; *1910:272*; *1917:39*; 'Göteborgs barnsjukhus', *Göteborgs Handels- och Sjöfarts-Tidning* 24 Nov. 1903. See also Isberg, 'Barnavård', 69;

and governors of the Municipal Maternity Hospital and the Children's Hospital. In the late nineteenth century, the resources of these institutions were stretched to their limits. Increasing patient populations and the introduction of new technologies – medical and non-medical – had caused capital and operating costs to rise and finally forced the hospitals to seek more substantial public funding.

The director and the governors of the Municipal Maternity Hospital appealed several times in the late nineteenth century for funds to extend and modernize their institution. They argued that the hospital building had proved too small almost as soon as it had opened its doors in 1875. Gothenburg expanded rapidly in the late nineteenth century, resulting in greater numbers of poor maternity patients than the hospital had initially been intended for. Medical advances in maternity care exacerbated the situation, since they demanded the reorganization of the hospital's interior and encouraged a wider range of patients. As hospital deliveries became safer, hospital maternity care was sought not only by the poorest of the poor, but also by women factory workers and the wives of sailors, artisans and farmers.[68]

A temporary committee set up by the Gothenburg City Council in 1894 to consider the issue took the view that a modern maternity hospital was an essential part of municipal health care services. The City Council followed the recommendation and built a new maternity hospital, which was opened in 1900. However, almost immediately after the opening of the new building, the hospital board turned to the City Council again. The building had proved to be too small and needed to be extended.[69] At this stage the campaigners were able to refer to the international infant welfare movement to justify the demands they made on the public purse. For example, the director of the Maternity Hospital compared his hospital to other European institutions, seeking to convince the decision-makers that the Gothenburg hospital had always provided value for money. The rate of maternal mortality was lower among patients in the Gothenburg hospital than among patients in famous French and German institutions, and the high standard of treatment in Gothenburg was also reflected in the infants' survival. The rate of neonatal mortality due to birth injury was low.[70]

Apart from making international comparisons, the campaigners sought medical legitimacy for their plans to extend the Maternity Hospital and to increase the number of hospital confinements. The campaigners were aware that drawing firm conclusions about the relative safety of hospital versus home deliveries was difficult, since it was the women most at risk of dying who were usually admitted to hospital.

S. Johansson, 'Göteborgs barnsjukhus' historia', *Hygiea* **84** (1922), 454–67; L. Öberg, *Göteborgs Läkaresällskap: En historik* (Göteborg 1983), 223.

[68]   *GSH 1886:71*; *1894:14*; *1896:29*; A.H. Westman, 'Barnbördsanstaltens historia', in *Årsberättelsen 1900*, appendix; 'Minnesskrift: Carl Magnus Ullman', *Hygiea* **81** (1919), 987–9.

[69]   *GSH 1894:14*, and minutes 8 Mar. 1894, item 2, *1896:29*; *1896:55* and minutes 30 Apr. 1896, item 12; Westman, 'Barnbördsanstaltens historia'; K.J. Gezelius, 'Göteborgs stads hälso- och sjukvård', in N. Wimarson (ed.), *Göteborg: En översikt vid trehundraårsjubileet 1923* (Göteborg 1923), 369–71.

[70]   K.A. Walter, 'Barnbördshuset i Göteborg verksamhet under tiden från 1 Oktober 1875 till 1 Juli 1900', in *Årsberättelsen 1900*, appendix.

Consequently, they contented themselves with presenting some research findings which spoke in favour of institutional maternity care. Firstly, they pointed out that the death rate from puerperal fever was lower in the Gothenburg Maternity Hospital than among home deliveries. Secondly, they emphasized that women who had complications during pregnancy or during labour benefited from hospital care, since the techniques developed for the management of abnormal labour could not be applied properly in homes. Referring to these findings, the campaigners argued that it would have been extremely unwise to discourage women from seeking institutional maternity care.[71]

A similar kind of campaign was launched to secure more public funding for the Children's Hospital. This institution, although voluntarily run, was dependent on the municipality for financial support, and the hospital board had been answerable to the City Council since 1869. In the early twentieth century, the campaigners pointed out to the councillors that appropriations no longer kept pace with the growth of the population and with the demand for technologically intensive medical care. Another problem was that the admission patterns of the hospital were thoroughly outmoded: children from well-to-do homes and infants under two years of age were not admitted. In a modern hospital, the campaigners argued, the diagnosis rather than the social position of the patient should be the criterion for admission. The campaigners stressed that hospital treatment could especially benefit infants and small children suffering from non-pulmonary tuberculosis, diarrhoea, pneumonia and congenital defects. However, the reforms could be carried through only if the hospital budget was augmented by various forms of municipal support.[72]

The fact that medical practitioners knew little about congenital defects or bronchitis, for example, was not an insurmountable obstacle to starting a campaign against these diseases; after all, the authority of doctors was not based on their capacity to prevent and cure illnesses. In Gothenburg, the medical practitioners who worked for municipal hospitals or for the Health Department enjoyed a relatively high status in society. Their competence was not questioned, even though the reforms they carried through did not always bring immediate results. In Birmingham, the status of public health doctors was lower, and therefore they were constantly under pressure to prove themselves efficient.[73]

To conclude, an important reason why the Gothenburg campaign covered a broad spectrum of diseases was that the infant welfare movement habitually argued for more extensive institutional care not only for infants, but also for young children and mothers. Had the Gothenburg campaigners concentrated on preventing infantile diarrhoea, they would not have got far with their aim. In other words, while the

---

[71]   *GSH 1886:71*; *1896:29*. See also S. Vallgårda, 'Hospitalization of deliveries: the change of place of birth in Denmark and Sweden from the late nineteenth century to 1970', *Medical History* **40** (1996), 173–96.

[72]   *GSH 1903:122B*, no. 14; *1903:196*, 15–19; *1910:269*; Johansson, 'Göteborgs barnsjukhus' historia'; Gezelius, 'Göteborgs stads hälso- och sjukvård'. For the medicalization of the hospital, see C.E. Rosenberg, 'Community and communities: the evolution of the American hospital', in D.E. Long and J. Golden (eds), *The American General Hospital: Communities and Social Contexts* (Ithaca, NY 1989), 3–17.

[73]   See Chapters 1 and 3.

Birmingham authorities sought to find a way to bring down alarmingly high infant mortality and to introduce order and hygiene to the slums, the Gothenburg campaigners worked for the expansion of publicly funded medical care and for the further enhancement of the status of medicine and medical practitioners. In their letters to the Gothenburg City Council, the campaigners emphasized that effective treatments could be made more widely available and that the international standing of Swedish obstetrics and paediatrics could be ensured only if the municipality allocated more resources to the hospitals.[74]

Reconciling Divergent Interests   Since local government funding was crucial for the Gothenburg hospitals, one can appreciate the eagerness of the hospital doctors and governors to define health problems as medical matters. It is also easy to understand why the Gothenburg Health Committee was sympathetic to this line of thinking. Until the 1930s, about 30 per cent of the Health Committee members were medical practitioners, and other professionals such as architects, engineers and lawyers were also well represented on the Committee. The strong position of established professions meant that health problems were often seen as technical questions best resolved by professionals on the basis of scientific criteria.[75] In early twentieth-century Birmingham it was a different story. The Birmingham Health Committee usually included only one medical practitioner among its eight members, and on the Public Health and Housing Committee, which replaced the Health Committee in 1912, medical practitioners were conspicuous by their absence. Both Birmingham committees were dominated by local business interests.[76]

The Gothenburg city councillors, though sometimes hesitant to invest large sums of money in hospitals, clearly recognized the importance of medical services. One reason for their favourable attitude was that the policy of making medical services more widely available was in line with traditions. Although the Swedish health authorities had failed to deliver in the nineteenth century, in theory they had been responsible for providing medical care for seriously ill patients. Accordingly, in the early twentieth century the debate did not centre on the question of *whether* the municipal authorities were responsible for providing hospital beds for babies with life-threatening bronchitis or diarrhoea. The controversial question was *when* they could afford to provide services of this type.[77]

Another reason for the popularity of the medical approach among the policy makers was that it was oblivious to the context in which patients had fallen ill. By emphasizing the role of medical practitioners, policy makers kept the problem

[74] *GSH 1903:122B*, no. 14; *1903:196*, 15–19; *GSH 1910:269*; Walter, 'Barnbördshuset i Göteborg verksamhet'.

[75] *Årsberättelser 1888–39*. See also S. Edvinsson and J. Rogers, 'Hälsa och hälsoreformer i svenska städer kring sekelskiftet 1900', *Historisk Tidskrift* **121** (4) (2001), 547–8.

[76] In Birmingham, medical practitioners comprised 0–20 per cent of the Health Committee/Public Health and Housing Committee/Public Health Committee members in the years 1900–39, with the exception of the years 1908–10, when their proportion was higher, at 25 per cent. See also E.P. Hennock, *Fit and Proper Persons: Ideal and Reality in Nineteenth-century Urban Government* (London 1973), 37, 48–9.

[77] See, for example, *GSH 1903:196*.

of disease prevention in laboratories, clinics and hospitals, and managed to avoid discussing the social causes of diseases such as defective housing and poverty. In fact, some policy makers saw hospitalization as a way of managing the housing problem. They assumed that an increase in the number of hospital beds could, to an extent, compensate for bad housing conditions. When maternity cases or patients suffering from tuberculosis or other infectious diseases were removed from overcrowded homes to hospitals, the health and welfare of the poorest of the poor would improve, even though they still lived in insanitary houses.[78]

Irresponsible Parents   Another response provoked by the question of child welfare in Gothenburg focused on the incompetence and negligence of parents. This debate was initiated by social reformers who were concerned that inadequate parenting would undermine the efforts to reform society and to enhance national efficiency. If the modernization of Swedish society was to succeed, the governmental and voluntary agencies should ensure a proper childhood for every child, and especially those of the poor, by protecting them from adult cruelty, indifference and incompetence.[79]

At first glance, the way in which the Gothenburg health authorities responded to these demands was similar to the policies pursued by the Birmingham authorities in the 1910s. In both cities, the authorities argued that mothers' ignorance and fathers' negligence were important contributory factors to infant mortality. Furthermore, instilling a sense of responsibility into parents was an aim which these authorities shared. However, beyond that basic goal, the campaigns differed in many characteristics. In Birmingham, the families living in the slum areas were defined as being the problem. Their poor personal and household hygiene, their ignorance of safe methods of infant care and their deviation from 'normal' gender roles, so it was argued, led to high infant mortality. Therefore, one of the main goals of the campaign was to create 'well-ordered homes', where the presence and influence of 'a capable mother' was felt in manifold ways.[80] In Gothenburg, where illegitimacy was common, the blame for high infant mortality was laid on single mothers and absent fathers. Their failure to maintain their children and to prevent them from falling into the hands of bad foster parents or other unscrupulous adults was defined as the largest obstacle to improving infant welfare. Accordingly, the Gothenburg authorities concentrated on ensuring that the parents of illegitimate children accepted their responsibility to maintain and protect their offspring. Less attention was paid to household hygiene, safe methods of infant care and gender roles.

The Gothenburg authorities often perceived absent fathers as the main culprits for the plight of illegitimate children, but since the authorities had few effective ways of dealing with the problem of absent fathers, they usually targeted single mothers instead.[81] Particularly sharp criticism was levelled at women who denied

---

[78]   For further discussion about hospitalization and housing, see Chapter 5.

[79]   Ohrlander, *I barnens och nationens intresse*.

[80]   Robertson, *Report on Industrial Employment*, 15–16.

[81]   See also, H. Bergman, '"En feministisk konspiration": kvinnors politiska aktivism för barnavårdsmannainstitutionens införande i 1910-talets Sverige', in C. Florin and L. Kvarnström (eds), *Kvinnor på gränsen till medborgarskap: Genus, politik och offentlighet*

their motherhood. Until 1917, mothers who gave their newborn babies away could remain anonymous. A survey conducted in Gothenburg in 1912 showed that approximately eighty unmarried mothers exercised this right annually. The vast majority of them sought care within private maternity homes, and the midwives who delivered them also arranged for their children to be placed in foster homes or orphanages. Almost without exception, these children were bottle-fed and therefore exposed to diarrhoeal diseases, but many of them were also wilfully neglected and abused. What also concerned the authorities was that mothers who remained anonymous could easily evade their responsibility for maintaining their children, which meant that many of these children eventually ended up in the care of the poor law authorities. The Gothenburg health authorities demanded an amendment to the law that allowed mothers to remain unknown.[82]

The vast majority of unmarried mothers, about 90 per cent, did not exercise the right to remain anonymous. However, the health authorities were quick to point out that this was of little comfort, as long as the authorities were unable to intervene in a meaningful way even in cases where the child's health was endangered. They called for immediate steps to improve the situation. Firstly, the greatest evil affecting the welfare of unmarried mothers and illegitimate children was the unwillingness of absent fathers to support their children. The health authorities argued that fathers managed to evade their responsibility partly because ignorant and inexperienced mothers rarely made an effort to gain legal recognition of paternity or any financial assistance from the fathers. Prompted by the desire to improve the situation of illegitimate children and the determination to keep them and their mothers off public funds, the health and poor law authorities recommended that the City Council provide legal advice for mothers. Non-supporting fathers were not to be tolerated.

Secondly, the health authorities were aware that even though fathers would pay maintenance for their illegitimate children, most unmarried mothers would still have to work outside the home. To help single mothers and other poor women reconcile motherhood with paid work, the Gothenburg authorities adopted a favourable attitude to nurseries. This approach did not provoke strong criticism in Gothenburg, where the textile and food processing industries were keen to employ female labour and where male trade unionists were not too concerned about the competition from women for jobs, since the labour market was thoroughly sex-segregated.[83] The difference from the policy pursued by the Birmingham authorities was clear. The Birmingham authorities stressed the importance of full-time motherhood to

---

1800–1950 (Stockholm 2001), 172–191; B. Hobson and M. Takahashi, 'The parent–worker model: lone mothers in Sweden', in J. Lewis (ed.), *Lone Mothers in European Welfare Regimes: Shifting Policy Logics* (London 1997), 121–39.

[82]   *GSH 1912:18*; *1912:273* and minutes 31 Oct. 1912, item 8. See also E. Elgán, 'Le législateur au secours de la mère célebataire: la solution de la responsabilité individuelle', in M.C. Nelson and J. Rogers (eds), *Mother, Father, and Child: Swedish Social Policy in the Early Twentieth Century* (Uppsala 1990), 55–67.

[83]   *GSH 1909:252*; *1912:18*; *1912:273*. See also J. Gröndahl, 'Single mothers and poor relief in a Swedish industrial town (Gävle) at the beginning of the twentieth century', and Elgán, 'Le législateur au secours de la mère célebataire', in Nelson and Rogers, *Mother, Father, and Child*, 31–53 and 55–67.

the well-being of children, and working mothers were denounced in no uncertain terms. The Gothenburg authorities, while admitting that a too hasty return to work by new mothers was inadvisable, did not consider maternal occupation as such to be deleterious to infant welfare. Similarly, the Gothenburg authorities adopted a more flexible attitude to bottle-feeding than their Birmingham counterparts. The First City Physician, Karl Gezelius, and other doctors campaigning for milk depots in Gothenburg by no means belittled the benefits of breast-milk. On the contrary, they suggested that voluntary societies instruct mothers in infant care and, if necessary, help them maintain breast-feeding by providing modest economic assistance. However, if these measures failed, voluntary and municipal agencies should ensure that uncontaminated cow's milk was available (Figure 4.5).[84] Bottle-feeding, the Gothenburg authorities argued, could be safe if prepared in the right conditions. This was the prevailing orthodoxy in Gothenburg until the mid-1920s.[85]

Thirdly, the Gothenburg health authorities focused their attention on foster care. They pointed out that unmarried mothers often handed their children over to unscrupulous foster mothers who exposed the infants to death and disease. Since many foster mothers were clearly unreliable and profited shamelessly at the expense of illegitimate children, the municipal authorities were to step in.[86] The Gothenburg authorities did not criticize unmarried mothers for giving their children away; on the contrary, they seemed to think that many illegitimate children were better off fostered or adopted, without their natural parents. However, the foster arrangements needed to be supervised by experts.

The focus on illegitimate children and their parents was justified by referring to the high infant mortality among children born out of wedlock. For example, in the years 1908–12 the mortality rate for legitimate infants was about 64 per thousand live births, and the rate for illegitimate babies was 127.[87] However, although the authorities were quick to link infant mortality with unmarried motherhood, the problem was by no means restricted to the children of single mothers. Both legitimate and illegitimate infants whose families were living in poverty were exposed to fatal diseases.[88] The Gothenburg authorities were aware of a close association between

---

[84]   *GSH 1909:252*, 3–5, 11–14, 25–6 and minutes 7 Jan. 1910, item 6; *1910:59*; *1911:27*, in particular 3–9. See also 'K.J. Gezelius', in M. Fahl, *Göteborgs Stadsfullmäktige 1863– 1962*, vol. II: *Biografisk Matrikel* (Göteborg 1963).

[85]   A. Wallgren, 'Barnavårdscentraler och deras förebyggande verksamhet i spädbarnsåldern: en betydelsefull social-medicinsk uppgift', *Social-Medicinsk Tidskrift* **11** (1934), 165–71; C.G. Sundell, 'Effectivare spädbarnsvård och spädbarnskontroll', *Social-Medicinsk Tidskrift* **6** (1929), 232–40.

[86]   For unscrubulous foster parents, see *Årsberättelsen 1906*, 2; *1907*, 2; Göteborgs stadsarkiv (GSA) Göteborgs Hälsovårdsnämnd, I avdelningen (HVN I) minutes 23 Mar. 1917, item 58; 4 Apr. 1917, item 61. For the definition of the problem, see *GSH 1912:18*; *1912:273*; *1917:109*; *1917:284*.

[87]   Å. Brodin, 'Spädbarnsdödligheten i Göteborg tiden 1908–1937', *Nordisk Medicin* (1939), 3,659–70. See also Isberg, 'Barnavård', 69–71; Lindman, *Dödligheten*, 23–6; Almquist, *Allmän hälsovårdslära*, 792–3; *GSH 1917:109*; *1917:284*.

[88]   For poverty and infant mortality, see for example Lindman, *Dödligheten*, 20–23; I. Jundell, 'Moderskydd', *Social Tidskrift* (1908), 52.

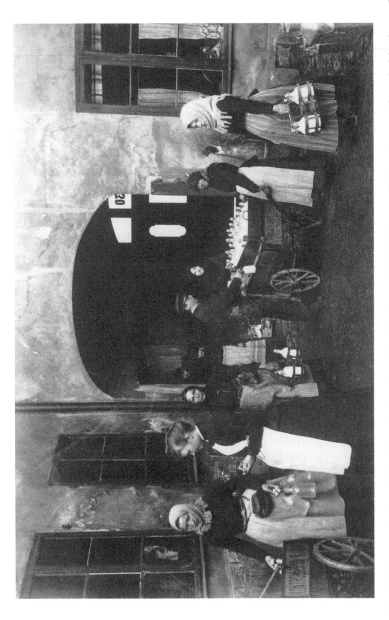

Figure 4.5 Milkshop Audumbla in Norrlandsgatan, Stockholm, *c.* 1895. Before milk depots were founded in the early years of the twentieth century, 'controlled' milk was available in some milkshops. However, the relatively high price of the controlled milk put it beyond the means of the poorest people.

Source: Stockholm City Museum.

poverty and infant mortality, but were ready to deal with the poverty problem only by indirect means, for example by advising unmarried mothers and by supporting nurseries and milk depots. One of the main aims of these measures was to help, or force if necessary, both fathers and mothers to provide for their children and therefore to restrict the burden imposed on the taxpayers.[89] The next section examines as to how the ideas on infant welfare were implemented in Gothenburg and Birmingham and how they were re-interpreted in the 1920s and 1930s.

Infant Welfare Campaigns and Urban Politics

Birmingham

Convinced that the solution to infant mortality lay in the education of mothers and in the reinforcement of the 'natural' gender roles, the Birmingham authorities concentrated on providing educational health services, and in particular health visiting and infant consultations. These services, which promoted healthy habits and conformity to norms of femininity and masculinity, represented continuity in the Birmingham campaign from the early twentieth century to the late 1930s. However, the campaign also underwent important changes. Firstly, its socio-spatial orientation changed over time. The Birmingham authorities began the campaign among the poorest of the poor in the central wards, but shifted the focus towards working-class and lower-middle-class suburbs in the 1910s and 1920s. The shift reflected and reinforced changes in the political scene and in the relationship between social classes and urban space. The second important change concerned medical services. Initially, the Birmingham health officials took great care not to encroach upon the territory of general practitioners, but as time passed and the infant welfare campaign expanded, they occasionally ignored the protests of general practitioners and introduced some medical services.

Emphasis on Educational Health Services   Health visiting and infant consultation services in Birmingham followed the same pattern of development as in many other British cities, with the distinction that in Birmingham the emphasis placed on these educational services was stronger than in most other places.[90] The first municipal health visitors were appointed in Birmingham in 1899, a few years before the infant welfare campaign started in earnest, and by 1907 the sub-department had a staff of 14. In these early stages of the campaign, when insanitary environment and domestic dirt were still regarded as the major culprits in causing infant deaths, the majority of the health visitors were working-class women with a rudimentary grasp of the principles of hygiene. They worked in the 'unhealthy areas', trying to get people 'to clean their rooms, to open their windows and to unstop their chimneys', and

---

[89]   See, for example, *GSH 1909:252*, 11, 29; *1912:18*; *1917:284*.

[90]   C. Davies, 'The health visitor as mother's friend: a woman's place in public health, 1900–14', *Social History of Medicine* **1** (1) (1988); Lewis, *The Politics of Motherhood*.

in addition to matters of home hygiene, they gave advice on proper feeding and clothing of children.[91]

While the MOH and the Health Committee praised the visitors for improving the lives of the poor, they also deplored the difficulties 'in obtaining the services of the best class of Health Visitor'.[92] Sporadic criticism also came from outside the municipal apparatus. In his statement to the Royal Commission on the Poor Laws in 1907, Dr Albert Bycott of Birmingham doubted whether the visitors had achieved any improvement in the habits of the poor. 'I do not hear them much quoted by mothers,' he stated, urging the Health Department to employ 'a better class of women', and preferably trained nurses.[93] Moreover, the very definition of the problem of infant mortality was in the process of being revised. The focus was shifting away from insanitary environment and towards lack of mothering skills, so practical policies had to be brought into line with the new definition.

The Health Committee gradually upgraded the campaign by employing 'lady doctors' and trained nurses. The poorest mothers were to learn child care techniques not from health officers whose background was similar to their own, but from ones whose authority was based on formal qualifications and superior social position. In 1908, Dr Jessie Duncan and two experienced health visitors started their work in St George's and St Stephen's Wards, where traditional health visiting had not succeeded in reducing infant mortality. They specialized in infant welfare work, visiting the homes of newborn babies every week for the first five weeks, and then every month. Practically all the mothers and newborn babies in the two wards were reached, since the 1907 Notification of Births Act obliged fathers to notify the MOH of the birth within 36 hours.[94] Dr Duncan also organized 'infant consultations', where mothers were instructed in infant care and babies were weighed and examined. Convinced of the potential of the services, the Health Committee in 1912 formed three new special areas into which systematic home visiting and consultations were introduced. Moreover, infant welfare work undertaken by voluntary societies supplemented the local authority services. The societies formed their own special areas and employed doctors and health visitors, largely sharing the methods of the municipal campaign.[95]

The doctors and health visitors, while overtly concentrating on health care, also contributed to the everyday administration of social order. Commitment to healthy habits and conformity to social norms were promoted through regular contact with

----

[91]   BCA HC minutes 14 Feb. 1899, item 5559; 28 Mar. 1899, items 5666–7; 25 Jul. 1899, item 5896; 24 Jul. 1900, item 6418; 28. Jul. 1903, item 8187 (the quote); 26 Mar. 1907, item 474; *Annual Report 1899*, 34–9, *1900*, 28–33.

[92]   BCA HC minutes 26 Mar. 1907, item 472.

[93]   *Royal Commission on the Poor Laws and Relief of Distress, 1909*, appendix, vol. IV, Questions 43998 (26); 44590–44603.

[94]   BCA HC minutes 14 Jan. 1908, item 907; 11 Feb. 1908, item 974; 19 Feb. 1908, item 1001; *Annual Report 1907*, 17; Duncan, *Report on Infant Mortality*, 3; Robertson, *Report on Industrial Employment*, 2–6.

[95]   BCA PH&HC minutes 8 Mar. 1912, item 311; 22 Mar. 1912, item 364; 24 Oct. 1913, item 1785; *Report of the MOH on Child Welfare in 1913*, see in particular Chart F. See also *Annual Reports of the BIHS 1908–18* and Chapter 6.

the mothers. Any change, for better or worse, in infant care, in the cleanliness of the home, in the consumption of alcohol or in the division of labour within the family did not go unnoticed by health officers, and better compliance with the norms was encouraged by using various incentives and sanctions.[96] The services were primarily designed to help full-time mothers and to strengthen their commitment to motherhood and, in consequence, full-time mothers and their children usually benefited most from them. From the point of view of working mothers, the same services might look different. At best, the services ignored the difficulties these mothers faced in trying to reconcile motherhood with paid work, and at worst they created an additional burden for them. The families of working mothers were labelled as problem families, and their everyday life was kept under close scrutiny: a strategy which was adhered to, especially until the First World War, even though some individual officers, like Dr Jessie Duncan, questioned its benefits.[97]

Other policy decisions strengthened the key messages of the health education. For example, with the exception of the war years, the Birmingham authorities did not provide nurseries. Underlying the strict policy was the belief that some married women, if given any encouragement, would rather take a job than stay at home. The MOH warned in 1912 that '[i]f good, clean crèches were everywhere available', this 'would be an inducement to married women ... to leave the infants at the officially recognized crèche and go to work'.[98] Municipal nurseries established during the First World War were 'a purely war emergency measure', and the Committee stressed that they had 'no intention of engaging in this work in normal times'. They were as good as their word: the nurseries were closed at the end of the war. The only concession the Committee made was to subsidize a nursery receiving children whose mothers were undergoing hospital treatment.[99] The Committee also held firm in their stance against milk depots, although some city councillors and associations urged them to take action in the matter. The decision was justified by referring to the lack of accurate knowledge: the statistics illustrating the effect of milk depots in places like Liverpool and St Helens were misleading. Mortality among milk depot babies was low, mainly because 'the ignorant and careless parents [did] not go near' the depots. It was the careful parents who used the service.[100]

In addition to working and bottle-feeding mothers, mothers to whose health further pregnancies posed a significant risk fell outside the good mother ideal held up by the Birmingham campaign. Attention was drawn to these mothers in the 1920s, when the discussion about birth control intensified, and especially in 1930, when the Ministry of Health gave local authorities permission to give birth control advice in 'cases

---

[96]   *Annual Report 1912*, 18–26; *Report of the MOH on Child Welfare in 1913*, 9–10, 15–16.

[97]   *Annual Report 1906*, 17–9; *1912*, 18–26; *1914*, 14; Robertson, *Report on Industrial Employment*; Duncan, *Report on Infant Mortality*; Duncan, *Report on the Prevention of Infantile Mortality*; BCA M&CWSC minutes 7 Jan. 1916, item 19.

[98]   BCA PH&HC minutes 8 Mar. 1912, item 312.

[99]   BCA PH&HC minutes 8 Dec. 1916, item 4154; Birmingham Maternity and Child Welfare Committee (M&CWC) minutes 23 Apr. 1920, item 580.

[100]   BCA HC minutes 12 Mar. 1907, item 424; 25 Jun. 1907, item 631; 8 Mar. 1912, item 337; 22 Mar. 1912, item 364.

where further pregnancy would be detrimental to health'. Despite the pressure from the Ministry and some women's organizations, the Birmingham Maternity and Child Welfare Committee and Dr H.P. Newsholme, who had succeeded John Robertson as MOH in 1927, adopted a negative stance on establishing municipal family planning clinics, and even used the threat of dismissal to keep their staff in line. In 1928, the MOH demanded the resignation of Dr Clara Macirone, who was a medical officer at the Floodgate Street municipal infant welfare centre but who also worked for the voluntary family planning clinic in Castle Street. The MOH disapproved the 'dual appointment', especially since the Catholic clergy discouraged Catholic mothers from attending the municipal centre where Dr Macirone worked. In this case, the Maternity and Child Welfare Committee decided not to take action. However, in 1931 the Committee dismissed a health visitor, Mrs Waters, who admitted having mentioned to a Catholic mother with 13 children that there were 'facilities for women with large families to have advice in Castle Street'.[101] Until 1935, when the first municipal birth control clinics were opened, the Birmingham campaign concentrated on improving the health of expectant women and on safeguarding the health of mothers 'in relation to future pregnancies'. Birth control advice did not fit under this umbrella.[102]

From the Slums to the New Suburbia   In the early twentieth century, the Birmingham authorities directed their attention almost exclusively to the 'unhealthy areas' in the centre of the city. In the 1910s, however, some of the optimism with which the campaign had been launched in the inner-city districts gradually vanished. An assistant MOH, Alexandra MacCallum, deplored in 1913 that it was very difficult to induce the poorest mothers 'to do anything with care and regularity'.[103] In the following year, the MOH stated that while instructing 'mothers of the intelligent class of artisans' was comparatively easy, working among the feckless was 'one of the most depressing of occupations'.[104] The frustration was not surprising. In 1913, it was realized that in the inner-city areas where the special campaign had been launched in 1908, infant mortality had declined by only 4 per cent, whereas in the other areas – where only some or none of the services had been available – the reduction was far greater, varying from 16 to 28 per cent.[105]

Disappointed with the results that had fallen short of expectations, the Birmingham authorities changed the prime target group of their campaign. Since the best results from the work seemed to be 'obtained among the artisan classes rather than among the slum-dwellers', the MOH urged the Committee to establish

---

[101] BCA M&CWSC minutes 30 May 1928, item 2288; 14 Jan. 1931, item 369; 17 Jun. 1931, item 518; M&CWC minutes 8 Jun. 1928, item 1694; 22 Jun. 1928, item 1714; 23 Jan. 1931, item 519; 26 Jun. 1931, item 676; 10 Jul. 1931, item 691; 8 Apr. 1932, item 919. See also Chapter 6.

[102] BCA M&CWSC minutes 2 May 1928, item 2232; 14 Jan. 1931, item 369; M&CWC minutes 23 Jan. 1931, item 519; 8 Apr. 1932, item 919; *Annual Report 1935*, 148.

[103] BCA PH&HC minutes 24 Oct. 1913, item 1785.

[104] *Annual Report for 1914*, 17.

[105] *Report of the MOH on Child Welfare in 1913*, 5.

'up-to-date institutions' in respectable working-class areas.[106] The opportunity to widen the scope of the campaign opened up during the First World War, when there was renewed concern about the health and welfare of children. With the help of government grants, the Birmingham authorities extended the provision of health visiting and infant consultation services beyond the slum districts to areas like Hockley and Saltley inhabited by better-off artisans and the lower middle classes.[107] The focus of the campaign continued to move towards suburbs in the 1920s and 1930s, when the Health Department, together with voluntary societies, introduced infant welfare services into new council estates.[108] The slum-dwellers were not ignored, but much of the emphasis and energy of the campaign was now focused on the 'respectable' working classes and lower middle classes. Municipal services, whether council housing or child care advice, were increasingly meant for these politically important groups and designed to ensure that they were fully integrated into society and that they shared its fundamental values. This strategy had an impact on the disparity in infant mortality between different social groups. While the gap between the moderate-income groups and their social superiors narrowed, the gap between the moderate-income groups and the poorest people widened. Infant mortality was 24 per cent higher in the central wards than in the working-class and lower-middle-class suburbs in the early 1910s, and 36 per cent higher in the early 1930s.[109]

The new housing estates were ideal places to disseminate modern child care techniques. While in the slums women often turned to their mothers and neighbours for advice, in the new estates they were detached from the harmful influences of their relatives and former neighbours, and therefore in a good position to start from a clean slate. It was easy to attach them to 'acceptable' collectivities such as mothers' clubs, where they met their new neighbours and talked over their concerns under the watchful eye of a health visitor.[110] As the infant welfare campaign expanded, the range of services widened and the quality of facilities improved: infant consultations developed into modern child welfare centres. Church halls, unoccupied houses and corner shops, in which infant consultations had been initially arranged, were often replaced with purpose-built buildings (see Figures 4.6 and 4.7).[111]

---

[106] *Report of the MOH on Child Welfare in 1913*, 15.

[107] BCA PH&HC minutes 10 Jul. 1914, item 2503; 10 Sept. 1914, items 2601–2; 9 Oct. 1914, items 2686–7, 2722; 13 Nov. 1914, item 2785; M&CWSC minutes 3 Dec. 1915, item 8; 16 Jun. 1916, item 105; 'Report of the MOH on maternity and child welfare during 1916', see chart 'Maternity and Child Welfare'; G.E. Cherry, *Birmingham: A Study in Geography, History and Planning* (Chichester 1994), 90.

[108] See, for example, M&CWSC minutes 29 Feb. 1928, item 2185; 19 Feb. 1930, item 73; M&CWC minutes 11 Mar. 1927, item 1432; 25 Sept. 1931, items 752–3.

[109] *Annual Report 1933*, 99.

[110] *Annual Report 1910*, 20; *1914*, 16–17; *1923*, 53. See also C. Hall, 'Married women at home in Birmingham in the 1920s and 1930s', *Oral History* **5** (2) (1977), 62–83.

[111] See, for example, BCA PH&HC minutes 9 Oct. 1914, item 2687; M&CWSC minutes 2 Mar. 1927, item 1971; 28 Sept. 1927, item 2066; M&CWC minutes 25 Sept. 1931, items 752–3.

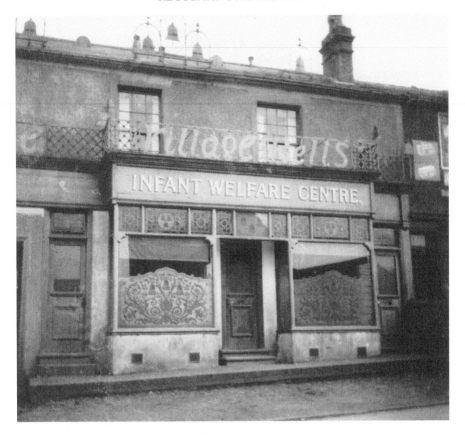

Figure 4.6   An infant welfare centre in Birmingham. The first infant welfare centres operated in very modest facilities in unoccupied houses, shops or church halls.
Source: Local Studies and History, Birmingham Central Library.

The new centres were imbued with an aura of medical authority, the architecture of the buildings contributing to the educational objectives of the campaign. For example, Dr Ethel Cassie praised the Carnegie Infant Welfare Institute, a model centre opened in 1924, for giving 'a satisfying effect of space and dignity ... The large hall is particularly successful in its effect, which has been heightened by a fine painting of a mother and child presented by Alderman W.A. Cadbury.'[112]

Health visiting and infant welfare centres continued to occupy the central place in the Birmingham campaign throughout the 1920s and 1930s. By the mid-1920s, the doctors and health visitors working under the Birmingham Maternal and Child Welfare Committee reached the vast majority of the infants and mothers living in Birmingham. About 75 per cent of the babies attended an infant welfare centre at least once, and no less than 90 per cent were visited by a health visitor. In 1934,

---

[112] *Annual Report 1924*, 59.

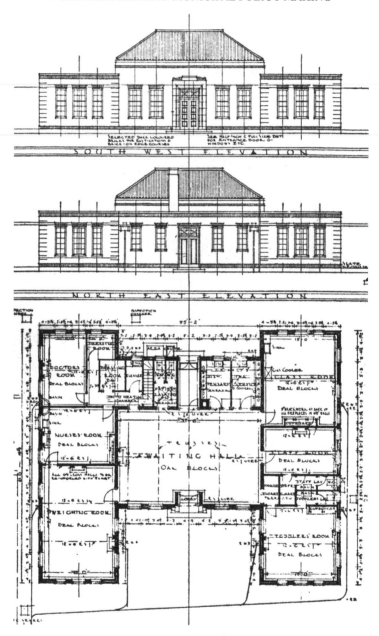

Figure 4.7   Plan of a new infant welfare centre from the 1920s, Warren Farm Estate, Kingstanding, Birmingham. The architecture of the new purpose-built infant welfare centres was to contribute to the educational objectives of the campaign.

Source: Local Studies and History, Birmingham Central Library.

when the Local Government Board recommended that local authorities appoint one health visitor per 250–280 births, Birmingham had already one visitor for every 140 births. For example Liverpool and Hull were lagging far behind: in Liverpool, health visitors had to cover 310 births, and in Hull, over 500 births.[113] The influence infant welfare centres exerted on the surrounding communities was considered to be so important that the centre was often among the first municipal services provided in the new council estates. This was the case, for example, in Kingstanding, the largest council estate in Birmingham, and in Weoley Castle, a more ambitious suburb, both built in the early 1930s.[114]

More Emphasis on Medical Services   The emphasis on individual responsibility in the Birmingham campaign was clearly at its strongest in the early 1910s. Environmental issues, which had been considered as part of the problem in the first decade of the century, no longer attracted attention, and the importance of medical care to the welfare of mothers and infants did not yet figure in the campaign. Medical services provided by the municipal health authorities for mothers and small children were minimal. Medical practitioners working for infant consultations were not allowed to provide medical treatment but were expected to refer cases of illness to family doctors or voluntary hospitals. As to the institutional maternity care, the Birmingham policy makers were convinced that their city, with its population of 500,000, managed with a small number of maternity beds provided by the poor law authorities and voluntary hospitals.[115] The large percentage of home deliveries would not have been a problem if the midwives had been trained. However, midwifery standards in Birmingham compared unfavourably with those of other large cities. In 1906, about 90 per cent of the certified midwives practising in Birmingham were untrained, and 30 per cent of them were illiterate and unable to take a patient's temperature. At the same time, in Manchester the percentage of untrained midwives was 35, and in Liverpool and London only 10. Voluntary hospitals took some measures to train midwives in Birmingham, but the change was slow to come.[116]

In reviewing their infant welfare services in 1916, the Birmingham authorities started to consider the possibility of increasing and improving the provision of medical care. Three members of the Maternity and Child Welfare Sub-Committee were sent

---

[113]   BCA PH&HC minutes 10 Sept. 1914, item 2602; 9 Oct. 1914, item 2687; 13 Nov. 1914, item 2785; M&CWC minutes 4 Oct. 1918, item 505; 11 Mar. 1927, item 1432; 'Report of the MOH on maternity and child welfare during 1916'; *Annual Report 1933*, 7, 17; Lewis, *The Politics of Motherhood*, 106; Marks, *Metropolitan Maternity*, 167–85.

[114]   BCA M&CWSC minutes 19 Feb. 1930, item 73; M&CWC minutes 25 Sept. 1931, items 752–3; Birmingham Public Health and Maternity and Child Welfare Committee (PH&MCWC) 9 Feb. 1934, item 4014; 13 Apr. 1934. For Kingstanding, see H. Meller, *European Cities 1890–1930s: History, Culture and the Built Environment* (Chichester 2001).

[115]   Jones, *History of the Hospitals*, 55–8; BCA PH&HC minutes 24 Oct. 1913, item 1785; 'Report of the MOH on maternity and child welfare during 1916'.

[116]   BCA HC minutes 11 Jul. 1905, item 9411; *Annual Report 1905*, 53–6; *1906*, 57–9; 'Report of the MOH on maternity and child welfare during 1916', 4; Jones, *History of the Hospitals*, 55–8. See also, L. Marks, *Model Mothers: Jewish Mothers and Maternity Provision in East London 1870–1939* (Oxford 1994), 97–9.

to acquaint themselves with the infant welfare programmes in London, Liverpool, Manchester and Bradford. They were particularly impressed by what they saw in Bradford. Apart from health visiting and infant consultations, the Bradford Health Department ran a milk depot and two hospitals for infants. Municipal maternity services were far more comprehensive than those in Birmingham, consisting of an antenatal clinic, municipal midwives and a maternity hospital with a modern operating theatre and an ambulance. Meals were supplied for pregnant and nursing mothers, and children's clothes were sold at cost price. Moreover, the Bradford authorities were seeking powers to compel factory owners to establish nurseries. Inspired by the Bradford campaign and prompted by the wartime preoccupations with national health, the Birmingham Committee started working on new ways to develop their campaign.[117]

The proposals submitted to the City Council were accompanied by the explicit acknowledgement that the campaign which had concentrated on combating diarrhoeal diseases had not come close to solving the problem of infant mortality. In particular, the MOH drew policy makers' attention to the high rates of neonatal mortality. Educational health services had not been effective in reducing mortality among newborn babies and therefore they needed to be supplemented by other services.[118] The MOH and the Maternity and Child Welfare Committee suggested that 100 hospital beds be provided for infants with 'wasting diseases' or rickets and that an emergency hospital be set up every summer for infants suffering from diarrhoea. The midwifery service was to be made more attractive to 'well trained and capable women' by municipalizing the service and by securing midwives a better remuneration. Moreover, the Committee wanted to enhance antenatal care and to provide 160 maternity beds by establishing maternity homes and by making a contract with a voluntary hospital.[119]

What facilitated the expansion of the work was the 1918 Maternity and Child Welfare Act, which conferred new powers on local authorities and made 50 per cent government grants available to them for the support of infant and maternal welfare services. However, the efforts to implement the new plans in Birmingham and in many other cities were hampered by the recession in the early 1920s. The development of antenatal care was one of the few plans which were not shelved during the years of financial austerity. As a result of the introduction of antenatal consultations, 35 per cent of women who were confined in Birmingham in 1926 had been seen by a doctor at one of the infant welfare centres before the confinement.[120] The implementation of the other plans was slower. In 1921, only 30 beds were reserved for babies suffering from wasting diseases, and in 1932 the number of beds was still below the target of 100 beds. In the mid-1920s, when pressures were mounting for maternity beds, the Maternity and Child Welfare Committee hesitantly started to co-operate with

---

[117] BCA M&CWSC minutes 3 Dec. 1915, item 9; 7 Jul. 1916, item 112; 1 Dec. 1916, item 163.

[118] BCA M&CWSC minutes 4 Jan. 1918, item 386.

[119] BCA M&CWSC minutes 4 Feb. 1916, item 36; 4 Oct. 1918, item 505; M&CWC minutes 23 Apr. 1920, item 580.

[120] BCA M&CWC minutes 11 Mar. 1927, item 1432.

the Poor Law Board to improve maternity care in the city. This arrangement, which meant that 'Council cases' – 'respectable' married working-class women – were treated in the same hospital buildings as 'Poor Law cases', many of whom were unmarried mothers, was strongly criticized by some members of the Committee.[121]

This discussion and other debates about to whom municipal services were made available reveals the plight of unmarried mothers. The needs of working mothers and bottle-feeding mothers were largely ignored in the Birmingham infant welfare campaign, but unmarried mothers were often entirely excluded from the mainstream campaign and openly discriminated against. In the eyes of the Birmingham authorities, illegitimacy was a 'foreign' phenomenon, and unmarried mothers, especially if allowed to mingle with respectable married mothers, were a threat to moral values and social order. The determination to protect 'the family' and married motherhood which were closely associated with the well-being of the nation meant that unmarried mothers were consigned to 'separate spaces', to separate institutions or hospital wards. They were often labelled as feeble-minded, and even mothers who managed to evade that label were often treated similarly to mentally deficient women, another group deemed unfit for motherhood and in need of protection and control.[122]

The Model City   Although the policy makers were fully aware that many of their plans had not been carried through, it came as a surprise to them in the late 1920s that no headway had been made in reducing neo-natal mortality. The hope that antenatal consultations would be effective in improving the well-being of infants and mothers proved too optimistic: the decline in neo-natal mortality had been small and maternal mortality appeared to have been rising in the 1920s. When the City Council urged the Maternity and Child Welfare Committee to rethink its strategies, the Committee responded that a large proportion of mothers did not attend antenatal consultations and many of those who did failed to follow the instructions. However, the Committee also admitted that there was room for improvement in medical services. The MOH recommended that the Health Department introduce post-natal examinations and provide more hospital beds for maternity cases and premature babies.[123] Again, some of these plans could not be implemented, since municipal spending had to be cut in the early 1930s.

The Birmingham authorities regarded financial difficulties as their greatest obstacle to improving health care provision, but there were also other factors that

---

[121]   BCA M&CWSC minutes 5 Oct. 1921, item 992; 1 Oct. 1924, item 1525; 3 Dec. 1924, item 1553; 2 Mar. 1927, item 1969; M&CWC minutes 12 Dec. 1924, item 1141; 9 Jan. 1925, item 1159; 13 Feb. 1925, items 1165 and 1167; 8 May 1925, item 1205; 9 Dec. 1927, item 1525; *Annual Report 1932*, 116.

[122]   BCA PH&HC minutes 8 Mar. 1912, item 312; M&CWSC minutes 1 Oct. 1924, item 1525; M&CWC minutes 14 Nov. 1924, item 1137; 9 Dec. 1927, item 1525; *Annual Report 1932*, 97–8; M. Thomson, *The Problem of Mental Deficiency: Eugenics, Democracy, and Social Policy in Britain c.1870–1959* (Oxford 1998), 21–2; M. Ladd-Taylor and L. Umansky, 'Introduction', in M. Ladd-Taylor and L. Umansky (eds), *'Bad' Mothers: The Politics of Blame in Twentieth-century America* (New York 1998), 1–28.

[123]   BCA M&CWSC minutes 28 Mar. 1928, item 2218; 2 May 1928, item 2232.

hampered the development of services. In Birmingham, medical services were often a battleground, where all parties – general practitioners, voluntary hospitals and municipal authorities – claimed to be acting in the best interest of the patient. The general practitioners accused the authorities of interfering in the relationship between the patient and her family doctor, whereas the municipal health officials pointed out that many working-class women could not afford to consult a general practitioner. The exact location of boundaries between the private and public health care remained a source of controversy in Birmingham throughout the period reviewed here.[124]

Although the Birmingham campaign did not accomplish all its goals, central government was clearly convinced that the Birmingham authorities were on the right path. In particular, the Birmingham authorities were applauded for concentrating on the essence: health education. In the early 1920s, after an investigation into the Birmingham maternity and child welfare scheme, the Ministry of Health praised Birmingham for its achievements: 'It is significant that both in Leicester and Birmingham, where very little treatment has been provided, better results have been obtained, so far as infant death rates are an indication, than in Bradford and Willesden, where in the past treatment has been provided on a large scale.' Finally, Birmingham was raised as an example for other authorities: 'The Maternity and Child Welfare Service is as far as practicable limited to preventive and educational work; treatment and relief are excluded to a greater extent than in most of the large districts.'[125]

Gothenburg

In early twentieth-century Gothenburg, health education was clearly a lesser priority than medical care. Instead of instructing mothers in infant care and domestic hygiene, the municipal health authorities were busy building hospitals and other health care facilities. The significant public investment in hospital infrastructure in Gothenburg was not an isolated case, but part of a national pattern – municipal authorities in many Swedish cities allocated more resources to improving mothers' and children's access to medical care. Nor were these investments in Gothenburg restricted to the early years of the century: the emphasis on medical services represented continuity in the maternity and child welfare campaign throughout the period reviewed here.[126] Another important continuity was the Gothenburg authorities' aspiration to control parenthood outside marriage. A growing number of municipal officers and voluntary workers were ensuring that the rights of illegitimate children were protected and

---

[124] BCA M&CWC minutes 12 Dec. 1930, document 97; 27 Feb. 1931, item 557. See also PH&HC minutes 14 Feb. 1913, item 1160; M&CWSC minutes 29 Sept. 1920, item 810; 'Medical fees in midwives' cases'; Bateman, 'Doctors in Parliament'.

[125] Public Record Office (PRO), Ministry of Health 52/231, Birmingham County Borough Council, 1922–25 Maternity and Child Welfare and Tuberculosis Services, Investigation and Report of Borough Health Services.

[126] W. Kock, 'Lasaretten och den slutna kroppsjukvården', and J. Ström, 'Den förebyggande barnavården', in W. Kock (ed), *Medicinalväsendet i Sverige 1813–1962* (Stockholm 1963), 188, 528; Vallgårda, 'Hospitalization of deliveries'. On public health expenditure in general, see Edvinsson and Rogers, 'Hälsa och hälsoreformer', 548–53.

that their parents accepted their responsibilities. Despite these continuities, there were also important new elements in the Gothenburg campaign in the 1920s and 1930s. The authorities gradually shifted away from their former focus on problem families and on the role of experts in reorganizing these families' everyday lives, and took steps towards universal coverage and a stronger emphasis on individual responsibility and preventive care.

Improved Access to Medical Care   In economic terms, the most important elements in the delivery of municipal health care services for mother and child in Gothenburg were the Municipal Maternity Hospital and the Children's Hospital. The new building of the Maternity Hospital, opened in 1900 and extended in 1908 and 1923, precipitated a significant increase in hospital deliveries. While in 1899 only 25 per cent of mothers in Gothenburg went to hospital to give birth, in 1918 half of the births took place in hospital, and in the 1930s the percentage of hospital deliveries rose to 85. In Birmingham, the percentage of births taking place in hospital was considerably lower, even though the number of maternity beds in poor law infirmaries, voluntary hospitals and private maternity homes was on the increase. Only 6 per cent of deliveries took place in institutions in 1920, and 33 per cent in the mid-1930s.[127] The rapid increase in hospital deliveries in Gothenburg reflected not only the general consensus prevailing among the leading politicians and health officers in favour of improving institutional maternity care, but also the willingness of mothers to use the service. One explanation for the popularity of hospital deliveries was overcrowding and poor housing conditions in working-class areas: mothers could not get adequate rest after childbirth in homes where a whole family lived in one or two rooms. Another reason why mothers actively sought in-patient care was that pain relief and post-natal care were more readily available in hospitals.[128]

The Gothenburg Children's Hospital, initially a voluntary institution, was gradually taken over by the municipal authorities in the first decade of the twentieth century. In 1903 the City Council allocated 100,000 crowns of donated funds for the campaign to erect a new up-to-date building for the hospital. The building was opened in 1909, and thereafter the running of the hospital was financed from public funds. With the public funding, the old image of the Children's Hospital as a charitable institution serving only the poor was replaced by a new image as a centre of scientific medicine functioning for the community at large. Owing to the increasing patient populations and the introduction of new technologies, the hospital wards were soon filled to overcapacity. The City Council approved the plan for the extension of the hospital in 1917, and in the early 1920s, when the new building was

---

[127] For Gothenburg, see Walter, 'Barnbördshusets i Göteborg verksamhet', 13; *Statistisk årsbok för Göteborg 1900*, 44; Brodin, 'Spädbarnsdödligheten', 3,662; Westman, 'Barnbördsanstaltens historia'; Gezelius, 'Göteborgs stads hälso- och sjukvård', 369–71; GSA Göteborgs Hälsovårdsnämnd, II avdelningen (HVN II) minutes 27 Nov. 1931, item 838. For Birmingham, BCA M&CWC minutes 23 Apr. 1920, item 580, 3; *Annual Report 1933*, 135.

[128] *GSH 1896:55*, 2; *1934:387*; Westman, 'Barnbördsanstaltens historia', 4. See also Vallgårda, 'Hospitalization of deliveries', 188–90; Marks, *Metropolitan Maternity*, 209–14; Lewis, *The Politics of Motherhood*, 117–39.

opened, the Children's Hospital had 240 beds, 36 of which were for infants. [129] At the same time in Birmingham, whose population was four times that of Gothenburg, the municipal and poor law authorities, together with the voluntarily-run Children's Hospital, provided approximately 400 hospital beds for children. [130]

During the period reviewed here, the Gothenburg authorities significantly improved mothers' and children's access to medical care and hospital beds, and the municipal provision was further supplemented by a publicly supported voluntary organization, *Föreningen Mjölkdroppen*, which provided infants with sterilized milk and medical care. [131] Although policy makers occasionally expressed their concern over the ever-expanding health expenses, the reforms were usually carried out in the overall climate of agreement that the whole society benefited from advances in medical and hospital services. In particular, the authorities were able to develop new medical services without fear that every measure they took would be scrutinized and criticized by general practitioners. For the Gothenburg policy makers, the solution to the problem of infant mortality lay primarily in the hands of experts who provided a wide arrange of medical and other related services but who also – as shown in the next section – adopted strenuous control measures.

Parenthood Outside Marriage   The reforms to improve the availability and quality of medical care were already under way when the Gothenburg authorities in the early 1910s decided to pursue another important challenge. In 1913, the Health Committee, together with the Poor Law Board and the Child Welfare Committee, established a Child Welfare Office in order to better safeguard the interests of illegitimate children and to promote their health and well-being. The Office inherited some old tasks such as the supervision of foster homes, but it was also given new responsibilities. The main functions were, firstly, to establish the identity of both parents of the child. The mother's and father's names were confirmed and, if necessary, the mother was advised on how to gain legal recognition of paternity and economic assistance from the father. Secondly, if the mother wanted to give her child away, the Office was to assist her in finding a good foster home. The third task was to campaign against child abuse and neglect, and in particular to ensure that foster children were provided with safe care and a proper moral upbringing. [132]

The initial enthusiasm for the Child Welfare Office waned in the following years, when the officers working for the unit realized how limited their chances of tackling the problems were. They were able to report some encouraging achievements, notably that the rate of infant mortality among foster children was low, but they had not had similar success, for example, in acting as intermediaries between unmarried

---

[129] *GSH 1903:196* and minutes 3 Oct. 1903, item 2; *1910:269*; 'Renströmska utdelningsfondens fördelning: beredningens förslag segrade', *Göteborgs Handels- och Sjöfarts-Tidning*, 4 Dec. 1903; *Årsberättelsen 1919, II del*, 28–9; Johansson, 'Göteborgs barnsjukhus' historia'; Gezelius, 'Göteborgs stads hälso- och sjukvård', 374–7.

[130] BCA M&CWSC minutes 5 Oct. 1921, item 992; 1 Oct. 1924, item 1525; Waterhouse, *Children in Hospital*, 67.

[131] *GSH 1909:252*, 3–5, 25–6; *1910:59*; *1911:27*; *1911:264*.

[132] *GSH 1912:18*; *1912:273* and minutes 31 Oct. 1912, item 8; *1919:156*, in particular 9–11.

mothers and potential foster homes. In 1916, it was reported that 80 unmarried mothers looking for foster homes had turned to the Office for help. In 30 cases, no action was taken, since the mother was unable to pay enough for the care of her child and therefore finding a reasonable foster home was practically impossible. Eventually, the Office managed to arrange for 18 children (23 per cent) to be placed in foster homes.[133]

Frustrated at their inability to deal with certain problem situations, the municipal authorities called for new legislation to confer on them new powers to 'protect' unmarried mothers and their children. The 1917 Illegitimate Children Act (*Lagen om barn utom äktenskap*) provided at least a partial solution to their concerns. The Act went some way towards improving the legal position of unmarried mothers and their children, enabling municipal authorities to put pressure on the father to pay child maintenance and to support the mother for six weeks before and after the birth. However, if the new legislation improved the economic situation of unmarried mothers and their children, it also subjected them to close and, in some cases, demeaning supervision. An unmarried woman who was expecting a child had to notify the Child Care Committee of her pregnancy three months before the confinement. After receiving the notification, the Committee appointed a 'guardian' (*barnavårdsman*) to advise the mother, to ensure that paternity was established and to protect the interests of the child. The guardianship was often a long-term commitment: the guardian followed the life of the illegitimate child and supervised the parents until the child came of age or was legitimated by marriage or by adoption.[134]

The disparity in mortality between illegitimate and legitimate children diminished over the years. The mortality rate for illegitimate infants was 98 per cent higher than that for legitimate babies around 1910, and only 43 per cent higher in the early 1930s.[135] However, there were still obstacles to overcome in improving the health of illegitimate children and their mothers. For example, the improvement in the economic situation of unmarried mothers was relatively small. The payments from fathers tended to be low or were not paid at all, which meant that even in the 1920s and 1930s a large proportion of unmarried mothers and their children suffered from poverty.[136] Self-sufficiency was simply beyond the reach of many lone mothers, since women's earnings were often below the subsistence level. Intervening in the labour market, however, was beyond the accepted sphere of municipal activity, therefore the Gothenburg health authorities did not even contemplate addressing the women's limited leverage in the workplace. What the authorities did to help unmarried and

---

[133] *GSH 1917:109; 1917:284; 1919:156.*

[134] *GSH 1919:156;* 'Tillämpningen av barnafaderns bidragsskyldighet gentemot modern enligt lagen om barn utom äktenskap', in *SOU 1929:28,* 100–104; Bergman, 'En feministisk konspiration'; Elgán, 'Le législateur au secours de la mère célebataire'; Ohrlander, *I barnens och nationens intresse,* 148–52.

[135] In the five-year period 1931–35, the mortality rate for infants born to married mothers was 35 per 1,000 live births, compared with 50 for infants born to unmarried mothers; *Statistisk Årsbok för Göteborg 1939,* 28–30.

[136] A survey conducted in Malmö in 1926 showed that only 65 per cent of the fathers who had been ordered to support the mother actually provided assistance. See 'Tillämpningen av barnafaderns bidragsskyldighet', in *SOU 1929:28.*

other poor mothers maintain their families was to support voluntary nurseries, which were praised for providing mothers 'with an opportunity to earn money and supplement the family income'.[137] The potentially harmful effects of mother's employment, which were thoroughly examined in numerous reports in Birmingham, received very scant attention from the Gothenburg Health Committee.[138]

While unmarried mothers were seen as problem mothers in Gothenburg, the authorities were convinced that many of them – with the help and close guidance of health and social workers – were capable of raising their children. This line of thinking reflected the way in which the Swedish authorities perceived unmarried motherhood. Unlike in Britain and many other European countries, where unmarried mothers were primarily defined in a gender-specific way as immoral women, in Sweden they were usually placed within the category of the ignorant and irresponsible poor.[139] Admittedly, single mothers were often labelled as bad mothers in Gothenburg, but at the same time they were given the opportunity to become good mothers. No such opportunity was granted to women diagnosed with mental illness, mental deficiencies, epilepsy or tuberculosis and who were considered to be likely to transmit these disorders or diseases to their children.

Mentally ill, mentally deficient and epileptic women were deemed unworthy to even bear children, and many of them were sterilized with or without their consent. During the seven-year period following the enactment of the Sterilization Act of 1934, over 3,000 people, mostly women, were sterilized in Sweden.[140] Women diagnosed with tuberculosis avoided the harsh fate which befell some 'feeble-minded' and epileptic women, but even they were seen as a major threat to the health of their newborns, and were often pressurized into placing their children in foster care.[141] In defining who was unsuitable to be a mother, the Gothenburg authorities, like their Birmingham counterparts, used both medical and non-medical rationalizations. However, given the strong emphasis on the medical approach in Gothenburg and in Sweden in general, it is hardly surprising that the authorities there often preferred to use medical and biological language in labelling someone as unfit for motherhood even when the real reasons for stigmatization had more to do with moral and social issues. Likewise, in tackling the problem, the Swedish authorities often used means

---

[137] *GHS 1909:252* (the quote is from p. 11) and minutes 7 Jan. 1910, item 6; *1926:192* and minutes 12 May 1926, item 24.

[138] At the national level, the question aroused more interest. After repeated calls for legislation to protect women and the next generation, four weeks' compulsory maternity leave was introduced in Sweden in 1900, and extended to six weeks in 1912. However, the law proved as ineffectual as its British counterpart. *SOU 1929:28*, 21–31; Isberg, 'Barnavård', 68; Ohlander, 'The invisible child?', 60–67.

[139] Hobson and Takahashi, 'The parent–worker model'; Bergman, 'En feministisk konspiration'.

[140] As the scope of the Act was expanded in 1941, the number of sterilizations rose significantly, reaching a peak in the late 1940s and early 1950s. G. Broberg and M. Tydén, 'Eugenics in Sweden: efficient care', in G. Broberg and N. Roll-Hansen, *Eugenics and the Welfare State: Sterilization Policy in Denmark, Sweden, Norway, and Finland* (East Lansing, MI 1996), 77–149. For comparison, see Thomson, *The Problem of Mental Deficiency*.

[141] See Chapter 5.

available in the 'medical' armoury, for example the separation of the mother and the child to break the chain of tubercular infection, or the sterilization of women diagnosed with serious hereditary disorders. The Birmingham authorities, who concentrated on educating people and instilling a sense of responsibility in them, placed more emphasis on moral characteristics, but also used medical and biological explanations. Single mothers, who were seen as the ultimate 'bad' mothers in Birmingham, were often placed under protection and control in refuges and homes on the grounds that they were both 'immoral' and 'feeble-minded'.

From Problem Families to Universal Services   The contacts between the authorities and city-dwellers became more frequent in both Gothenburg and Birmingham over the years, but the ways in which the authorities utilized the contacts were different. The Gothenburg authorities awakened to the possibilities of health education more slowly than their counterparts in Birmingham. In Gothenburg, providing guidance in motherhood skills was first left to voluntary organizations such as *Föreningen Mjölkdroppen*, which, in addition to providing infants with sterilized milk and medical care, also gave mothers advice on hygiene and 'rational' child care. In 1911, the health education delivered by the milk depots reached about 13 per cent of all mothers with newborn babies.[142] Educating working-class women to a more mature understanding of their duties as mothers was a cause with which many city councillors heartily sympathized, but it needed a serious crisis such as the food shortage of 1917 to actually put the question on the agenda of the Council. In discussing the effects of the food shortage, some councillors pointed out that in many families the mother and the youngest children were malnourished, since most of the food was given to the husband and older children.[143] Central government agencies and voluntary associations had allocated some funds to alleviate the food shortage, but the councillors were unanimous about the need for further measures. Of the alternatives under consideration, the proposal that working-class women should be advised as to how to manage their households attracted most support.[144]

Three domestic science teachers were appointed as municipal household advisers (*hem konsulent*) in August 1917. While one of them organized classes in cookery and household management, the others visited 'problem homes'. During the second half of 1917, they visited 54 homes and spent on average four days in each, instructing mothers in cooking and other household chores. A few weeks later, the adviser visited the family again in order to check whether her teaching was being put into practice. This service, which was introduced as an emergency measure, turned out to be very popular, and the municipality continued to provide it until 1923, when it was taken over by a voluntary association.[145]

---

[142]   *GSH 1909:252*, 25–6; *1910:59*; *1912:120A*; *1917:295*.

[143]   *GSH 1917:97* and the discussion 19 Apr. 1917, item 7.

[144]   *GSH 1916:285*; *1916:297*; *1916:313*; *1916:345*; *1917:24*; *1917:97* and minutes and discussion 19 Apr. 1917, item 7; *1917:489* and minutes and discussion 10 Jan. 1918, item 17.

[145]   *GSH 1919:546* and minutes 22 Dec. 1919 item 14; *1921:260*; *1921:484* and minutes 22 Dec. 1921, item 15; *1923:34*.

The City Council also set up a working party in 1917 to look into the problem of infant mortality. After consideration, the working party pointed out that mothers' ignorance of safe methods of infant care rather than poverty *per se* was the greatest obstacle to improving the health of infants. Consequently, they recommended that the Health Committee appoint a child care adviser (*barnvårdskonsulent*) to ensure that the poorest mothers would also have an opportunity to learn about mothering from an authoritative source. The Committee and City Council supported the proposal.[146] The child care adviser visited homes where mothers were experiencing difficulties with child care and, like the household advisers, she concentrated only on a small number of 'problem families', 100–200 annually.[147]

In the early 1920s, the focus of the infant welfare work gradually shifted from the close supervision of the problem families to the provision of health education to wider sections of society. In 1923, a governmental committee, which had been asked to consider ways of improving infant and child welfare in Sweden, proposed the new approach. They recommended that the Swedish health authorities should follow the example set by the British authorities and establish infant welfare centres which would reach a vast majority of mothers and infants.[148] At the same time in Gothenburg, milk depots were increasingly criticized for being an outmoded and inefficient way of tackling the problem of infant mortality (see also Figure 4.8). The consultant paediatrician of the Children's Hospital, Dr Arvid Wallgren, launched a campaign, the main aim of which was to turn the old milk depots into 'modern' infant welfare centres.[149] Like the public health officials in Birmingham, Wallgren attributed the high rates of infant mortality largely to mothers' ignorance and negligence. Instead of providing sterilized milk, the new infant welfare centres were to encourage breast-feeding; instead of concentrating on a small number of problem families, they would monitor the development of all children. Wallgren got his way. While in 1926 medical practitioners working for the milk depots examined only 11 per cent of all children born in Gothenburg, in 1935 the percentage of children attending infant welfare centres was already 54.[150]

---

[146] *GSH 1917:295; 1918:79* and minutes 28 Feb. 1918, item 33; *1918:169* and minutes 8 May 1918, item 17; GSA HVN I, minutes 3 Apr. 1918, item 71.

[147] GSA HVN I, minutes 20 Mar. 1918, item 66; 3 Apr. 1918; *GSH 1918:79, 1918:169* and minutes 8 May 1918, item 17; 5 Jun. 1918, item 108; 3 Jul. 1918, item 127; *Årsberättelser 1918–1928*.

[148] Sundell, 'Effectivare spädbarnsvård'. See also, U. Hjärne, 'Några drag ur engelsk barnavårdsverksamhet', *Nordisk Medicinsk Tidskrift* 2 (1930), 204–7.

[149] *GSH 1926:58*, 8–9; Wallgren, 'Barnavårdscentraler'; Sundell, 'Effektivare spädbarnsvård'.

[150] *Föreningen Mjölkdroppens barnavårdcentraler i Göteborg, Årsberättelser 1930; 1935*.

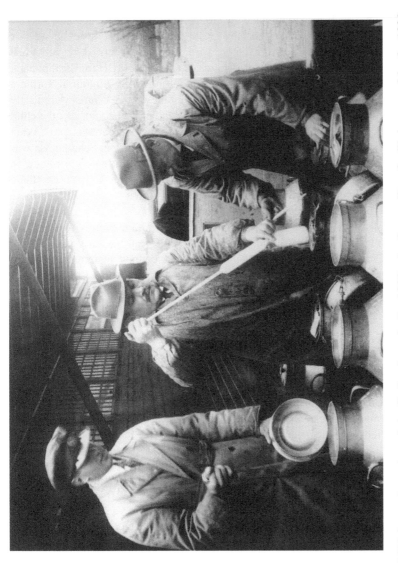

Figure 4.8   Milk inspectors at work in Gothenburg in the 1920s. As the quality of milk improved in the 1920s, milk depots gradually lost their significance.

Source: Gothenburg City Museum.

Conclusion

The Birmingham and Gothenburg infant welfare campaigns, which had been radically different in the early twentieth century, converged in many ways in the 1920s and 1930s. The Birmingham authorities defied the protests of general practitioners and introduced some medical services, and the Gothenburg authorities supplemented the medical services they already offered by establishing British-style infant welfare centres which concentrated on preventive care. However, there were still great differences in emphasis between the campaigns. An assistant MOH for Birmingham, Dr Ethel Cassie, analysed these differences upon returning from her tour in Northern Europe in 1930. She argued that the Birmingham infant welfare centres were vastly superior to the equivalent institutions abroad: in Scandinavian countries, 'the child welfare work (in the public health sense) is definitely behind our standard'. What compensated for the deficiencies in educational health services in Scandinavia was the cleanliness of cities and the good-quality medical and midwifery services. In Swedish and Danish cities, Cassie claimed, the standard of hygiene was high, 'there [was] little desperate poverty, the midwifery [was] of a high standard ... and there [was] a large provision of hospital beds for children'.[151]

It is hardly surprising if the Birmingham infant welfare centres were indeed superior to the equivalent institutions in Gothenburg. From the early years of the twentieth century, the Birmingham authorities had defined maternal ignorance and negligence as the major cause of infant death and had worked on new ways of helping and motivating mothers to achieve better standards of child care and housewifery. This campaign, the centrepiece of which was the lifestyle theory of disease causation, ran smoothly in upper-working-class and lower-middle-class suburbs, where mothers had means to put the teaching they received into practice. In these areas, the campaign not only safeguarded the health of the mothers and their children, but at best it also boosted the work the mothers performed and provided them with an opportunity to demonstrate their 'respectability', therefore giving them a sense of well-being. Moreover, promoting the implicit aims of the campaign, and in particular fostering responsible and self-reliant families in which the husband and wife had strictly complementary roles, was relatively easy in the moderate-income suburbs. The women living in these areas were more able and willing to concentrate on motherhood than their less fortunate sisters in the slums and than the more highly educated middle-class women, many of whom had an ambition to combine motherwork with unpaid or even paid work outside the home.

While the explicit and implicit objectives could be achieved at the same time in the moderate-income suburbs, in the central wards the Birmingham authorities were faced with difficulties. The poorer the area, the more the implicit aims interfered with the efforts to reach the explicit goal, improving the health of infants and mothers. Firstly, the campaign that emphasized personal control over disease could not recognize, let alone deal with, many problems confronting the poorest mothers

---

[151] BCA M&CWSC minutes 19 Mar. 1930, item 100. See also Hjärne, 'Några drag'; H.W. Pooler, 'Infant mortality work in Berlin: a visit to the third international congress on infantile mortality', *Midland Medical Journal* **12** (1) (1913), 1–7.

in insanitary slums. Secondly, by employing narrow definitions of what constituted a proper family and proper child rearing, the Birmingham campaign often added the hardships which many working mothers and bottle-feeding mothers already suffered, therefore the campaign could even contribute to the growing disparity in health between social groups. Although infant mortality decreased in all areas in Birmingham, it remained significantly higher in the central wards, so much so that the gap between the poorest areas and the moderate-income suburbs actually widened over the years. The situation of unmarried mothers and their children was, however, worst. The commitment to 'the family' meant that in Birmingham, unmarried mothers were often excluded from the mainstream health schemes and consigned, legally and socially, to 'separate spaces'. They were the ultimate 'bad' mothers who posed a threat to married motherhood and the family, and therefore to British society as a whole.

In improving mothers and infants' access to medical care, the Birmingham authorities performed a delicate balancing act. General practitioners, more or less concerned about their own livelihoods, were suspicious of plans to expand municipal health services, and often warned the Public Health Committee not to 'encroach' on their territory. At first, the Committee stuck to the principle that the health of infants and mothers could be secured without publicly funded medical care. In the late 1910s, this principle was partly abandoned and the Committee started to provide medical services, the scope of which, however, remained limited throughout the 1920s and 1930s. In this respect, the Gothenburg campaign offers a dramatic contrast. In Gothenburg, almost the entire medical profession saw public investments in health care as the best way of enhancing their professional prospects. Utilizing their access to the centres of policy making and building on the esteem they and other experts enjoyed in Swedish society, medical practitioners convinced other policy makers that the questions concerning infant health were primarily medical matters. Consequently, in the provision of hospital beds for children and mothers, the achievements of the Gothenburg municipal authorities clearly surpassed not only the efforts of their Birmingham counterparts, but also the combined efforts of the Birmingham municipal, poor law and voluntary agencies. The comparison of Gothenburg and Birmingham reveals the great extent to which the health care needs of infants and mothers were defined in the way that served the interests of the medical profession.

The Gothenburg authorities, too, sought to ensure that children were brought up in stable families. However, the Gothenburg and the Birmingham authorities had somewhat different views on what a 'stable' family consisted of and what was appropriate for its members to do. The Gothenburg health officials had very little option but to accept that, in many cases, it was impossible to place the whole responsibility for maintaining the family on the father. Many unskilled men did not make enough money to support their families, and the number of unmarried mothers maintaining their children entirely by themselves was high in Gothenburg. In other words, the family's responsibility to be self-supporting and the male-breadwinner family model were, to an extent, irreconcilable objectives, and in making the choice between these aims the authorities decided to encourage economic self-reliance. Instead of strongly emphasizing the complementary roles of mothers and fathers, the

Gothenburg authorities discussed how to ensure more *parental* responsibility. They took the view that not only fathers, but also mothers, if necessary, were responsible for maintaining their children, and that parents who evaded the responsibility were largely to blame for the high infant death rates.

The principle that mothers had the obligation to both maintain and care for their children placed many mothers, and especially single mothers, in a difficult position: Combining paid work with child care was a constant challenge for them, and their earnings were often so low that they were not able to support themselves, let alone their children. The Gothenburg authorities did not even consider addressing the inequalities on the labour market, but together with publicly-supported voluntary societies, they helped mothers to cope with some other problems by providing medical care, sterilized milk and nursery places, and by giving advice on health issues and the position of illegitimate children. Partly owing to these measures and partly for other reasons, infant mortality decreased both among legitimate and illegitimate children, and the gap between these two groups narrowed during the period reviewed here. The downside was that the 'welfare' services in Gothenburg, as in Sweden in general, were often combined with strict and elaborate control measures, and the tension between enhancing the life prospects of 'problem mothers and children' on the one hand and regulating their behaviour on the other often led to a victory of the latter concern. Unmarried mothers were supervised so closely that some of them, and especially those who were co-habiting, got married in order to avoid the constant control of child welfare officers and guardians. Women suffering from tuberculosis, epilepsy or mental disabilities, however, were subjected to even more stringent control measures. Their reproduction was considered to pose a serious threat to the health of the nation, and even to the (superior) Nordic race.

In the early stages of the infant welfare campaigns, the authorities in both Birmingham and Gothenburg sought to establish a contact with the most 'ignorant and irresponsible' sections of the population. With these contacts, the information about the poorest city-dwellers proliferated and the authorities were able to govern their cities more intensively and effectively. In the course of the 1910s and 1920s, the authorities gradually shifted their main focus from the poor to upper-working-class and lower-middle-class people, hoping to ensure that these politically important groups were now fully integrated into society. The general trend was similar in Birmingham and Gothenburg, but the actual ways in which infant welfare services were organized were different, reflecting and reinforcing the spatial and social structures of the cities. In Birmingham, where residential segregation was relatively high, infant welfare policies often served to exacerbate the socio-spatial segregation. The idea that the city was divided into 'unhealthy', 'less unhealthy' and 'healthy' areas affected the ways in which the problem of infant mortality were defined and responded to. The campaign was started by employing health visitors to monitor the people living in the 'unhealthy areas', and in the 1910s and 1920s the health visiting service reached out to 'less unhealthy areas'. In Gothenburg, where residential segregation was less pronounced, the authorities did not articulate the problem of infant mortality spatially. Instead, they used different information channels and sources to track down first the problem families, and in the 1920s and 1930s, also upper-working-class and lower-middle-class families with small children.

   Although the approaches chosen in Gothenburg and Birmingham were different
in many ways, the infant mortality rate was steadily declining in both cities (Figure
4.9). Accounting for the decline is difficult. In addition to the specific infant welfare
measures, there were a number of other factors such as environmental and nutritional
improvements which were likely to contribute to improving infant health. Be that
as it may, the health authorities in both Birmingham and Gothenburg hastened to
interpret the favourable development as a validation of their campaign. The approach
they had chosen was not only scientifically sound and rational, but also effective.

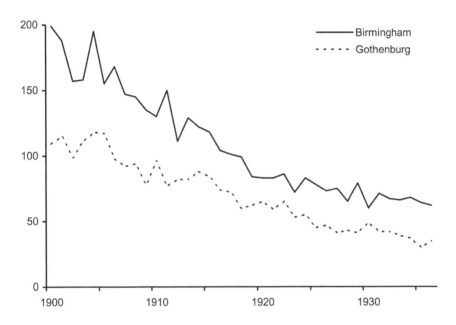

**Figure 4.9   Infant mortality per 1,000 live births in Birmingham and
                Gothenburg, 1900–1936.**
*Source: Annuals Report of the MOH for Birmingham 1900–1936; Statistiska årsböcker för
Göteborg 1900–1936.*

CHAPTER 5

Shaping Urban Society: Campaigns Against Tuberculosis, 1900–1940

In the early twentieth century, tuberculosis impinged on the public consciousness to a far greater extent than ever before.[1] The disease, which had been a major cause of death and chronic illness throughout the nineteenth century, eventually assumed the dimensions of a public, political problem. Health authorities in both Britain and Sweden attributed the sudden awakening of interest mainly to new, accurate knowledge about the disease. For decades they had recognized tuberculosis as 'a catching disease', but disagreement over the finer details about its transmission and behaviour had 'prevented action being taken in the past'.[2] Robert Koch's identification of the tubercle bacillus in 1882 and subsequent experiments by him and other researchers had finally put an end to these deep-seated conflicts. The experiments had shown that, in the majority of cases, the tubercle bacillus was transmitted from person to person by droplet infection and that it depended on the infected persons' power of resistance whether they developed disease or not. These new indisputable facts, so it was argued, equipped public health authorities to deal with the problem by prescribing the direction and form which an effective anti-tuberculosis campaign was to take.[3]

---

[1]   In this chapter, and in the book in general, the term 'tuberculosis' is used as a synonym for pulmonary tuberculosis. When the scope of discussion is widened to include the non-pulmonary forms of tuberculosis, this is expressly stated.

[2]   The quotes are from *Special Report by the Medical Officer of Health on Further Measures for the Prevention of Consumption in the City of Birmingham* (hereafter *Special Report by the MOH on Consumption*) (Health Department, Birmingham 1906), 8.

[3]   For Gothenburg and Sweden, see *Göteborgs Stadsfullmäktiges Handlingar* (hereafter *GSH*) *1903:141*; *Betänkande och förslag af den utaf Kungl. Maj:t den 20 oktober tillsatta kommitté för verkställande af utredning angående åtgärder för människotuberkulosens bekämpande* (hereafter *Betänkande och förslag*) *I* (Stockholm 1907); G. Dovertie, 'Öfversikt öfver striden mot tuberkulos i Sverige och utlandet', 3, in *Betänkande och förslag I*; B. Buhre, 'Svenska Nationalföreningen mot tuberkulos, dess uppkomst, medel och mål', *Social Tidskrift* (1906), 12. For Birmingham and Britain, see G.B. Dixon, *Lectures on the Prevention of Consumption Delivered to the Birmingham and Derbyshire Tuberculosis Visitors* (Derby *c.* 1910), 3; *Annual Report of the Medical Officer of Health for Birmingham* (hereafter *Annual Report*) *1898*, 28–30; *1903*, 27; G. Newman, *The Health of the State* (London 1907), ch. 7; H. Sutherland, 'The extent of the disease and the sources of infection', in H. Sutherland (ed.), *The Control and Eradication of Tuberculosis: A Series of International Studies* (Edinburgh 1911), 5–23. For further discussion about the nineteenth-century conceptions of the causes

Another important reason for launching the campaign in the early years of the twentieth century, so health authorities claimed, was the severity of the problem: the high death rates from tuberculosis and the pre-eminence of the disease among major killers. In Gothenburg, much cause for concern was given by comparative studies showing that Gothenburg suffered considerably higher death rates from pulmonary tuberculosis (almost 3 per thousand population) than many other large cities in Northern Europe.[4] Moreover, the First City Physician for Gothenburg, Dr Karl Gezelius, drew policy makers' attention to the high percentage of deaths caused by tubercular diseases. In 1900, pulmonary tuberculosis accounted for no less than 19 per cent and the other forms of the disease 7 per cent of all deaths in the city.[5] In Birmingham, pulmonary tuberculosis was responsible for 9 per cent and other forms of the disease for 3 per cent of all deaths in 1901. As a major cause of death, tubercular diseases were exceeded by another group of diseases: bronchitis, pneumonia and pleurisy.[6] Yet in the public health debate, tuberculosis assumed a far greater importance than these leading destroyers of life. While bronchitis usually killed elderly people and infants, pulmonary tuberculosis was a disease which 'uniformly attacks young adults … on whose education and training much money has been spent'.[7] Birmingham's death rates from pulmonary tuberculosis (about 1.4 per thousand of the population) compared favourably with those for many other European cities, but they were higher than the average for England and Wales.[8]

Many present-day writers have challenged the account given by the early twentieth-century health authorities of the first phase of the anti-tuberculosis movement. These writers have shown that the high death rates from tuberculosis and Koch's identification of the tubercle bacillus were by no means the only motivating forces behind the anti-tuberculosis campaigns.[9] Indeed, although the death rates from

---

of pulmonary tuberculosis, see D.S. Barnes, *The Making of a Social Disease: Tuberculosis in Nineteenth-century France* (Berkeley, CA 1995), 23–73; F.B. Smith, *The Retreat of Tuberculosis 1850–1950* (London 1988), 25–55; B. Puranen, *Tuberkulos: En sjukdoms förekomst och dess orsaker: Sverige 1750–1980* (Umeå 1984), 19, 73–98.

⁴   J.E. Johansson and R. Moosberg, *Lungsotsdödligheten i Sverige enligt prästerkapets anteckningar i dödböckerna 1901–1905* (Stockholm 1908), 18–19, 22–3; Dovertie, 'Öfversikt'. See also G. Kearns, 'Zivilis or Hygaeia: urban public health and the epidemiologic transition', in R. Lawton (ed.), *The Rise and Fall of Great Cities: Aspects of Urbanization in the Western World* (London 1989), 102.

⁵   *Göteborgs hälsovårdsnämnds årsberättelse* (hereafter *Årsberättelsen*) *1900*, 43–4; GSH 1900:104.

⁶   *Annual Report 1900*, 6–8; *1901*, 46–7.

⁷   *Special Report by the MOH on Consumption*, 2. See also A. Hardy, 'Reframing disease: changing perceptions of tuberculosis in England and Wales, 1938–70', *Historical Research* **76** (194) (2003), 535–8.

⁸   *Annual Report 1912*, 38; *Special Report by the MOH on Consumption*, 4–5; Kearns, 'Zivilis or Hygaeia', 102.

⁹   See, for example, L. Bryder, *Below the Magic Mountain: A Social History of Tuberculosis in Twentieth-century Britain* (Oxford 1988), 2, 15–22; G. Kearns, 'Tuberculosis and the medicalisation of British Society, 1880–1920', in J. Woodward and R. Jütte (eds), *Coping with Sickness: Historical Aspects of Health Care in a European Perspective* (Sheffield 1995); Barnes, *Social Disease*, 13–20; G.D. Feldberg, *Disease and Class: Tuberculosis and*

tuberculosis made depressing reading in early twentieth-century Birmingham and Gothenburg, both cities had experienced much higher rates in the preceding decades (Figure 5.1).[10] Moreover, the authorities were well aware of the downward trend in the tuberculosis death rates. The Medical Officer of Health (MOH) for Birmingham, Dr John Robertson, claimed that the chart showing the decline in tuberculosis mortality in the late nineteenth century was 'one of the most satisfactory that can be produced as showing a real improvement in the public health during recent years'.[11] Similarly, the governmental Tuberculosis Committee that considered different approaches to the problem of tuberculosis in Sweden firmly dismissed the popular assumption that tuberculosis was on the increase.[12] It is understandable that tuberculosis mortality began to figure more prominently among contemporary concerns, since many epidemic killers such as typhus and cholera ceased to be significant causes of death in the course of the nineteenth century. Yet in absolute terms, death rates from tuberculosis in early twentieth-century Birmingham and Gothenburg were well below the levels that had prevailed in the preceding century.

As to the effect of Koch's discovery, the relationship between knowledge and action was far more complex than the authorities would admit. This was clearly revealed, for example, by the considerable time lag between Koch's discovery and its practical application. At the local level, for example in Gothenburg and Birmingham, almost twenty years elapsed between the discovery of the tubercle bacillus and the launching of the anti-tuberculosis campaigns. Admittedly, the blame for the delay did not necessarily lie with public health officers, who – as discussed in Chapter 1 – were actively involved in creating a social and political setting in which the solutions that Robert Koch and other bacteriologists could offer appeared important and efficient. Without this setting, the hunt for germs would not have attracted so many able minds in the late nineteenth century.[13] However, the enthusiasm of some health officers

---

the *Shaping of Modern North American Society* (New Brunswick, NJ 1995), 36–80; Puranen, *Tuberkulos*, 315.

[10] Comparing tuberculosis death rates across national borders or over time in a single country is extremely problematic, since the understanding of the disease, the methods of record-keeping and incentives to conceal the occurrence of a tuberculosis death in the family varied from society to society and changed from one period to another. A. Hardy, '"Death is the cure of all diseases": using the General Register Office cause of death statistics for 1837–1920', *Social History of Medicine* **7** (3) (1994), 473–92; L. Bryder, '"Not always one and the same thing": the registration of tuberculosis deaths in Britain, 1900–1950', *Social History of Medicine* **9** (2) (1996), 253–65.

[11] *Special Report by the MOH on Consumption*, 4.

[12] Dovertie, 'Öfversikt', 3; Johansson and Moosberg, *Lungsotsdödligheten*, 19, 24–6. See also C. Runborg and G. Sundbärg, 'Dödligheten af lungtuberkulos i Sveriges städer, åren 1861/1900', *Statistisk Tidskrift* (1905), 198–224.

[13] See also B. Latour, *The Pasteurization of France* (Cambridge, MA 1988); R.J. Evans, *Death in Hamburg: Society and Politics in the Cholera Years* (London 1990), 264–75; K. Johannisson, 'Folkhälsa: det svenska projektet från 1900 till 2:a världskriget', *Lychnos: Årsbok för idehistoria och vetenskapshistoria* (1991), 139–45.

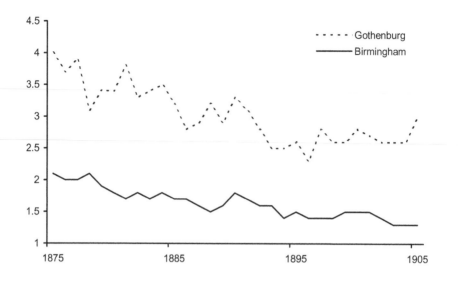

Figure 5.1   Tuberculosis mortality per 1,000 population in Gothenburg and Birmingham, 1875–1905.

Note: The figure shows the death rate for the Birmingham registration districts (Birmingham, King's Norton and Aston), not for the City of Birmingham. See *Special Report by the MOH on Further Measures for the Prevention of Consumption in the City of Birmingham* (Health Department, Birmingham 1906), 4–5.

Source: Annual Reports of the Registrar General of Births, Deaths and Marriages in England and Wales 1875–1901; E. Almquist, 'Dödorsakerna i Göteborg 1861–85', in *Göteborgs helsovårdsnämnds årsberättelse 1888*, 90–91; *Göteborgs helsovårdsnämnds årsberättelser 1885–1901*; *Statistisk årsbok för Göteborg 1939*, 9–10.

alone failed to transform new scientific ideas into practical campaigns. It needed serious political and social concerns to actually put tuberculosis on the agenda.

A major reason why health authorities took action at the turn of the century was, as in the case of the infant welfare movement, the growing concern over national inefficiency. In a climate of intensifying international rivalry, a concerted campaign to deal with tuberculosis, primarily a disease of young adults, came to be seen as an essential part of a nation's efforts to uphold its interests in the international arena. Equally important, albeit less publicized, was the role that the anti-tuberculosis campaigns were to play in the management of social problems and in mediating urban conflicts at home. In the late nineteenth century, the techniques of analysis and intervention which bacteriology provided came to be seen as an efficient and value-free way of dealing with urban problems, and thus indispensable to the governance of large industrial cities. It is the latter role as a mediator, facilitator and legitimizer that is of greatest interest here.

Owing to close international links between medical practitioners working in the field and to specialized journals and conferences through which new research findings were disseminated, there were many universal features, for example, in Swedish, British, German and French anti-tuberculosis movements. Yet all these campaigns also had national characteristics which distinguished them from each other. The new 'truth' about tuberculosis clearly allowed different definitions of the disease and left ample room for disagreement on what measures would be the most appropriate to address the problem. In this chapter, the Birmingham and Gothenburg anti-tuberculosis campaigns are compared and their differences and similarities are analysed to show the ways in which definitions of the problem and responses to it were bound to the social and political aims the Birmingham and Gothenburg policy makers sought to advance.

The comparison between Gothenburg and Birmingham reveals very clearly the health authorities' tendency to accept unquestioningly those aspects of the new 'truth' that supported their own preconceptions of the problem and to selectively ignore research findings that challenged their understanding. Some public health officers concentrated their attention on the tubercle bacillus, seeking to create an impression of tuberculosis as a medical problem, devoid of deep societal roots. For them, the campaign against tuberculosis was basically a scientific battle against the bacillus led by experts on medicine and public health. Others emphasized the importance of the research findings, which indicated that only a small percentage of people who had at some time suffered tubercular infection actually developed full-blown tuberculosis. These experts argued that the approaches concentrating on the bacillus did not come close to explaining tuberculosis, since the disease was a consequence of unhealthy habits that weakened the body's own defence mechanism. The only effective way of combating the disease was health education. Yet others focused on social and environmental factors such as poverty and defective housing, which were believed to make people susceptible to diseases, and called for changes in the economic order. The Birmingham and Gothenburg anti-tuberculosis schemes, like most anti-tuberculosis campaigns in Western countries, combined the three approaches, fighting the bacterial, behavioural and environmental causes of tuberculosis at the same time. In reports published by the health authorities, all of these approaches could easily coexist, and might even come and go in the course of the text. Yet the authorities had a tendency to give preference to one line of reasoning and to play down the others, depending on policy legacies and on wider political and social aims behind the health policy.

Chapter 4 discussed how 'scientific' infant welfare campaigns served to regulate urban family life. In contrast to infant mortality, which was related to dysfunctional families, tuberculosis was viewed as a more public problem and was associated with a wider range of social contacts and with public space as well as homes. This chapter examines, firstly, the way in which the question of defective housing was integrated into the official conception of tuberculosis in Birmingham and Gothenburg. The debates about housing and tuberculosis reveal sharply the conflicting demands that were imposed upon municipal health authorities by the operation of their conflicting roles. Authorities were not only combating tuberculosis, but also sought to maintain social order and to regulate the local economy. In both Birmingham and Gothenburg, authorities used scientific knowledge about tuberculosis, albeit in different ways, to legitimize municipal *interventions* in homes and to justify sometimes *intervention* and sometimes *non-intervention* in the housing market.

Secondly, this chapter examines how the strategies that aimed at shaping the relations between the sick and the healthy served to regulate urban society in general. Tuberculosis was one of the 'social diseases' that were constituted not only in the individual body, but also in the social body. Hence, in order to control tuberculosis, health authorities did not confine themselves to controlling individuals, but they also sought to regulate the relationships between different social classes, between parents and children, and between the state and the family. Thirdly, the chapter discusses the extent to which anti-tuberculosis campaigns were products and prisoners of the interests of the medical profession. The theme has already been examined in the preceding chapter, which showed that the structure of the health care system – and in particular the relative importance of public and private sectors – had a marked impact on the direction which the infant welfare campaigns took. Tuberculosis, however, was a 'second-class disease', which never was of great interest to British general practitioners and voluntary hospitals. Consequently, in Birmingham, as in Gothenburg, the public health authorities took most of the responsibility for dealing with the problem. The question explored here is whether the Gothenburg health officers, who held a relatively strong position within the medical profession and in society in general, and the Birmingham officers, who did not enjoy the same status, were inclined to define the problem of tuberculosis differently. Can the different policies, again, be explained in terms of the professional manipulation of power and status?

Homes and Habits: Two Definitions of Tuberculosis

Gothenburg

What public health authorities saw when they examined the problem of tuberculosis depended very much on what they expected or wanted to see. The Gothenburg health authorities were clearly determined to concentrate their attention on unhygienic flats, attics and cellar dwellings. They viewed tuberculosis, first and foremost, as a 'dwelling-disease' (*bostadssjukdom*) most likely to affect those living in overcrowded, ill-ventilated, dark and squalid homes.[14] This view of tuberculosis was shared by many key figures in the national anti-tuberculosis campaign. Dr Ernst Almquist, Professor of Hygiene in Stockholm, emphasized time and again that poor housing conditions rather than poverty *per se* were what lay behind the high incidence of tuberculosis in large Swedish towns.[15] Similarly, the governmental Tuberculosis Committee,

---

[14]   *GSH 1900:104*; *1902:2*; *1908:252*; *Årsberättelsen 1902*, 40; *1911*, 10–13; *1912*, 10–13; G. Göthlin, 'Några bostadshygieniska reformkrav', *Hygiea* **79** (21) (1917), 1,152–6.

[15]   E. Almquist, *Allmän hälsovårdslära med särskildt afseende på svenska förhållanden för läkare, medicine studerande, hälsovårdsmyndigheter, tekniker m. fl.* (Stockholm 1897), 740–43; E. Almquist, *Hälsovårdslärans framsteg under senaste åren* (Stockholm 1902), 26–9. See also G.H. von Koch, 'Bostadsfrågan', in G.H. von Koch (ed.), *Social Handbok* (Stockholm 1908), 79.

which published a report in 1907–8, was convinced that bad housing conditions were largely to blame for the high death rates from tuberculosis.[16] In defining the problem of tuberculosis, the Swedish health authorities clearly wanted to focus on defective housing, and they paid relatively little attention to other consequences of poverty such as malnutrition and overwork.

Unhygienic Homes   As proof of the link between defective housing and tuberculosis, the Gothenburg health authorities cited investigations conducted in Sweden and abroad. In France, as in Sweden, housing problems were closely integrated into the medical and social understanding of tuberculosis, therefore the Chief Tuberculosis Officer for Gothenburg, Dr Gösta Göthlin, often invoked French research to support his arguments.[17] However, there was also an abundance of evidence available from other countries which backed up the Gothenburg authorities' conclusion: the worse the housing conditions, the higher the death rate from tuberculosis. In particular, studies showing a clear correlation, firstly between house size and the incidence of tuberculosis, and secondly between overcrowding and tuberculosis gave the Gothenburg authorities much cause for concern.[18] A large proportion of the inhabitants of Gothenburg lived in small, overcrowded flats. In 1910, about 63 per cent of the homes in the city had only one room or one room and a kitchen, and 38 per cent of the inhabitants lived at a density of more than two persons per room.[19]

The leading health officers were convinced that improved housing would be an effective remedy against tuberculosis. Indeed, many proposals that the First City Physician, Karl Gezelius, and the Chief Tuberculosis Officer, Gösta Göthlin, put forward in the early twentieth century rested on the explicit acknowledgement that the problem of tuberculosis *could not be solved* without radical housing reform. Göthlin argued that the private housebuilding sector was unequal to the task of meeting the demand for decent housing, therefore more active municipal intervention in the housing market was necessary. The municipality should not only control the private building and renting sectors and support co-operative enterprises, but also build houses. Göthlin pointed out that the social hygienic study of housing conducted in Gothenburg in 1911 corroborated his view: tenants were not solely to blame for poor housing conditions. The problem revolved around two core issues: the conservatism of poor city-dwellers and the conservatism of decision-makers. While the former

---

[16]   *Betänkande och förslag I*, 3–16 and *II* (Stockholm 1908), 47–9; K. Petrén, 'Tuberkuloskommitténs betänkande', *Social Tidskrift* (1908), 110–16.

[17]   For references to French or Swedish studies, see *GSH 1908:252*; *1913:337*; *Årsberättelsen 1911*, 10–13; *1912*, 10–13; Göthlin, 'Reformkrav', 1,153–4. For the French discussion about the housing–tuberculosis connection, see Barnes, *Social Disease*, 112–37.

[18]   Göthlin, 'Reformkrav', 1,151–69. See also Almquist, *Hälsovårdslärans framsteg*, 26–7; G. Stéenhoff, 'Kampen mot tuberkulosen i England', *Hygiea* **79** (1917), 794–5; Dovertie, 'Öfversikt', 101–6.

[19]   *Statistisk årsbok för Göteborg 1925*, 99, 103, 105; A. Attman, *Göteborgs Stadsfullmäktige 1863–1962*, vol. I.1: *Göteborg 1863–1913* (Göteborg 1963), 278–9. The figures presented here are different from those in Attman's book. Attman has looked only at the flats/houses with less than five rooms and the section of the population which lived in these houses. See also Chapter 2.

were unwilling to abandon their old unhygienic habits, the latter stuck to their traditional ways of dealing with social problems.[20] In order to convey this message to the key policy makers and to promote the case for municipal housing, Göthlin worked his way onto the Housing Committee in 1911.[21]

The leading health officers campaigned for housing reform throughout the first two decades of the twentieth century, but at the same time they were realistic enough to know that housing problems in a badly overcrowded city such as Gothenburg could not be solved overnight. For one thing, in the early twentieth century the majority of the city councillors in Gothenburg continued to cling to the view that municipal intervention in the housing market should be kept to a minimum. Private builders and co-operative enterprises were to build houses, and the role of the municipality was, at most, to support these agencies. The housing strategies that the City Council was ready to adopt thus merely scratched the surface of the problem.[22] Furthermore, even if the City Council had embarked on a programme of radical housing reform, putting an end to overcrowding would have taken years. The health officers were acutely aware that an anti-tuberculosis campaign concentrating exclusively on improving housing conditions was not a realistic option.

The Tubercle Bacillus   The problem was solved by manipulating the presentation of the housing–tuberculosis problem. In examining the role which housing conditions played in the pathogenesis of tuberculosis, public health experts in Gothenburg invoked ideas of 'soil' and 'seed'. Defective housing was doubly to blame. Firstly, it was pointed out that poor housing conditions rendered the human soil receptive. Living in damp, mouldy, ill-ventilated and squalid houses gradually diminished the body's capacity to fight off the infection and thus paved the way for the active disease.[23] This aspect failed, however, to attract widespread interest among public health experts in Gothenburg or in Sweden in general, and the discussion was usually determinedly steered into the seed, the tubercle bacillus. The risk of infection and of recurring re-infection was considered to be high in insanitary, overcrowded houses. Not only were tubercle bacilli transmitted easily from person to person when people lived huddled together in small rooms, bacilli were also believed to thrive in filth, darkness and stale air.[24]

The Chief Tuberculosis Officer cited a number of French studies showing that the lighting of a house greatly affected the bacilli. In bright daylight, tubercle bacilli

---

[20]   *GSH 1908:252; 1909:197* and minutes 28 Oct. 1909, item 5, *1911:216*, 12–13; *1913:337*; Göthlin, 'Reformkrav'.

[21]   *Göteborgare 1923: Biografisk uppslagsbok* (Göteborg 1923), 118; L. Öberg, *Göteborgs Läkaresällskap: En historik* (Göteborg 1983), 138.

[22]   *GSH 1917:14; 1923:113* and minutes and discussion 5 Apr. 1923, item 13. Göthlin, 'Reformkrav'; B. Nyström, 'Åtgärder till förbättring av de mindre bemedlades bostadsförhållanden i vissa städer', in *Statens Offentliga Utredningar (SOU) 1935*:2, Appendix I, 11–14.

[23]   *GSH 1908:252*. See also von Koch, 'Bostadsfrågan', 79, 82.

[24]   *Årsberättelsen 1902*, 40; *1911*, 13; *GSH 1902:2; 1913:337*, 2–3; Göthlin, 'Reformkrav', 1,152–3; Almquist, *Allmän hälsovårdslära*, 740–43; Almquist, *Hälsovårdslärans framsteg*, 26–7; B. Buhre, 'Tuberkulosens bekämpande', in von Koch, *Social Handbok*, 325–32.

were estimated to die within three days; in dark and mouldy cellars, they survived for weeks or even months.[25] The scientific evidence used by the authorities to substantiate their argument that stale air contributed to the proliferation of bacilli was more fragmentary. In most cases, the simple reasoning behind this argument was that stale air was 'disgusting' and 'intolerable', and therefore unhealthy. The way in which dirt affected the incidence of tuberculosis was again discussed in more detail. For example, Professor Ernst Almquist argued in his textbooks that dirt protected bacilli from sunlight and therefore enabled them to survive longer.[26]

The emphasis on the tubercle bacillus allowed the Gothenburg health officers to present the housing–tuberculosis problem in such a way that a solution to the problem was within their grasp. They emphasized that the tubercle bacillus, not defective housing, was after all the *real* cause of tuberculosis. Poor living conditions contributed to the prevalence of tuberculosis by *facilitating* the proliferation and transmission of bacilli, but were not the fundamental cause. Once the tubercle bacillus had been identified as the main culprit, it was relatively easy to find remedial responses that were within the bounds of the accepted value framework. The health officers recommended two strategies. Firstly, they argued that the spread of the tubercle bacillus could be contained by tracking down infectious tubercular patients living in small insanitary flats and by segregating them from their families and neighbours. Secondly, they suggested that the authorities should introduce a system of housing inspection as a prop until private enterprise met the housing demand. The officers were convinced that the proliferation and transmission of tubercle bacilli could be curbed by urging landlords to carry out necessary repairs and by instructing tenants in domestic hygiene. In developing the two strategies, the Gothenburg authorities shifted the focus of the tuberculosis debate away from poor living conditions and towards disease-causing micro-organisms, away from environmental reform and towards bacteriological solutions.

Breaking the Chain of Infection   The first strategy, the segregation of people suffering from infectious advanced tuberculosis, was given much emphasis in the early phases of the campaign. The Gothenburg health officers stressed that it was very difficult to contain the spread of tuberculosis in poor families in which one or more family members suffered from the disease. Therefore, it was of utmost importance to remove advanced tubercular patients into hospitals, especially if there were small children in the family.[27] The segregation of the sick and the healthy also appealed to many city councillors, for practical and political reasons. Apart from

---

[25]   *Årsberättelsen 1911*, 13; Göthlin, 'Reformkrav', 1,153–4; Almquist, *Hälsovårdslärans framsteg*, 18.

[26]   Almquist, *Hälsovårdlärans framsteg*, 18, 25. For further discussion about the processes by which certain smells, behaviours and filth came to be considered as unhealthy and insanitary, see A. Corbin, *Pesthauch und Blütenduft: Eine Geschichte des Geruchs* (Frankfurt am Main 1988); N. Elias, *The Civilizing Process: The History of Manners & State Formation and Civilization* (Oxford 1994).

[27]   *Årsberättelsen 1902*, 2; *1906*, 44; *GHS 1902:90*, 3–5; *1926:258*; Göteborgs stadsarkiv (GSA) Göteborgs Hälsovårdsnämnd, I avdelningen (HVN I) minutes 4 Dec. 1918, item 228. See also G. Kjellin, 'Bekämpandet av tuberkulosen bland barnen', *Hygiea* **79** (1917), 1,331–

being relatively cheap, this policy accommodated conflicting interests and promoted order and harmony in society. The strategy was a kind of compromise: while it included a tacit admission that the housing situation was extremely difficult, it gave policy makers an excuse to postpone the discussion of housing problems.

Some of the eagerness to institutionalize 'advanced' tubercular patients stemmed from changing attitudes to death. Dying at home – and in particular dying of tuberculosis – was increasingly seen as inconvenient and unhygienic. Initially, health authorities directed their attention mainly to houses where tubercular patients had died and to furniture, bedding, clothing and personal belongings that the patients had used while they were ill. Everything was to be disinfected before being used by other members of the family or before being taken to a pawnbroker or sold.[28] However, the focus of attention soon shifted from patients' personal belongings to the dying patients themselves. Advocates of institutional care argued, explicitly or implicitly, that the lingering death of a tubercular patient was 'unhygienic' and 'unmanageable' at home, and that advanced tubercular patients posed a considerable danger to the health of their family members and friends. They were highly infectious and often incapable of taking any necessary precautions or looking after themselves. Hence they were completely dependent on their family members and friends, who in turn often lacked both the discipline and resources to take care of patients properly and to protect themselves from infection.[29]

The importance of institutional care – both sanatorium and hospital care – was also emphasized by the governmental Tuberculosis Committee in 1907–8. The Committee argued that in large towns, local authorities should provide about as many hospital beds for tubercular patients as there were deaths annually from the disease. According to the report, Gothenburg, where 447 people died of tuberculosis in 1905, would have needed about 390 beds.[30] The Committee recommended hospitalization chiefly on the grounds that medical doctors were in favour of this approach and that foreign examples seemed to show that the isolation of infectious tubercular patients alleviated the problem of tuberculosis. It is interesting that England was used as an example illustrating the advantages of institutionalization. It was argued that in England, the death rates from tuberculosis were low mainly because so many people – including many infectious tubercular patients – died in institutions.[31] However, in late nineteenth-century Birmingham, only about 15 per cent of deaths took place in hospitals or other institutions, while at the same time in Gothenburg, 20–25 per cent

---

40; A. Aronson, 'Dispensärna och tuberkuloskampen', *Social-Medicinsk Tidskrift* 1 (1924), 210–13.

[28]   *GSH 1900:104.*

[29]   *GSH 1902:90; 1903:122C* no. 17.

[30]   *Betänkande och förslag I,* 4–6.

[31]   Dovertie, 'Öfversikt'. The Swedish Tuberculosis Committee was not alone in arguing that the low tuberculosis mortality in England could be ascribed to the institutional segregation of tubercular patients. See also A. Newsholme, 'An inquiry into the principal causes of the reduction in the death-rate from phthisis during the last forty years, with special reference to the segregation of phthisical patients in general institutions', *Journal of Hygiene* 6 (1906), 304–84.

of deaths occurred in institutions.[32] This example illustrates how 'flexibly' health authorities used foreign examples to legitimize the policies they were determined to pursue.

The second strategy adopted by the Gothenburg authorities was to regularly inspect all small flats and houses. In other words, instead of intervening in the housing market, the municipal authorities would intervene in the homes of the poor. The housing inspectors would deal with problems such as insufficient sunlight and ventilation, which were believed to make houses hospitable to the tubercle bacilli. Public health experts usually took the view that the lack of sunlight was largely due to the structural defects of cellar dwellings and of flats facing small backyards. Poor ventilation, by contrast, was considered to be almost entirely the fault of the inhabitants. The Chief Tuberculosis Officer argued that only 10 per cent of poorly ventilated houses in Gothenburg had structural defects preventing effective ventilation, and therefore in 90 per cent of cases poor ventilation was due to ignorance and neglect. The want of cleanliness was attributed partly to the structural defects of houses and partly to the negligence of the inhabitants. These two factors, structural defects and people's indifference and ignorance, were inextricably interwoven into the housing–tuberculosis debate: houses were cold or over-heated, draughty or poorly ventilated, and difficult to keep clean or then occupied by people who did not take proper care of their homes. To further illustrate the level of indifference, the Chief Tuberculosis Officer pointed out that in almost 50 per cent of all homes with a tubercular patient, the children were not properly looked after.[33]

The way in which the housing–tuberculosis connection was delineated in Gothenburg set forth a rational basis for active official intervention. Firstly, by emphasizing that tubercle bacilli were easily transmitted from person to person in small, overcrowded rooms, the authorities were able to define all small flats as problems and to justify intervention in the everyday lives of all city-dwellers living in them, whether they suffered from tuberculosis or not. Secondly, by establishing a connection between a number of ultimately separate phenomena – tuberculosis, squalor, lack of sunlight, indifference, ignorance, neglect of children and even alcoholism – they created a generalized picture of the home of a tubercular patient. In so doing, they justified the principle that all aspects of tubercular patients' and their family members' everyday lives could be subjected to close surveillance.

Birmingham

The Birmingham public health authorities, like their counterparts in Gothenburg, were convinced that housing conditions affected the incidence of tuberculosis. In 1901–2, the MOH, Dr Alfred Hill, drew policy makers' attention to wide variations in tuberculosis mortality between the run-down central quarters and the suburban residential areas. In 'the older, poorer and less sanitary' areas such as St Mary's and St Bartholomew's wards, death rates from the disease were three times higher than those reported in the

---

[32]   *Annual Report 1899*, 5; *Statistisk årsbok för Göteborg 1900*, 46, 68–73.
[33]   *GSH 1900:104*; *1913:337*; *Årsberättelsen 1911*, 8–13; *1912*, 9–13; *1913*, 13–17.

healthiest wards, Edgbaston and Balsall Heath.[34] Hill's successor, Dr John Robertson, also considered the question of insanitary housing and tuberculosis in his special report on the unhealthy conditions of the Birmingham slum districts in 1904.[35] However, the way in which Hill and Robertson examined the housing–tuberculosis connection was somewhat different from the approach chosen by the Gothenburg authorities.

Unhealthy Areas   Firstly, in Birmingham, the more privacy the family enjoyed, the more hygienic and healthy their home environment was assumed to be. Sharing space and facilities with neighbours, so it was argued, inevitably brought about health problems. Not only were shared water taps and communal privies associated with insanitary conditions and with low resistance to diseases such as tuberculosis, but also shared yards or stair wells were commonly considered to be unhygienic. Robertson attributed the problem to people's (natural) disinclination to take care of communal space or facilities: 'what is everybody's duty is nobody's duty'.[36] By linking shared facilities and communal space with ill health, he provided legitimization for the Birmingham municipal housing and city planning policies, one aim of which was to promote working-class suburban migration. The MOH claimed that the health of the population could be vastly improved if the working classes 'spread themselves over a much wider area' and lived in self-contained houses 'with sufficient space around or near' them.[37] Rather than arguing, the MOH took it for granted that reinforcing middle-class ideals of privacy and seclusion in society would promote the health of the population. In Gothenburg, where not only the majority of working-class people but also many middle-class people lived in flats, communal space – yards, entrances and stair wells – and shared facilities were not necessarily regarded as unhealthy or unhygienic.[38]

Secondly, the fact that residential segregation was relatively high in Birmingham had an impact on how the Birmingham authorities perceived the tuberculosis–housing connection. Tuberculosis, like infant mortality, was closely associated with a few problem wards, known as unhealthy areas, where a high proportion of people lived in old, ramshackle back-to-back houses. In death-rate tables, these municipal wards were consistently at the top, and in maps they were always shaded black, as shown in Figure 5.2. Light colours were reserved for the healthy middle-class suburbs,

---

[34]   Birmingham City Archives (BCA) Birmingham Health Committee (HC) minutes 11 Mar. 1902, item 7319; *Annual Report 1901*, 20–22.

[35]   *Report of the MOH on the Unhealthy Conditions in the Floodgate Street Area and the Municipal Wards of St. Mary, St. Stephen and St. Bartholomew* (Health Department, Birmingham 1904).

[36]   *Report of the MOH on the Unhealthy Conditions*, 13.

[37]   *Report of the MOH on the Unhealthy Conditions*, 23; *Annual Report 1912*, 6.

[38]   H. Wallqvist, *Bostadsförhållandena för de mindre bemedlade i Göteborg: Studie sommaren 1889* (Stockholm 1891), 7–11. However, large tenements which were divided into numerous small flats and where the standard of facilities was low were considered to be unhealthy places to live. Moreover, some writers regarded housing policy pursued by the state and local authorities in England as a relevant model for Swedish housing policy. E. Heyman, 'Bostadsfrågans betydelse ur sanitär synpunkt', *Hygiea* **52** (1890), 329–50; von Koch, 'Bostadsfrågan', 82–7.

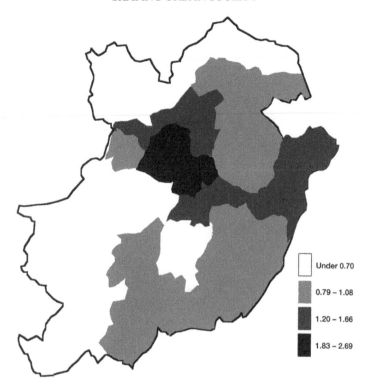

| Under 0.70 |
| 0.79 – 1.08 |
| 1.20 – 1.66 |
| 1.83 – 2.69 |

Figure 5.2 **Tuberculosis map, Birmingham, 1912. By comparing tuberculosis death rates in different wards, the Birmingham authorities defined the 'unhealthy areas'.**

Source: Annual Report of the MOH for Birmingham 1912.

and between these two extremes were the grey wards inhabited mainly by lower-middle-class and 'respectable' working-class families.[39] This interpretation of the problem not only reflected, but also reinforced the social and spatial arrangements in the city. The division between the unhealthy, less unhealthy and healthy areas made by the authorities inevitably took a strong imaginative hold on people, serving to promote residential and social differentiation. The Gothenburg authorities, too, gave a spatial expression to the problem of tuberculosis, but it was rather different from the Birmingham one. In Gothenburg, the degree of spatial separation of social groups was more moderate, and the authorities, instead of defining unhealthy areas, directed their attention to low-rent houses and flats scattered in the socially mixed city centre and in working-class areas. For example, the authorities pinpointed the precise location of all houses where someone had died of tuberculosis, as shown in Figure 5.3.[40]

---

[39]   *Annual Report 1898*, 8–15, 34–9; *1901*, 6–8, 21–2; *1910*, 4; *1912*; *Report of the MOH on the Unhealthy Conditions*, 5–14.
[40]   *GSH 1908:252* and minutes 10 Dec. 1908, item 18; *1909:197* and minutes 28 Oct. 1909, item 5; Wallqvist, *Bostadsförhållandena*, 4–11, 72–5; G. Lönnroth, 'Stadsbilden

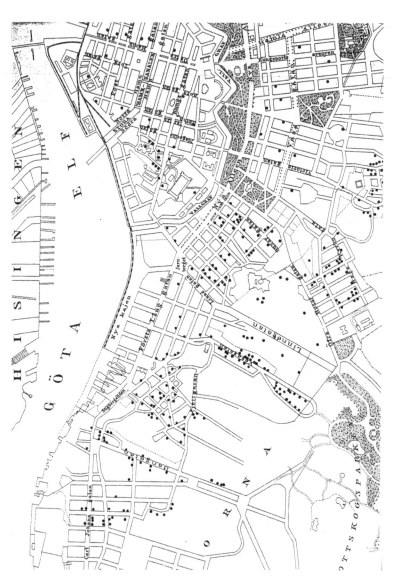

Figure 5.3 Tuberculosis map, Gothenburg, 1904. Instead of defining 'unhealthy areas', the Gothenburg authorities focused their attention on individual buildings.

Source: Göteborgs Hälsovårdsnämnds årsberättelse för 1914.

Unhealthy Way of Life   The concept of the unhealthy area maintained its significance as a major tool for understanding the problem of tuberculosis in Birmingham, even though the focus of attention soon turned from insanitary houses to other aspects of slum-dwellers' everyday lives – their social contacts, bodily maintenance, diet and treatment of illnesses. In 1906, the MOH, John Robertson, determinedly looked at the question from the new perspective. While he still admitted that insanitary housing took its toll on people's health, he argued that poor housing conditions were not the *main* contributory factor to the problem of tuberculosis in Birmingham.[41]

The Birmingham authorities stressed that the disease was not only spreading in homes inhabited by poor tubercular patients, but the danger was also lurking in any public space – in streets, tram-cars, trains and public houses – where careless patients had been spitting and coughing. The germs of consumption lived in fine dust, 'which the slightest breath of air, the foot of a passer-by, the whisk of a lady's skirt, or a crawling infant distributes broadcast to be drawn into the lungs of all who are unfortunate enough to come in contact with it'. Moreover, tuberculosis was highly contagious: anyone could contract it, and everyone was potentially ill.[42]

As tuberculosis was believed to be ubiquitous in the city and rampant in the unhealthy areas, it did not seem sensible to start hunting down bacilli. The Birmingham authorities maintained that the isolation of advanced cases was not an effective way of preventing the spread of tuberculosis. In fact, isolation measures could aggravate the situation by encouraging a false sense of security. The measures that concentrated on building up people's resistance to the disease, on making their bodies repellent to infection, would yield much better results. However, the Birmingham authorities made it clear that their own role in building up people's resistance would inevitably be limited. The authorities could instruct people in domestic and personal hygiene and carry out some environmental reforms, but ultimately the choice between healthy and unhealthy ways of life would be up to the people themselves. Indeed, during the preceding decades the Birmingham Public Health Department had already done much in regard to reducing the number of susceptible people by improving housing and working conditions, by dealing with environmental problems and by checking the quality of food.[43] What had largely been lacking, argued Robertson in 1906, was a change in people's attitudes and behaviour. Instead of keeping themselves 'in such a condition of health as will enable them to resist the invasion of the germ', people increased their susceptibility to infection by their unhealthy way of life.[44]

Bad workshop conditions and drinking in pubs were regarded as major culprits in spreading tuberculosis in Birmingham. These factors were believed to render

---

– praktfulla palats och usla kåkar', in *För hundra år sedan – skildringar från Göteborgs 1880-tal* (Göteborg 1984), 27–62; M. Åberg, *En fråga om klass? Borgarklass och industriellt företagande i Göteborg, 1850–1914* (Göteborg 1991), 132–7; O. Wetterberg and G. Axelsson, *Smutsguld och dödligt hot: Renhållning och återvinning i Göteborg 1864–1930* (Göteborg 1995), 118–20.

[41]   *Annual Report 1906*, 62–3; *Special Report by the MOH on Consumption*, 5–7.

[42]   The quotes are from Dixon, *Lectures on the Prevention of Consumption*, 4–5; *Special Report by the MOH on Consumption*, 8–9.

[43]   *Annual Report 1903*, 27.

[44]   *Special Report by the MOH on Consumption*, 9.

human soil hospitable to infected seeds and to increase the number of seeds to which individuals were exposed. Firstly, by working in poorly ventilated, dark and damp factories and by 'soak[ing] themselves with drink every day', people weakened their resistance to infection. Secondly, in workshops, where people worked in cramped conditions, and in pubs, where they coughed over one other and shared glasses, the risk of infection was believed to be extremely high. Indeed, the MOH suggested that drinking combined with ignorance and negligence played a more important part than bad housing and poverty in causing tuberculosis and many other illnesses.[45]

The Birmingham authorities also pointed out that people had only themselves to blame for their disease if they spent all their days indoors. '[B]y having an abundance of fresh air, which even in the centre of the city costs nothing and is of good quality' they could, in most cases, have prevented tuberculosis, claimed the MOH in his report in 1912.[46] Yet he never elaborated on the fortifying properties of 'fresh air', let alone the ways in which these properties assisted the body's defence mechanism in fighting against tuberculosis. Nor did he make any attempt to prove that the air in the city centre was of good quality. In fact, he claimed in another report that numerous factories and workshops, which were interspersed among houses in the central wards, made the atmosphere 'smoky and gloomy, and therefore comparatively sunless'.[47]

A more analytical approach was taken by the Medical Officer of the General Dispensary, Dr A. Carver, who argued that bad marketing and ignorance of nutrition paved the way to full-blown tuberculosis in many working-class families in Birmingham. By comparing the weekly diets of 40 healthy families and of 40 families in which one or more persons suffered from tuberculosis, he was able to show that families with tubercular patients did not have as nutritious a diet as healthy families at the same income level. Families with tubercular patients, he concluded, had spent their money on expensive articles such as beef instead of buying cheap, nutritious food, and in consequence, both the overall energy value and the carbohydrate and fat content of their diet had been too low to protect them from tuberculosis. The value of his research finding was diminished by the fact that his conclusion was based on rather small groups of families and, more importantly, that the families were not randomly selected.[48]

Building Up People's Resistance to Infection   The Birmingham health authorities drew on the same scientific results as their Gothenburg counterparts: overcrowding, lack of sunshine and fresh air, want of cleanliness, and malnourishment contributed to the high incidence of tuberculosis. Yet they put a very different interpretation on these findings. Instead of concentrating their attention on the tubercle bacillus and

---

[45]   *Report of the MOH on the Unhealthy Conditions*, 17–18; *Annual Report 1906*, 62–3; *1912*, 44–5; *Special Report by the MOH on Consumption*, 5–7.

[46]   *Annual Report 1912*, 6.

[47]   *Report of the MOH on the Unhealthy Conditions*, 5.

[48]   A.E. Carver, *An Investigation into the Dietary of the Labouring Classes of Birmingham, With Special Reference to Its Bearing upon Tuberculosis* (Birmingham 1914). See also D.E. Lindsay, *Report upon a Study of the Diet of the Labouring Classes in the City of Glasgow Carried out During 1911–1912* (Glasgow c. 1912).

pinning their hopes on the isolation of infectious tubercular patients, the Birmingham authorities stressed the role of unhealthy attitudes and behaviours in causing tuberculosis. They argued that tuberculosis was a consequence of unhealthy habits which weakened the body's own defence mechanism, and that the most effective way of combating the disease was health education.

Education appealed to the public health officers and the Health Committee members for a variety of reasons. Not only were educational measures cheap, but they also had the additional benefit of improving the health of the population and strengthening the moral fabric of society. Health and social reforms could be combined. To justify educational measures, many of which were intrusive, health authorities cited examples of ignorance and negligence: many tubercular patients seemed to be completely ignorant that their sputum spread the infection, they shared their bed with one or more healthy persons, and they were even selling food in shops.[49] The way in which the problem of tuberculosis was defined legitimized municipal intervention in homes, in people's everyday lives. At the same time, it justified non-intervention or selective intervention in the housing market. Providing houses for the poorest of the poor would not necessarily make these people healthier, since the main problem behind their ill health was ignorance and negligence.

Environmental problems such as defective housing and industrial waste were never left completely out of the picture, but even these problems were often defined in individualistic terms. Pervading the public health debates in Birmingham was the conviction that market forces – and in the 1920s and 1930s, the partnership between the market and the public sector – provided solutions to environmental and housing problems.[50] What inhibited improvements, so it was argued, were the individuals involved, who did not make informed choices. The MOH argued that many people were used to their insanitary houses and did not seize the opportunities offered by the new working-class suburbs. If only these people actively sought better homes and surroundings, insanitary houses near polluting factories and workshops would become impossible to let. Similarly, many people worked in an unhealthy environment, although working conditions were 'more or less under the control of the individual. If he thinks his workplace or the character of the work is likely to affect his health he has a remedy in his own hands by leaving the work.'[51]

Not only were people expected to keep themselves fit to fight off infection, but they were also responsible for managing the cure if they developed tuberculosis. In this respect, the Birmingham campaign differed clearly from its Gothenburg counterpart. In Gothenburg, where a strong current of medical paternalism pervaded the anti-tuberculosis scheme, tubercular patients were often considered to be almost incapable of improving their situation. Experts, and particularly medical doctors and nurses, went to great lengths to reorganize people's everyday lives. In Birmingham,

---

[49]   *Annual Report 1905*, 65.

[50]   See, for example, J. Robertson, *Housing and Public Health* (London 1919); J. Robertson, 'The slum problem', *Journal of the Royal Sanitary Institute* **51** (1930–31), 279–84. See also P. Garside, '"Unhealthy areas": town planning, eugenics and the slums, 1890–1945', *Planning Perspectives* **3** (1) (1988), 24–46.

[51]   *Annual Report 1912*, 5–6. The quote is from *Annual Report 1924*, 29.

health officials consistently emphasized that people themselves were responsible for taking care of their health. The basic tenet of the campaign was that the disease could be arrested or cured if patients consulted their doctors as soon as the first symptoms appeared and followed medical advice carefully. This line of reasoning clearly understated the degree of difficulty tubercular patients faced. Many of them were likely to lose their battle against tuberculosis whatever they did. If they left their jobs they would be too poor to buy nutritious food, and if they continued working they would be exhausted.[52]

The Birmingham health authorities were determined to seek both prevention and cure by transforming people's attitudes and behaviour. Yet they were under no illusion that education would succeed in putting everyone's life in order. The question of how to deal with individuals who ignored the advice and whose behaviour placed their family or other people at risk gave rise to serious consideration. The public were encouraged to be vigilant. If a tubercular patient was neglectful, his friends or neighbours were expected to 'either caution him or complain to the authorities of his bad habit'. In the most serious cases, the health authorities were allowed to use coercive powers to protect the healthy.[53]

Anti-tuberculosis Campaigns and Urban Politics

Gothenburg

In Gothenburg, the campaign against tuberculosis started out as a straightforward fight against the tubercle bacillus. The authorities pursued two different tactics to control the spread of bacilli: the institutionalization of infectious tubercular patients, and the systematic inspection of small houses and flats. Scientists, medical practitioners, nurses and housing inspectors were to fight against disease-bearing micro-organisms in hospitals and in the homes of tubercular patients. In the 1910s and 1920s, the scope of activities was gradually widened, but even then the campaign was essentially mounted using medical and bacteriological strategies.

Separating the Sick from the Healthy   The first municipal tuberculosis hospital in Gothenburg, *Hemmet för lungsotssjuka*, was opened in 1902. The institution was designed for 'incurable' tubercular patients who had to be isolated because their

---

    [52]   BCA HC minutes 22 Sep. 1908, item 1358; 19 Apr. 1910, item 2383; 26 Apr. 1910, item 2397; G.B. Dixon, 'The care of the consumptive in the home', reprint from the *Journal of the Royal Sanitary Institute* **25** (1914); Dixon, *Lectures on the Prevention of Consumption*; *Special Report by the MOH on Consumption*.
    [53]   The quote is from *Annual Report 1924*, 28. See also BCA HC minutes 23 Mar. 1909, item 1723; 12 Oct. 1909, item 2018; 23 Nov. 1909, item 2088; 22 Feb. 1910, item 2248; 10 Jan. 1911, item 2790; 26 Sep. 1911, item 3272; Birmingham Public Health and Housing Committee (PH&HC) minutes 11 Jul. 1913, item 1615; Birmingham Public Health Committee (PHC) minutes 8 Apr. 1927, item 10392; 13 Apr. 1934, item 4215; *Report on the Spread of Tuberculosis by Indiscriminate Spitting* (Health Department, Birmingham 1909); *Annual Report 1905*, 64–7; *1912*, 39–40.

illness was highly contagious and because their housing conditions were such as to increase the risk of other people being infected. A large proportion of the patients, 30–35 per cent annually, died during their stay in the hospital, but about 20 per cent were discharged from the 'death house' in better health and capable, to some extent, of working and supporting themselves.[54] Furthermore, the Poor Law Board, which was responsible for the poorest tubercular patients, opened a special tuberculosis ward for advanced cases in 1906. Children suffering from advanced pulmonary tuberculosis were treated in the fever hospital after 1909.[55]

The Gothenburg public health officials were clearly of the opinion that institutionalization served both the collective and individual good. While the healthy members of society were protected against the killer disease, seriously ill tubercular patients were provided with the treatment they needed during the last months of their lives. Death in hospital was increasingly associated with positive values and qualities. Not only was it humane and hygienic, it was also manageable and well managed. Medical doctors working in tuberculosis hospitals were the best people to determine how to treat the serious complications afflicting many dying tubercular patients and to decide when it was no longer worthwhile to treat them.[56] As Philippe Ariès has pointed out, death in hospital came to be seen as 'a technical phenomenon obtained by a cessation of care, a cessation determined in a more or less avowed way by a decision of the doctor and the hospital team'.[57] Constant medical supervision, professional nursing care, a hygienic environment and ever-improving hospital technology guaranteed the optimal death.

A major problem, the First City Physician argued in 1910, was that only 46 per cent of all people who died of tuberculosis in Gothenburg were able to avail themselves of this 'opportunity'.[58] Many tubercular patients seemed to share his view. The queue for hospital beds was long, and only a very small proportion of patients discharged themselves from hospital against the advice of the Medical Officer.[59] The quarantine policy was also popular among the public. Many townspeople were suspicious of tubercular patients and sympathetic to the health authorities' persistent attempts to remove as many patients as possible from cramped dwellings and densely built residential areas.[60]

Medical Care The isolation of advanced cases of tuberculosis remained an important part of the Gothenburg anti-tuberculosis campaign until the 1940s and 1950s, but this strategy was gradually combined with other policies. After 1907, the focus of the debate expanded to encompass the possibility of providing a cure for

---

[54]   *GSH 1900:104* and minutes 6 Dec. 1900, item 11; *1902:2* and minutes 23 Jan. 1902, item 3; *1902:90* and minutes 5 Jun. 1902, item 2; *1902:158* and minutes 30 Oct. 1902, item 6; *Årsberättelsen 1902*, 2–3; *1903*, 2; *1904*, 2, 34–5; *1905*, 2; Dovertie, 'Öfversikt', 21–2.

[55]   *Årsberättelsen 1906*, 46; *1909*, 32; *1910*, 2.

[56]   *GSH 1902:90*; *1903:122C* no. 17, *1910:105*; *Årsberättelsen 1906*, 42–4.

[57]   P. Ariès, *Western Attitudes Toward Death from the Middle Ages to the Present* (London 1994), 88–9.

[58]   *GSH 1910:105*.

[59]   *Årsberättelsen 1906*, 42–4.

[60]   *GSH 1902:90*, 6–8; GSA HVN I minutes 2 Apr. 1930, item 62 and documents K, L.

tuberculosis or, at least, of increasing patients' life expectancy and working ability. The Medical Officer of the tuberculosis hospital, Dr G. Carlström, initiated the discussion that precipitated the revision of the tuberculosis strategy in Gothenburg. He argued that the tuberculosis hospital was not the place for patients in need of long-term care. These patients might live for months or even for years, since the progress of their disease was arrested, but they would never be able to work and support themselves again. Carlström suggested that they should be moved back home or, if there were small children in the family, to the poor law infirmary. Only dying patients, those with serious complications or those who were responding to the treatment and getting better could be allowed to occupy scarce hospital beds. Patients who did not benefit from medical intervention in any way should seek care elsewhere.[61]

Further impetus to the revision of the strategy was given by people's mixed reactions to the anti-tuberculosis campaign. On the one hand, the Gothenburg health authorities were able to report good results of their anti-tuberculosis propaganda. As early as 1900, the First City Physician, Karl Gezelius, praised the public for acting more rationally. An increasing number of people contacted the Public Health Department on their own initiative, asking health officers to disinfect their houses after a member of the family had died of tuberculosis.[62] On the other hand, the alarmist anti-tuberculosis propaganda also brought some serious problems in its wake. The campaign instilled fear into the people, contributing to the stigmatization of the victims of the disease.[63] Gezelius and his colleagues realized that their anti-tuberculosis propaganda needed some modifications in order to ensure the public's co-operation. Although it was important to fight complacency, sometimes by shock tactics, the public had to be convinced that the health authorities had the problem under control. Shifting the focus towards the prospect of providing a cure was one way of making the campaign appear more effective.[64] In the tuberculosis hospital, more emphasis was gradually placed on medical care, and in 1910 the General Hospital allocated 50 beds for 'acute' cases of tuberculosis. Furthermore, the new tuberculosis hospital, *Sjukvårdsanstalten å Kålltorp*, which opened its doors in 1913, admitted not only advanced cases of tuberculosis, but also 'early' and 'intermediate' cases who were provided with sanatorium care (Figure 5.4).[65]

Around 1910, when the Gothenburg authorities and other local authorities in Sweden started to provide treatment for 'curable' cases, conservative therapies consisting of rest and open-air treatments, healthy diet and a rigid sanatorium regime had already lost some of their credibility in Sweden. The cold winter weather frustrated the plans to offer open-air treatment year-round, and in Gothenburg

---

[61]   *Årsberättelsen 1906*, 44.

[62]   GSH *1900:104*, 5–6; 'Smittoförande kläder', in *Göteborgs Handels- och Sjöfartstidning*, 14 Jul. 1900.

[63]   *Årsberättelsen 1900*, 44. See also Buhre, 'Tuberkulosens bekämpande', 328; V. Berglund, 'Försäkring mot tuberkulos', *Social Tidskrift* (1908), 258–9.

[64]   GSH *1904:189*, 10–12; *1907:115*.

[65]   GSH *1903:122C* no. 17; *1903:196*, 22–6, 46–9 and minutes 3 Dec. 1903, item 2; *Årsberättelsen 1913*, 9; 'Sjukvårds-anstalten å Kålltorp. Göteborgs stads lungsotssjukhus. Historik', in *Årsberättelsen 1914*, appendix.

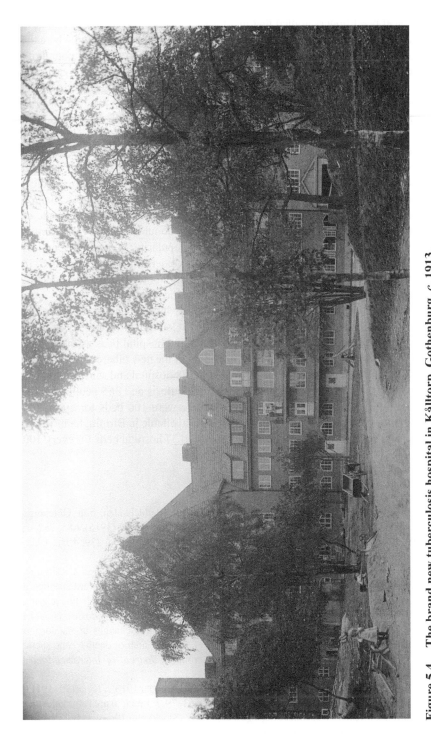

Figure 5.4   The brand new tuberculosis hospital in Kålltorp, Gothenburg, c. 1913.
Source: Gothenburg City Museum.

some medical practitioners argued that this form of therapy was impossible even in summertime, since the municipal sanatorium had been built on marshland where the air was damp. Another reason why the conservative therapies were losing popularity in Sweden was that tuberculosis specialists were keen on extending the conventional medical model into the field of tuberculosis treatment. By introducing new treatments that required specialized skill, they were able to strengthen their own authority in the matter. Furthermore, many tubercular patients who had failed to respond to conservative measures were eager to try technologically advanced therapies.[66] Under these pressures, the distinction between the sanatorium treatment and the hospital treatment of tuberculosis became blurred in Sweden.[67] The enthusiasm for surgical intervention, collapse therapy, illustrates the increasing interest in orthodox medical model among tuberculosis specialists and among their patients. Collapse therapy was introduced into Gothenburg and into Sweden in general in the first decade of the century, and although there were serious doubts about its efficacy and ample evidence of the great risks involved, it soon gained popularity. In the 1920s, no less than 60–70 per cent of Swedish sanatoria patients underwent this treatment.[68] In Britain, collapse therapy became widely available only in the late 1920s and 1930s, when the Ministry of Health encouraged local authorities to provide it.[69]

The Gothenburg health authorities also believed in the benefits of extensive hospital provision. The governmental Tuberculosis Committee recommended that Swedish cities should provide as many sanatorium and hospital beds as there were deaths from tuberculosis annually. With the opening of the new tuberculosis hospital in 1913, Gothenburg achieved the target. In 1914, 388 hospital and sanatorium beds were available for the treatment of pulmonary tuberculosis and 365 people died of the disease during that year.[70] In other words, there were 106 beds for every 100 deaths from the disease. Markedly fewer beds were available in Birmingham, where municipal and poor law authorities together provided 57 hospital beds for every 100

---

[66] *Årsberättelsen 1906*, 42–3; *1909*; 35; *1914*, 50; 'Meddelanden från Göteborgs Läkaresällskaps förhandlingar', *Hygiea* **73** (1911), appendix; *Hygiea* **77** (1915), 685, 752–4; *Hygiea* **78** (1916), 563–79. See also GSA HVN I minutes 2 Nov. 1921, item 239; 4 Jan. 1922, item 20: HVN Samfällda nämnden, minutes 7 Feb. 1928, item 9.

[67] GSH 1907:115; 1910:161; *Årsberättelsen 1909*, 9; 'Sjukvårdsanstalten å Kålltorp'; 'Årsberättelser från hemmet för lungsotssjuka' and 'Årsberättelser från Sjukvårdanstalten å Kålltorp', in *Årsberättelser 1919–1924 II*; G. Neander, 'Anti-tuberkulosarbetets financiering i Sverige. Återblick. Översikt. Önskemål', in *Det Fjärde Nordiska Tuberkulosläkarmötet i Stockholm, 25–27 augusti 1925* (Stockholm 1926), 106–8. For the changes in sanatorium treatment, see also F. Condrau, '"Who is the captain of all these men of death?": the social structure of a tuberculosis sanatorium in postwar Germany', *Journal of Interdisciplinary History* **32** (2) (2001), 244–5.

[68] 'Meddelanden från Göteborgs Läkaresällskaps förhandlingar 1910', *Hygiea* **73** (1911), appendix; *Hygiea* **77** (1915), 752–4; *Hygiea* **78** (1916), 563–79; J. Lundquist, 'Tuberkulosen', in W. Kock (ed.), *Medicinalväsendet i Sverige 1913–1962* (Stockholm 1963), 395–7.

[69] Bryder, *Magic Mountain*, 173–84.

[70] *Årsberättelsen 1913*, 9; *1919*, 19.

deaths from pulmonary tuberculosis.[71] In the 1920s and 1930s, neither city improved its sanatorium provision for adults, but in Gothenburg a large number of new beds were provided for children. In the early 1930s, the difference between the cities was very clear. In Gothenburg there were 175 sanatorium and hospital beds per 100 deaths, while in Birmingham there were only about 60 beds per 100 deaths.[72] Tuberculosis services in both Gothenburg and Birmingham were subsidized by central government grants.[73]

The important role which medicine played in the Swedish anti-tuberculosis campaign can be partly traced to the strong social position held by the leading public health officers. They had access to the centres of policy making and they enjoyed a relatively high status within the medical profession, within the state bureaucracy and within their own local communities. Achieving good results – reducing the death rate from tuberculosis – was important for them, but their status in society gave them considerable latitude. They were able to experiment, to introduce new specialized treatments and technologies, and even make mistakes. Hence it is hardly surprising that they sometimes overestimated the effectiveness of their measures and underestimated the risks involved, belittling research findings which were embarrassing to them.

Studies conducted in the 1930s suggested that the optimism about the new forms of therapy had been largely misplaced. For example, a study of 6,000 tubercular patients who had been treated in the Gothenburg sanatorium during the years 1910–34 made for rather depressing reading. Firstly, the study showed that long-term survival rates were poor. More than half of the patients had died within three years after having been diagnosed with active tuberculosis. Two-thirds had died within five years of diagnosis, and no less than three-quarters within ten years. More depressing, perhaps, was the second result, that patients' prospects of recovery had not improved during the period 1910–34 despite the vastly increased access to medical care and the introduction of surgical methods. The sharp decline in tuberculosis mortality from 3 per thousand population in 1900 to 0.9 in 1934 was, according to this study, entirely due to the fact that fewer people developed active tuberculosis.[74] However, these research findings did not undermine the Gothenburg anti-tuberculosis campaign nor the authority of the public health experts. The hospital and sanatorium treatments may have failed to provide a cure for tuberculosis, but the Gothenburg health authorities were still able to claim the credit for the declining tuberculosis mortality. They argued that in many cases they had managed to break the chain of infection, for example by isolating infectious tubercular patients, and therefore they had protected a large number of people from the disease.

---

[71]   In Birmingham, 633 beds were available for the treatment of pulmonary tuberculosis and 1,107 people died from the disease in 1916; *Annual Report 1916*, 22.

[72]   *GSH 1910:105* and *161*; 'Sjukvårdsanstalten å Kålltorp'; GSA HVN I minutes 4 Dec. 1918, item 229; *Årsberättelsen 1929 I*, 20–21; *1931 I*, 20; *Annual Report 1933*, 72, 87.

[73]   *Årsberättelsen 1910*, 2.

[74]   Öberg, *Läkaresällskap*, 143.

Inspection of Small Flats Another strategy pursued by the Gothenburg health authorities to tackle the problem of tuberculosis was the inspection of small houses and flats. In 1910, the City Council established a system of housing inspection and appointed two female inspectors to visit houses and a Chief Sanitary Inspector to deal with more complicated cases requiring expert knowledge. The purpose of the new municipal agency was twofold. Firstly, the inspectors kept a record of small houses and flats (1–2 rooms), carried out routine inspections of them and gave advice to the inhabitants as to how to look after their homes. Secondly, the inspectors instructed people suffering from tuberculosis in the necessary precautions and persuaded their family members to seek medical advice and be tested.[75] However, keeping all small dwellings and all poor tubercular patients under surveillance soon proved too ambitious an aim for the small organization with three health officers. In the following years, new female inspectors and a medical doctor specializing in tuberculosis were appointed, and in 1915 the Housing Inspection Office and the Tuberculosis Office were separated.[76]

The Tuberculosis Office developed into a dispensary, a centre of diagnosis and observation from which patients were referred to the most appropriate place, home, sanatorium or hospital. The office also provided outpatient treatment and advised tubercular patients and their families. The treatment and advice provided in the dispensary were supplemented by frequent home visits: tubercular patients were visited by a nurse at intervals of two weeks or several months, according to their needs.[77] The nurses collected a considerable amount of information about patients and their circumstances, but they also often went to great lengths to reorganize the everyday lives of the patients and their families. As the Chief Tuberculosis Officer, Gösta Göthlin, noted: 'the purpose of these visits is to organize all possible aspects of the patients' life, whether they concern the dwelling, household, child care, finances, employment, treatment or anything else'.[78] Dispensary staff also made determined efforts to track down consumptives who ignored or tried to conceal early symptoms of the disease. The Gothenburg authorities were convinced that the close supervision of home conditions and the active pursuit of early cases was an effective way of controlling and eradicating tuberculosis. However, what also made this approach attractive to many public health officials was that it provided an 'apolitical' means of managing social problems such as poverty, overcrowding and defective housing.

The role that the Tuberculosis Office played in the anti-tuberculosis campaign became increasingly important over the years.[79] The Housing Inspection Office, by

---

[75] *GSH 1908:252* and minutes 10 Dec. 1908, item 18; *1909:197* and minutes 28 Oct. 1909, item 5; *Årsberättelsen 1911*, 8–13; *1912*, 9–13.

[76] *Årsberättelsen 1915*, 14; *1916*, 22; GSA HVN I minutes 3 Oct. 1917, item 201; 12 Sep. 1923, item 483.

[77] *GSH 1908:252; 1909:197* and minutes 28 Oct. 1909, item 5; *1917:348*, 2–4; *Årsberättelsen 1911*, 10–13; *1912*, 10–13; *1916*, 21–4; *1917 I, 32–4; 1927 I*, 14–17; *1928 I*, 19–25; *1933*, 21–3.

[78] *Årsberättelsen 1912*, 11.

[79] *Årsberättelsen 1915*, 14, 16–18; *1927 I*, 15–17; K.J. Gezelius, 'Göteborgs stads hälso- och sjukvård', in N. Wimarson (ed.), *Göteborg. En översikt vid trehundraårsjubileet 1923* (Göteborg 1923), 353.

contrast, was faced with an impossible task, especially in the 1910s, and was able to do very little to alleviate the plight of the poor. The Chief Tuberculosis Officer argued that the housing problem developed from 'acute' in 1913 to 'catastrophic' by 1917.[80] The deterioration of the housing situation manifested itself very clearly in the everyday lives of many tubercular patients. If the standard of less than 15 cubic metres per adult and 7.5 per child was used to signify overcrowding, the percentage of tubercular families living in overcrowded accommodation rose from 28 to 52 in the years 1913–16.[81] However, housing inspectors could not prohibit landlords from letting out insanitary houses, since in many cases tenants had no other place to go. The gravity of the crisis is clearly illustrated by the fact that in 1916, the housing inspectors were able to close only two houses.[82]

In 1919, the Finance Committee and the Housing Department acknowledged that to resolve the prevailing housing crisis, a net increase of 6,500 flats or single-family houses was needed during the following five years, 1920–24. Both private and co-operative housebuilding being at a virtual standstill, success in easing the housing shortage depended largely on the City Council, which in turn dissipated its time and energy in fierce debates over whether municipal intervention was appropriate or not.[83] During the five-year period 1920–24, the public and private sectors together built 3,092 houses. At the same time, 447 houses and flats were demolished, so that the net increase was 2,645 flats and houses. The housing reform was failing even by its own standards (See Table 5.1).[84] When the Social Democrats managed to consolidate their power in the mid-1920s, public efforts to deal with the housing problem were somewhat intensified. However, only few policy makers campaigning for more active public intervention viewed municipal housebuilding as an answer to the problem of tuberculosis.[85] The factors which primarily prompted the Gothenburg City Council to accept municipal intervention in the housing market were more immediate considerations of class conflict and political circumspection, while the concerns about tuberculosis and poor health in general were clearly of secondary importance. The new council houses were not designed for the section of the population among whom the death rate from tuberculosis was highest, but for more affluent working-class people.

---

[80] *GSH 1913*:337; Göthlin, 'Reformkrav'.

[81] *Årsberättelsen 1916*, 23; *GSH 1917:129*.

[82] *GSH 1909:197*; *Årsberättelsen 1916*, 10–11.

[83] See, for example, *GSH 1917:14* and minutes and discussion 25 Jan. 1917, item 21; *1917:129*; *1923:113* and minutes and discussion 5 Apr. 1923, item 13; *1923:328* and minutes and discussion 13 Sep. 1923, item 13.

[84] *Statistisk årsbok för Göteborg 1925*; *GSH 1923:113*, 5.

[85] *Statistisk årsbok för Göteborg 1925*, 111–12; *1939*, 111; Nyström, 'Åtgärder', 1–16.

	New houses	Demolished houses	Net increase	Target
1920	125	52	73	1300
1921	783	75	708	1300
1922	301	74	227	1300
1923	783	77	706	1300
1924	1100	169	931	1300

Table 5.1   Housebuilding in Gothenburg, 1920–1924.
Source: Statistisk årsbok för Göteborg 1925; GSH 1923:113, 5.

Housing problems were less intense in the late 1920s and in the 1930s than they had been in earlier decades, but they were still of such proportions that housing inspectors encountered great difficulties in enforcing regulations. In 1930, small houses and flats still constituted 57 per cent of the housing stock and 25 per cent of the population lived in overcrowded accommodation.[86] The inspectors often had to confine themselves to collecting information about small houses and to keeping problem houses under constant surveillance. On a number of occasions, inspectors were accused of treating negligent landlords too leniently, but even their fiercest critics admitted that inefficient inspection was not the core of the housing problem.[87]

Birmingham

In the Birmingham anti-tuberculosis campaign, which was motivated by a strong desire to change habits and attitudes, dying patients did not figure prominently. Provision of isolation facilities for people suffering from advanced tuberculosis was not raised as an issue until the 1920s, and even then its importance remained minor. Instead of evoking images of isolation wards, the Birmingham campaign emphasized individual responsibility. The Birmingham authorities were to carry on the Chamberlain tradition and to give people a better chance of leading a healthy way of life, for example by providing them with useful information and by building new working-class suburbs. However, the success of the campaign ultimately depended on whether the individuals seized these opportunities and adopted new attitudes and ways of behaving.

Educational Sanatorium Treatment   The main focus of the Birmingham anti-tuberculosis strategy was sanatoria, where incipient cases of tuberculosis were fortified by various therapies and reformed by health education and orderly, regulated sanatorium life. While in Gothenburg there was no clear line of demarcation between

---

[86]   *Statistisk årsbok för Göteborg 1939*, 103–7; W. Göranson and G. Rosander, 'Vad siffrorna säga om göteborgarens sätt att bo', in *Katalog för Göteborgs stads bostadutställning 'Bo bättre', 1 Maj–1 Juni 1936* (Göteborg 1936), 25–4.

[87]   GSA HVN I minutes 6 Feb. 1929, item 35; 2 Apr. 1930, item 62. *GSH 1923:328* and minutes and discussion 13 Sep. 1923, item 16; *1923:113* and minutes and discussion 5 Apr. 1923, item 13.

sanatorium treatment and hospital treatment of tuberculosis, the Birmingham authorities clearly distinguished sanatoria from hospitals. The main function of the sanatorium treatment in Birmingham was to inculcate in people an orderly, hygienic way of life.[88] Ideally, a sanatorium was in a rural setting, 'in clean bracing country air, away from the smoke of towns and the dust of main roads, sheltered from cold and boisterous winds, elevated, and on a dry soil'. It was at a considerable distance from the city and any railway station, since it was 'undesirable to have too many visitors at a sanatorium, as they unwittingly upset their friends'.[89] The most commonly used therapeutic methods were open-air treatment, healthy abundant diet, tuberculin injections and graduated exercise and labour which were believed to improve both the patients' general health and their lung condition. Another essential part of treatment was strict regulation of life: sticking to the timetable, obeying doctors' instructions and even avoiding profane language.[90]

In Birmingham, the discussion about the value of sanatorium treatment began in earnest in 1905–6, when the City Council urged the Health Committee to take the matter into consideration. After visiting several institutions, the MOH, John Robertson, and the Health Committee came up with the proposal, and the Council approved the establishment of a sanatorium in 1907.[91] While the Birmingham decision-makers were considering the sanatorium question, a heated debate was raging in medical journals about the treatment. In both the *British Medical Journal* and the *Lancet*, many writers cast doubts on the efficiency of the 'mere routine of feed and freeze'. They also strongly criticized the way in which the open-air treatment and establishment of sanatoria were justified in Britain, arguing, for example, that 'there is no good in importing German statistics into the discussion unless a German climate can also be imported'.[92]

The medical profession in Britain was clearly divided over the value of this treatment, and neither side had conclusive scientific evidence to support its position. Predictably, the treatment was usually endorsed by public health officers and by tuberculosis experts who worked in private sanatoria, while the blistering attacks

---

[88]   See, for example, *Annual Report 1923*, 26–7; M. Worboys, 'The sanatorium treatment for consumption in Britain, 1890–1914', in J.V. Pickstone (ed.), *Medical Innovations in Historical Perspective* (London 1992), 47–71; Bryder, *Magic Mountain*.

[89]   *Special Report by the MOH on Consumption*, 26.

[90]   BCA HC minutes 27 Oct. 1908, item 1436; *Special Report by the MOH on Consumption*, 15; *Salterley Grange Sanatorium* (Health Department, Birmingham 1908), 5–7; *Annual Report 1912*, 43–4; H. Thomson, *Pulmonary Phthisis: Its Diagnosis, Prognosis and Treatment* (London 1906), 77–96. For sanatorium life, see also Condrau, '"Who is the captain of all these men of death?"'.

[91]   BCA HC minutes 9 Dec. 1902, item 7782; 11 Apr. 1905, item 9233; 26 Sep. 1905, item 9466.

[92]   A. Don, 'The sanatorium treatment of consumption: is it worthwhile?', *British Medical Journal*, 22 Jul. 1905, 214. See discussion, for example, the letters from F. Bushnell, E. Marriott and E.W. Diver, *British Medical Journal*, 15 Jul. 1905; from T. Dudfield, *British Medical Journal*, 22 Jul. 1905; from J.H. Dally and R. Macfie, *British Medical Journal*, 29 Jul. 1905; 'The sanatorium and the treatment of pulmonary tuberculosis: the question considered in its therapeutical and economic aspects', *Lancet*, 6 Jan. 1906.

came from outsiders, from medical practitioners who were not involved in work among tubercular patients and who would have liked the limited resources to be invested elsewhere.[93] Both the advocates and opponents of the sanatorium treatment were selective, invoking statistical material for their own political purposes.

The Birmingham MOH was an ardent advocate of the treatment. He side-stepped the criticism in the medical journals by arguing that he was well aware of the reasons why the results of sanatorium treatment had been inconclusive in the past. Firstly, in sanatoria treating paying patients, proper records were not usually kept, since 'such a class of people do not like their cases tabulated'. Secondly, working-class sanatoria, where cases were documented, admitted patients at practically every stage of disease, therefore the results could never be good. Robertson claimed that he knew 'of no sanatorium in this country or abroad which is worked on as good lines as it will be possible to work a municipal sanatorium in Birmingham'.[94] The MOH and the Health Committee were not alone in advocating the establishment of a municipal sanatorium in Birmingham. Many local medical practitioners were in favour of the reform, the poor law authorities were more than willing to leave the municipal authorities to accommodate infectious tubercular patients, and the Friendly Societies also urged the Health Committee to provide sanatorium beds.[95]

Salterley Grange, which was the first sanatorium in England entirely owned and managed by a municipality, was finally opened in Birmingham in 1909. This institution admitted only such early cases of tuberculosis who were likely to derive permanent benefit by the treatment offered, and the greatest care was taken to exclude all 'incurable' patients. Most patients stayed in the sanatorium for a short time, usually three months.[96] In 1910, the former smallpox hospital was converted to accommodate 'intermediate' cases of tuberculosis which were not eligible for admission to Salterley Grange Sanatorium, and after central government's generous capital and maintenance grants became available in 1912, the bed provision was extended further. The Tuberculosis Officer argued that by providing sanatorium treatment for 'intermediate' cases of tuberculosis, health authorities prolonged these patients' working lives by years and greatly reduced their capacity to spread infection.[97] The majority of patients in both sanatoria were discharged 'much improved'.[98]

The rate of increase in sanatorium beds, accelerated by central government's favourable attitude and generous grants, peaked in Birmingham in the years 1910–15 and then slowed down during the second half of that decade. The sanatorium treatment was the most important – and certainly the most expensive – element

---

[93]   Worboys, 'The sanatorium treatment'.

[94]   *Special Report of the MOH on Consumption*, 11. See also, Thomson, *Pulmonary Phthisis*, 76–7.

[95]   BCA HC minutes 11 Feb. 1902, item 7275; 11 Mar. 1902, item 7319; 11 Apr. 1905, item 9233; 11 Jul. 1905, item 9395.

[96]   BCA HC minutes 8 Jan. 1907, item 280; 12 Jan. 1909, item 1575; 8 Feb. 1910, item 2229; *Salterley Grange Sanatorium*, 4–5; *Annual Report 1910*, 4–5.

[97]   BCA HC minutes 22 Feb. 1910, item 2249; 26 Apr. 1910, item 2397; 11 Oct. 1910, item 2632.

[98]   BCA HC minutes 12 Jul. 1910, item 2536.

of the municipal anti-tuberculosis campaign in Birmingham.[99] Since the belief in sanatorium treatment had never been based on irrefutable evidence of its efficacy, it could not be eroded by reports suggesting that the treatment was unproductive. Hence sanatoria remained an integral part of British anti-tuberculosis strategies until the introduction of chemotherapy in the 1950s.

Pressure to Achieve Good Results   In Birmingham, the health authorities were clearly under considerable pressure to achieve good results. This was one reason why tubercular patients were so strictly categorized. Salterley Grange Sanatorium rejected patients who were not expected to benefit permanently from the treatment or who had many tubercular cases in their families. By operating a strict admission policy, the health authorities made the results look promising. Intermediate cases or early cases who did not respond well to the treatment were treated in Yardley Road Sanatorium. In this institution, the aim was only to prolong patients' working lives, and the authorities could again show that this goal was achieved.

Conveying an impression that the sanatorium scheme worked well was important, because patients had to be motivated to obey the strict sanatorium regime. Many early cases were still capable of leading a relatively normal life. Persuading them to stay for three months in a sanatorium was far more difficult than to convince dying or seriously ill patients (in Gothenburg) that the best place for them was a hospital. Only three months after the opening of Salterley Grange Sanatorium, the medical superintendent of the institution was asked to report on why patients left the sanatorium before their treatment was completed. The reasons given were domestic troubles, fear of losing employment, and inability to adapt to sanatorium life. To alleviate the financial problems of sanatorium patients, the Board of Guardians was asked to grant as liberal allowances as it could to the dependents of sanatorium patients. The Boards of Guardians promised to be generous, and adopted a Standing Order which made full compliance with the recommendations of the public health authorities a condition for granting relief.[100] This measure did not help. After six months, the medical superintendent again reported that almost 20 per cent of sanatorium patients left before the completion of their treatment. Furthermore, after the First World War, health officers had great difficulty in convincing ex-servicemen suffering from tuberculosis that they would benefit from sanatorium treatment. In Birmingham, 7 per cent of them refused point blank to go to a sanatorium and 11

---

[99]   BCA PH&HC minutes 12 Jan. 1917, item 4167; PHC minutes 16 Jan. 1924, item 7991; 8 Jan. 1932, item 2094; 15 Jan. 1932, item 2134; *Annual Report 1910*, 56–7; *1916*, 22; *1923*, 26; *1933*, 87–8; J. Jones, *History of the Corporation of Birmingham*, vol. V, Part I (Birmingham 1940), 202–3. For the sanatorium provision in other British cities, see Worboys, 'The sanatorium treatment'; N. McFarlane, 'Hospitals, housing, and tuberculosis in Glasgow, 1911–51', *Social History of Medicine* **2** (1) (1989), 59–85; J.V. Pickstone, *Medicine and Industrial Society: A History of Hospital Development in Manchester and Its Region, 1752–1946* (Manchester 1985), 225–35.

[100]   BCA HC minutes 12 Mar. 1909, item 1694–5; 23 Mar. 1909, items 1723 and 1731.

per cent left the institution before completion of the period for which they were referred.[101]

Secondly, good results were crucial from the tuberculosis officers' point of view. The status of the Birmingham tuberculosis officers – and that of public health officers in general – was nowhere near that enjoyed by their Gothenburg counterparts. The career of the tuberculosis officer was not prestigious, and poor results would easily have been taken as proof of their professional incompetence and failure. Furthermore, since the occupational status was low, very few medical doctors in Birmingham or in Britain in general took the job of a tuberculosis officer with a view to specializing in tuberculosis. In consequence, they were not particularly interested in developing the speciality and introducing new therapies.[102] The problems caused by low status were also discussed in the medical journals. One writer argued that '[u]nless sanatorium doctors are put in a satisfactory professional position, as in other countries, the sanatorium movement in Britain will continue to result in economic waste, in ill-digested statistics, and in growing public scepticism'.[103]

As in Gothenburg, a sense of disillusion and disappointment began to invade the minds of the Birmingham health authorities in the 1920s and 1930s. The Chief Tuberculosis Officer for Birmingham, who evaluated the results of the municipal anti-tuberculosis programme in 1928, stated that 'there is no indication either for extreme pessimism or excessive optimism'.[104] With the benefit of hindsight, it is tempting to conclude that neither in Gothenburg nor in Birmingham were the results of sanatorium and hospital treatment good. However, the Birmingham authorities claimed that, although sanatorium treatment did not usually ensure a cure for tuberculosis, it could arrest the advance of the disease and prevent people from becoming sources of infection. Furthermore, the sanatorium treatment had promoted a healthy way of life in the tubercular families and in society in general.[105] Hence the campaign had contributed to the decline in tuberculosis mortality, from 1.4 per thousand population in 1900 to 0.7 in 1934.

With Education Comes Control   The Birmingham health authorities' determination to build sanatoria did not stem only from the desire to provide treatment for early cases of tuberculosis: sanatoria were considered to be intrinsically useful, and a means to a greater end. They were powerful symbols of the healthy, rational and regulated way of life, and their influence was expected to extend far beyond the group of people who were actually treated in them. The MOH argued in 1907 that '[p]atients would be returned to the City every year well informed as to the proper treatment of the disease and public attention would be more and more directed to the

---

[101]   BCA HC minutes 15 Jul. 1909, item 1911; G.B. Dixon, 'The discharged soldier and sanatorium treatment', reprint from the *British Journal of Tuberculosis* (*c.* 1921).

[102]   Bryder, *Magic Mountain*, 72–5.

[103]   R. Macfie, 'The sanatorium treatment of consumption: is it worthwhile?'.

[104]   G.B. Dixon, 'Progress made in combatting tuberculosis', *Journal of the Royal Sanitary Institute* **48** (1928). See also Hardy, 'Reframing disease'.

[105]   *Special Report by the MOH on Consumption*, 9–14.

beneficial effect of fresh air, proper feeding and sanitary surroundings'.[106] Sanatoria served to strengthen the very fabric of society.

Alongside sanatorium treatment, which ranked high in the Birmingham anti-tuberculosis programme, the public health authorities developed some outpatient services. The first tuberculosis inspector was appointed in 1905, and the municipal Anti-tuberculosis Centre was established in 1910. The Centre or Dispensary, as it was often called, provided a relatively limited range of services during its first ten years, but in the course of the 1920s, when more rigid centralism was built into the municipal tuberculosis programme, the scope of the services provided by the dispensary was widened.[107] In Birmingham, as in Gothenburg, the municipal dispensary acted as a clearing house where tubercular patients were selected for publicly owned sanatoria and hospitals. The dispensary was also an outpatient clinic providing medical assistance and advice for a large number of poor patients, and in particular for women and children. In the late 1920s and 1930s, nurses annually visited 6,000–7,000 homes where someone was suffering or was thought to be suffering from tuberculosis or be 'predisposed' to it.[108] Tubercular patients who were being treated by a general practitioner were not usually visited by the municipal inspectors.

In Birmingham, the health instruction given to tubercular patients and their family members was made more efficient by ensuring that health visitors and medical officers were invested with authority derived not only from their expert knowledge, but also from the law. In 1911, the Birmingham City Council approved a by-law which prohibited spitting in streets and other public places.[109] The MOH explained that this regulation, modelled on American by-laws, was aimed at limiting 'spitting on streets, etc. by consumptives who are in infectious condition. In doing this it appears to me that opportunity should also be taken of reducing at the same time the unwholesome and dirty habit of promiscuous spitting on our foot walks.'[110] In order to show that the by-law was not a dead letter, proceedings were taken against a tubercular patient soon after the law had been passed.[111] Furthermore, from 1913, the health authorities were able to confine tubercular patients who 'wickedly spread the infection amongst other members of the household' to a hospital.[112]

To direct educational measures at the patients who needed advice and to intervene in situations where negligent and ignorant patients clearly endangered other people's health, the Public Health Department started to register and card-index patients from an early date. In 1903, it was estimated that about 10 per cent of tuberculosis

---

[106] BCA HC minutes 8 Jan. 1907, item 280.

[107] BCA HC minutes 14 Feb. 1905, item 8956; 22 Sept. 1908, item 1357; 28 Sept. 1909, item 1969; 14 Feb. 1911, items 2877–8; 13 Jul. 1911, item 3231 and the Report to the City Council, 10–11; PHC minutes 12 May 1922, items 6885–6; 28 Mar. 1924, items 8151–2; 14 Dec. 1928; 8 Jan. 1932, item 2094.

[108] *Annual Report 1933*, 76; *1935*, 88.

[109] BCA HC minutes 26 Sept. 1911, item 3272.

[110] *Report on the Spread of Tuberculosis by Indiscriminate Spitting.*

[111] BCA PH&HC minutes 10 May 1912, item 481; 14 Jun. 1912, item 556.

[112] BCA PH&HC minutes 11 Jul. 1913, item 1615.

cases came to the knowledge of the Department through health visitors.[113] These cases were patients who lived in the 'unhealthy areas' where health visitors worked. Voluntary notification was introduced in 1904, and in the following year the MOH estimated that the Department was notified of about 20 per cent of tubercular patients. Almost all of these cases belonged to the 'ignorant and careless' section of the population. From 1908 notification was compulsory for the patients of Poor Law institutions, and from 1912 for all cases.[114] Despite compulsory notification, many patients in Birmingham managed to conceal their disease with the connivance of their 'sympathetic' doctors who did not divulge the confidences entrusted to them. Concealing the disease was even easier in Gothenburg, where the health authorities did not introduce compulsory notification. In 1927, the Chief Tuberculosis Officer for Gothenburg reported that 25 per cent of people who died from tuberculosis had not been on the dispensary's register.

In Birmingham, as in Gothenburg, control measures caused some problems. The Chief Tuberculosis Officer for Birmingham deplored that tubercular patients were often 'treated as lepers of old, shunned by acquaintances, and refused work by employers of labour from a fear of infection'.[115] If the social consequences of sickness caused greater suffering than the disease itself, people took pains to conceal their illness, and thus hampered the campaign. To allay anxieties, the Birmingham authorities endeavoured to qualify their message by conveying an impression that the problem of tuberculosis, albeit complicated and imperfectly understood, was manageable. Tubercular patients whose habits were 'hygienic' and who lived in a 'hygienic' environment did not pose a serious risk to their families, friends and the public. Patients 'with dirty habits', by contrast, were described as always being a danger, as though their disease *per se* was more infectious.[116]

For or Against the BCG Vaccination?

The last section of this chapter examines the Birmingham and Gothenburg campaigns in the context of the international anti-tuberculosis movement. Most studies of tuberculosis campaigns tend to focus on the formulation of policies at national level, making little attempt to integrate national strands into international developments.[117] Yet early twentieth-century campaigns against tuberculosis in Europe and North America were truly an international undertaking. International conferences, journals and study tours, which became commonplace in the late nineteenth and early twentieth centuries, played an important role in the adoption or rejection of innovations. In these forums, some controversial research findings, procedures and therapies such as sanatorium treatment were hailed as important innovations, and

---

[113] *Annual Report 1903*, 28.

[114] BCA HC minutes 22 Dec. 1908, item 1544; 23 Feb. 1912, item 286; *Annual Report 1912*, 39–44.

[115] Dixon, 'The care of the consumptive', 500.

[116] Dixon, *Lectures on the Prevention of Consumption.*

[117] For studies that place national experience into an international context, see Worboys, 'The sanatorium treatment'; Feldberg, *Disease and Class.*

at the same time alternative procedures which could have been equally or more 'effective' were ignored. Likewise, some scientists and research institutes received more than their fair share of publicity and acclaim, whereas others whose research work might have been of equal merit failed to gain positions of influence.[118]

Innovations that commanded respect in the international arena did not always sweep through all countries in Europe and North America. On the contrary, it was sometimes in the interests of public health officials to show that the policy they pursued was not influenced by foreign examples. Scientific nationalism along the lines of 'only American science could resolve American problems' particularly informed policy making in the United States but was by no means restricted to that country.[119] Moreover, the prejudices springing from nationalist sentiments or, for example, from professional enmities were not the only factors that made health authorities wary of certain innovations. Sheer prejudice was usually connected to practical political concerns. If an innovation was clearly incompatible with the local policy legacies or with the broader political and social goals which health policy was expected to further, health authorities were likely to reject it, no matter how much empirical evidence was marshalled to prove its efficiency in reducing death rates.[120]

One important innovation that many health authorities found incompatible with their policies and aims in the first half of the twentieth century was the BCG vaccine. While some countries introduced the vaccine in the 1920s amid uncertainty and controversy, others still rejected the innovation in the 1930s and 1940s, when there was powerful evidence that the vaccine lowered the death rate from tuberculosis. This chapter discusses the motives of the Gothenburg health authorities, who introduced the vaccine to protect children from tuberculosis, and the motives of their Birmingham counterparts, who also sought to protect children, but who rejected the new technological option and clung to their educational approach until the 1950s.[121]

In both Birmingham and Gothenburg, public health officers had an active interest in the international anti-tuberculosis movement. Especially in Gothenburg, travel reports and studies that described anti-tuberculosis measures in other countries formed the core of the 'knowledge' on which decision-makers built their policies. The plans which were put before the Gothenburg City Council served as proof of the health authorities' commitment to follow the lead of, or if possible, to catch up with

---

[118]   For the uptake and rejection of medical innovations, see J.V. Pickstone, 'Introduction', and L. Granshaw, '"Upon this principle I have based a practice": the development and reception of antisepsis in Britain, 1867–90', in Pickstone, *Medical Innovations*, 1–46. See also M. Hietala, *Services and Urbanization at the Turn of the Century: The Diffusion of Innovations* (Helsinki 1987).

[119]   The quote from Feldberg, *Disease and Class*, 138.

[120]   Feldberg, *Disease and Class*; Pickstone, 'Introduction'. For scientific nationalism and foreign innovations, see also I. Dowbiggin, 'Back to the future: Valentin Magnan, French psychiatry, and the classification of mental diseases, 1885–1925', *Social History of Medicine* **9** (3) (1996), 383–408.

[121]   See also, L. Bryder, '"We shall not find salvation in inoculation": B.C.G. vaccination in Scandinavia, Britain and the U.S.A., 1921–60', *Social Science and Medicine* **49** (1) (1999), 157–67.

the most 'progressive' countries.[122] In Birmingham, the attention health authorities gave to ideas that had commanded respect in the international anti-tuberculosis movement was also fairly favourable. Importing foreign innovations into municipal anti-tuberculosis schemes seemed to coincide with the interests of the leading health officers.[123] However, their receptivity to foreign ideas was often checked by city councillors and central government's more sceptical attitude, as the debate about the BCG vaccine shows.

BCG Vaccine and Different Responses

In 1908, the French bacteriologists Albert Calmette and Camille Guérin made a breakthrough that, thirteen years and two hundred trials later, won them the battle for primacy in the development of a tuberculosis vaccine. The public announcement about their success in developing a safe attenuated strain of the bacillus was made in 1921, and in the following year BCG vaccine (Bacillus Calmette-Guérin) was administered to newborn babies at La Charité Hospital in Paris. The news about the vaccine and the apparently successful tests conducted on infants brought Calmette and Guérin instant recognition in France and much favourable publicity, for example, in French-speaking Canada, in Germany and in Scandinavia.[124]

In Gothenburg, the BCG vaccine was introduced in 1927 by Dr Arvid Wallgren, a consultant paediatrician at the Municipal Children's Hospital, who had visited the Pasteur Institute to observe vaccine trials first-hand.[125] Wallgren began work with infants born to families with one or more tubercular patients. These infants were in imminent danger of infection. Within the next few years, as the evidence of BCG's

---

[122]   The Medical Officer of the tuberculosis hospital visited Berlin to study Dr Friedmann's vaccine in 1914. Dr Arvid Wallgren, a consultant paediatrician at the Municipal Children's Hospital, visited the Pasteur Institute in the early 1920s and Anders Wassén, the First City Bacteriologist, in 1926 to follow BCG vaccine trials. The Chief Tuberculosis Officer, Gösta Göthlin, studied tuberculin treatment in Germany in 1921. Nurses Hilda Öhberg and Ruth Hellgren visited dispensaries in London and Amsterdam in 1928. 'Meddelanden från Göteborgs Läkaresällskaps förhandlingar', *Hygiea* **77** (1915), 685; *Årsberättelsen 1914*, 50; GSA HVN I minutes 2 Nov. 1921, item 239; 4 Jan. 1922, item 20; 4 Apr. 1928, item 60; *GSH 1926:258*.

[123]   The MOH, John Robertson, visited the United States in 1922 to familiarize himself with measures to guarantee a pure (tuberculosis-free) milk supply in 1922. The Chief Tuberculosis Officer, Godfrey Dixon, studied the light treatment of tuberculosis in Copenhagen in 1924 and preventive measures in the United States in 1927. The Assistant Medical Officer of the TB dispensary visited Denmark in 1927 and the MOH, H.P. Newsholme, made a tour in the Nordic countries in 1931. BCA PHC minutes 26 May 1922, item 6915; 22 Feb. 1924, item 8140; 8 Apr. 1927, item 10370; 24 Jun. 1927, item 10550; 3 Oct. 1930, item 835; 8 Jan. 1932, item 2094.

[124]   C. Guérin, 'Early History' and S.R. Rosenthal, 'The history of BCG in the United States as a tuberculosis vaccine', in S.R. Rosenthal, *BCG Vaccine: Tuberculosis – Cancer* (Littleton, MA 1980), 35–9; Smith, *The Retreat of Tuberculosis*, 194–203.

[125]   *GSH 1926:258* and minutes 1 Jul. 1926, item 20; A. Wallgren, 'Intradermal vaccinations with BCG virus', *Journal of the American Medical Association* **91** (1928), 1,876–81; Öberg, *Läkaresällskap*, 140.

efficacy and safety mounted, the vaccination programme was extended to include a number of newborn babies and children who were not considered to be high-risk cases. The results of these studies, which Wallgren published in the *Journal of the American Medical Association* in 1934, backed up Calmette's claim that the BCG vaccine was an effective means of reducing tuberculosis mortality.[126]

In 1939, when the Gothenburg health officers reviewed their vaccination programme, all 1,069 children and young adults vaccinated during the period 1927–37 were recalled for check-ups. The evidence that the BCG vaccine worked was impressive, but not entirely conclusive. Firstly, 9 per cent of the vaccinated children could not be traced, 5 per cent were apparently healthy but unable or unwilling to attend for check-up and 1 per cent had died from causes other than tubercular diseases. In consequence, the Tuberculosis Officers actually examined only 85 per cent of the vaccinated children. Secondly, the control group was too small, consisting 'at most of some ten [children]' whose parents had not given their consent to vaccination. While conceding the problems in their study design, the Tuberculosis Officers emphasized that these weaknesses did not detract from the significance of their main result. All 905 cases examined, including 400 children from high-risk families, 'were found to be in good health and without any signs of progressive tuberculous disease'.[127] This research, albeit not conclusive in the eyes of steadfast opponents, convinced the Gothenburg authorities that their decision to start vaccination trials in 1927 had saved a large number of children and young adults from tuberculosis and that it was justifiable to introduce a more general vaccination policy. During 1939 alone, over 600 people were vaccinated.[128]

While Calmette and Guérin had 'found warm friends' among Swedish public health officials, they did not meet similar success everywhere.[129] Much of the staunchest opposition to the BCG vaccine came from American and British medical experts who seized on serious flaws in Calmette's study designs as a weapon against him and his vaccine. While Calmette might have been rigorous in his laboratory work, the unsystematic way in which he conducted vaccination trials on infants and presented his results left him vulnerable to severe methodological criticism. Even Arvid Wallgren, who was to become one of the most vociferous advocates of the BCG vaccine, initially criticized the shaky premises on which Calmette built his arguments, and warmed to the idea of vaccination only when further evidence of

---

[126] A. Wallgren, 'Le rôle de la vaccination anti-tuberculeuse dans la lutte contre la tuberculose infantile' and discussion, *Acta Pædiatrica* **11** (1930), *The Transactions of the Second International Pediatrics Congress, Stockholm August 1930*, 410–13; A. Wallgren, 'Value of Calmette vaccination in prevention of tuberculosis in childhood', *Journal of the American Medical Association* **103** (1934), 1,341–5; H. Anderson and H. Belfrage, 'Ten years' experience of B.C.G.-vaccination at Gothenburg', *Acta Pædiatrica* **26** (1939), 1–5; *Årsberättelsen 1934*, 22.

[127] Anderson and Belfrage, 'Ten years' experience of B.C.G. vaccination', 1–11; *Årsberättelsen 1939*, 24.

[128] *Årsberättelsen 1939*, 24; Lundquist, 'Tuberkulosen', 389–91.

[129] Guérin, 'Early history', 35; T. Dormandy, *The White Death: A History of Tuberculosis* (New York 2000), 339–49.

BCG's efficacy and safety was provided by other researchers.[130] For British and American health officials, who deemed the vaccine incompatible with their anti-tuberculosis campaigns, Calmette's scientifically ill-formulated results and poor statistics provided an excuse not to consider the possible benefits of the vaccine. The trials conducted by Calmette, they argued, were so seriously flawed as to render the results meaningless.[131]

Thus, while health authorities in Gothenburg allocated both money and other resources to the BCG vaccine, sending health officers to France to observe trials, modifying Calmette's study designs and conducting tests on infants, their Birmingham counterparts hung back. In Britain, civil servants in the Ministry of Health and the prominent members of the medical community took either an extremely cautious or openly hostile view of the BCG vaccine, and the Birmingham health officers, for their part, did not see any reason to question this negative attitude. Writing in the *British Medical Journal* in 1931, the Chief Tuberculosis Officer for Birmingham, Dr Godfrey Dixon, summarized the sentiments of many British public health officers, noting that although 200,000 infants had already been vaccinated world-wide, 'Calmette's views as to the freedom from danger of this method of treatment have not been universally accepted. Fears have been expressed that an avirulent strain of bacilli, when injected into the human body, might regain its virulence.'[132]

All Children Under Supervision

Such a marked contrast between the British and Swedish anti-tuberculosis movements was somewhat surprising in view of their many common features. In the 1920s and 1930s, both British and Swedish campaigns were shaped by growing concern about tuberculosis among children. The shift in focus from adults suffering from pulmonary tuberculosis to children who were either suffering from the disease or 'predisposed' to it was motivated by the same line of reasoning that had paved the way for the introduction of infant welfare services and school medical inspection some years earlier. It was argued that health measures which concentrated on providing medical care for sick adults were treating symptoms rather than the root causes of problems. If the health authorities were to succeed in improving the health of the population, they should step up efforts to protect children's bodily health and the morality of their minds.[133]

The principal difficulty health authorities faced in preventing and treating pulmonary tuberculosis in children lay in the absence of agreed criteria as to who were 'predisposed' to tuberculosis and who actually had the disease. The tuberculin

---

[130] *GSH 1926:258*; A. Wallgren, 'Observations critiques sur la vaccination antituberculeuse de Calmette', *Acta Pædiatrica* **12** (1927–28), 120–37.

[131] Feldberg, *Disease and Class*, 125–75; Smith, *The Retreat of Tuberculosis*, 194–203; Bryder, *Magic Mountain*, 138–42.

[132] G.B. Dixon, 'Pulmonary tuberculosis in childhood', reprint from the *British Medical Journal*, 25 Apr. 1931.

[133] H. Hendrick: *Child Welfare: England 1872–1989* (London 1994), 93–128. See also *GSH 1922:398*, 3; Dixon, 'Pulmonary tuberculosis'.

skin tests and autopsies indicated, according to a report which was published in 1913, that about 90 per cent of the urban population in Britain had at some time suffered tubercular infection. Another frequently cited survey, published in 1930, reinforced this view, suggesting that in European cities an average of 20 per cent of children had been infected by the age of 2 and not less than 90 per cent by the time they were 15. An investigation conducted in Gothenburg during the years 1927–38 indicated that 40 per cent of children had been infected before they reached the age of 10.[134]

Clearly, infection with tuberculosis was not synonymous with the development of full-blown disease. But answers to interconnected questions such as who of those infected would eventually develop full-blown disease and what the most important factors were in transforming latent tuberculosis cases into active cases were never to be known with certainty. Nor was this all; tuberculosis officers and other doctors were also hard pressed to define the point at which the infection became a disease. Distinguishing between children who already had incipient tuberculosis and children who did not have tuberculosis but who tested positive and who were weak, pale and undernourished was sometimes even beyond the capacity of experienced specialists. A comprehensive study made in Stockholm's municipal primary schools in 1908 reveals the scale of this problem. According to this research, 1.6 per cent of the schoolchildren showed some signs of active disease, and 2.2 per cent were suspected of having tuberculosis, but the diagnosis could not be confirmed. A decade later, in 1919, the Gothenburg authorities did not seem to have any clearer view of the problem.[135] In 1931, the Chief Tuberculosis Officer for Birmingham published an article in the *British Medical Journal* in which he analysed the difficulties of diagnosing tuberculosis in early childhood.[136]

In public health rhetoric, knowledge was usually equated with the ability to control diseases and with the justification for intervening in homes and in the private world of the family. But, if necessary, lack of knowledge could also be used to justify intrusive measures. Health authorities in both Birmingham and Gothenburg took the view that drawing a definite demarcation line between children who were already suffering from tuberculosis and delicate children who would possibly be affected by it later in life was not only extremely difficult, but also completely unnecessary. It was in the interests of the community to keep all these children under supervision, to examine them from time to time, and to provide them with appropriate treatment. In order to justify the continuous supervision of children who did not have any specific disease and who had not even necessarily been infected with tuberculosis, health authorities introduced a new clinical category. In Birmingham, children who were

---

[134] S. Delepine, *Astor Committee Final Report* 2, 1913, 27 (cited in Bryder, *Magic Mountain*, 3–4); Evans, *Death in Hamburg*, 183; Anderson and Belfrage, 'Ten years' experience of B.C.G. -vaccination'. See also L. Bryder, '"Wonderlands of buttercup, clover and daisies": tuberculosis and the open-air school movement in Britain, 1907–39', in R. Cooter (ed.), *In the Name of the Child: Health and Welfare, 1880–1940* (London 1992), 72–6.

[135] *GSH 1919:34*, 3–5; Kjellin, 'Bekämpandet', 1,332.

[136] Dixon, 'Pulmonary tuberculosis'.

thought to be 'predisposed' to tuberculosis were often labelled as 'pre-tuberculous', while the Gothenburg authorities classified them as 'children susceptible to TB'.[137] In both cities, the definition of this category was basically the same as that used by the British Ministry of Health in its circular of 1927. Pre-tuberculous children were 'delicate children who, owing to family history or environment, may be thought to be predisposed to the disease, but who are not definitely diagnosed as suffering from tuberculosis and are not suspected to be actually so suffering'.[138]

This vague definition opened the floodgates for municipal intervention, often with unclear objectives and lack of concern for the social and emotional consequences of this policy for families. Decision-makers in both Birmingham and Gothenburg were presented with three potential avenues for controlling the spread of tuberculosis among children. Firstly, infants and young children who still tested negative could be protected from infection by removing them from the environment where the danger of infection was imminent or by vaccinating them. Secondly, more emphasis could be placed on the research finding that infection was not synonymous with active disease and that only a small fraction of those infected eventually fell ill. From this perspective, it seemed sensible to mount a concerted campaign to strengthen the bodily resistance of all children – and in particular of those who tested positive and were weak – so that they would grow up healthy and not develop the disease. Thirdly, more hospital and sanatorium beds could be provided for those children who were already suffering from tuberculosis.[139] Although the order of priorities in Birmingham was again different from that in Gothenburg, policy makers in both cities deemed all these three avenues worth exploring. With this decision, they gave considerable power to health officers, who in the name of protecting children from tuberculosis could intervene in many families' everyday lives as they saw fit. The extent to which anti-tuberculosis schemes extended and enlarged health officers' authority over all (poor) children can be illustrated by comparing these schemes to the systems for child care and juvenile justice. Authorities did not only deal with children who were ill, who had shown signs of disturbance or who had committed a crime, but also with children who had not yet fallen ill (pre-tuberculous), who had not yet shown signs of disturbance (pre-psychotic) and who had not yet committed crimes (pre-delinquent).[140]

Technological Solution or Education

While the Birmingham and Gothenburg authorities shared the aim of keeping both tuberculous and pre-tuberculous children under supervision, there were important

---

[137] BCA PHC minutes 27 Jan. 1928, item 10921; 17 Feb. 1928, item 11003; *Årsberättelsen 1916*, 22–3; *1927*, 16.

[138] BCA PHC minutes 8 Apr. 1927, item 10392.

[139] *GSH 1922:398*, 3; Dixon, 'Pulmonary tuberculosis'.

[140] R. Dingwall, J.M. Eekelaar and T. Murray, 'Childhood as a social problem: a survey of the history of legal regulation', *Journal of Law and Society* **11** (2) (1984), 207–32; J. Walker, 'Interventions in families', in D. Clark (ed.), *Marriage, Domestic Life and Social Change* (London 1991), 188–213.

differences in the approaches that explain why the Gothenburg authorities followed France in adopting the BCG vaccine, and why the Birmingham authorities chose a different path. The Gothenburg authorities defined the problem of 'susceptible children' in a way that enabled them to solve it by official action and medical intervention. At first, in the 1910s and 1920s, health officers saw segregation as by far the best means of tackling the problem, since they considered it an impossible task to protect children in families with tubercular patients living in small flats.

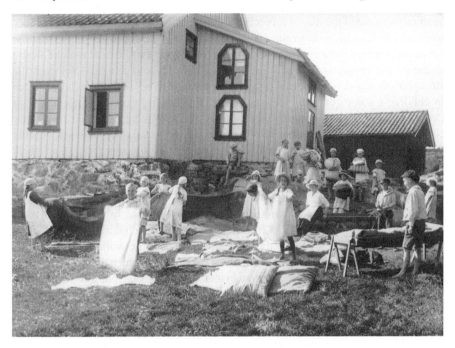

Figure 5.5   Summer colony for children from deprived homes in the 1920s.
Source: Gothenburg City Museum.

These children, they argued, would be infected at some point no matter how hygienic the homes were.[141] The primary strategy was to remove the member of the family suffering from tuberculosis to an institution. In many cases, however, the tubercular patient stayed at home and children who did not have the disease were boarded out in foster-homes in the country or were sent, temporarily or permanently, to a colony or a children's home (Figure 5.5). The purpose of the latter strategy was often twofold – to remove children from continuous exposure to infection in the home, and to fortify their resistance to infection in a 'healthy' rural environment.[142] In the late 1920s, the municipal dispensary annually arranged holidays for no less than 500–600 pre-tuberculous children and for 150 tuberculous children. More importantly,

---

[141] Aronson, 'Dispensärna och tuberkuloskampen'; G. Kjellin, 'Tuberkuloskampens organisation i större stadssamhällen', *Social-Medicinsk Tidskrift* **6** (1929), 224–7.

[142] GSA HVN I minutes 4 Dec. 1918, item 228.

150–250 delicate children from high-risk families were sent to permanent settlements or to children's homes each year. Health officials went about solving this problem in a very systematic way, especially in cases in which the mother was suffering from tuberculosis. From the 1920s, mothers were routinely tested in Stockholm's maternity hospitals, and babies of tuberculous mothers were sent to children's homes or fostered out. This policy was soon adopted by other municipal authorities in Sweden.[143]

The policy of removing children from families with tubercular patients and keeping them out of the way of tubercle bacilli continued to dominate the Gothenburg tuberculosis strategy even in the 1930s. Its popularity stemmed not only from the health authorities' concern over the spread of the disease, but also their desire to ensure the proper socialization of children born to poor families. Yet even the strongest advocates of segregation policy were ready to admit that placing children in children's homes or in the custody of healthy foster-parents was not always a perfect solution. Some mothers categorically refused to be separated from their children, and a growing number of policy makers supported these mothers, arguing that public health measures should seek to preserve family ties rather than break them.[144] These considerations had prompted Swedish public health experts to follow vaccine trials in Germany and France throughout the 1910s and 1920s.

Another important attraction of the BCG vaccine, in the eyes of the public health officers, was that it clearly strengthened the role of science in the Swedish anti-tuberculosis scheme. Modifying Calmette's method of vaccination and conducting trials on infants added significantly to the body of scientific work on tuberculosis, widening the knowledge gap between medical doctors and laymen. In the Gothenburg City Council the proposal to introduce this technological solution was readily adopted, for it satisfied the practical needs of a large number of decision-makers who wanted to save both lives and money.

The Birmingham public health authorities would have liked to follow, to an extent at least, the same path that the Gothenburg authorities had chosen. The Chief Tuberculosis Officer, stressing that the segregation of infectious tubercular patients and young children would go a long way towards breaking the vicious circle of infection within families, was clearly in favour of more extensive hospital bed provision. Moreover, he argued that some arrangements should be made to remove children – and in particular those who tested positive – 'from continuous exposure to infection in the home'.[145] After a study trip to the United States in 1927, he pursued his aim by proposing that the Health Committee should establish a 'preventorium' where children from high-risk families could be sent. Although the Ministry of Health did not approve the plan for grant purposes, the Committee decided to proceed with it. However, a month later the plan was rejected, and the Committee decided to follow the Ministry's guidelines, which clearly stated that pre-tuberculous children as well as tuberculous children who did not need sanatorium treatment 'should be dealt

---

[143] *Årsberättelser 1920–29*; Kjellin, 'Tuberkuloskampens organisation', 225.

[144] Kjellin, 'Bekämpandet', 1,331–40; Kjellin, 'Tuberkuloskampens organisation', 225.

[145] *Annual report 1916*, 23; *1926*, 80; Dixon, 'Progress made', 404; Dixon, 'Pulmonary tuberculosis', 10.

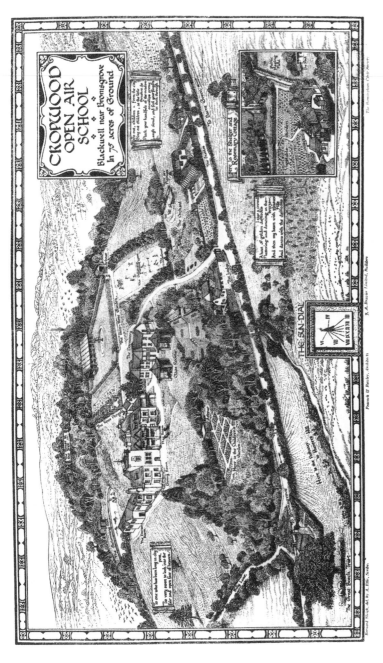

Figure 5.6 Cropwood open-air school in Birmingham. In the 1920s, the Cadbury family donated Cropwood House and acres of surrounding land to be used as an open-air school for children from deprived areas of Birmingham suffering from chest and heart conditions.

Source: Local Studies and History, Birmingham Central Library.

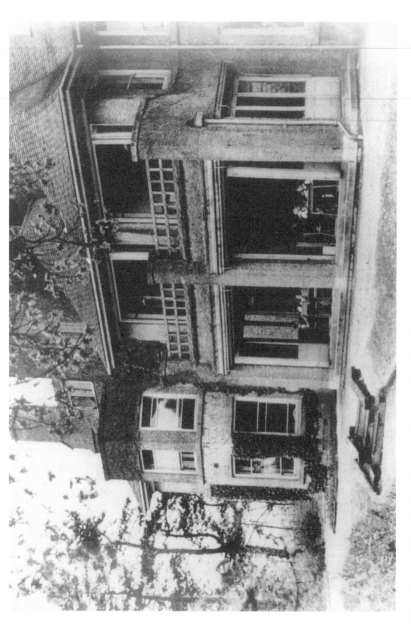

Figure 5.7 A school day in the Cropwood open-air school.
Source: Local Studies and History, Birmingham Central Library

with by Local Education Authorities at Open Air Schools' (Figures 5.6 and 5.7).[146] Holidays for delicate children were arranged by voluntary associations, but these activities were not connected to the municipal anti-tuberculosis schemes.

Had the Chief Tuberculosis Officer and other health officers in Birmingham managed to implement the policy, which placed more emphasis on the segregation of the sick and the healthy, the BCG vaccine would probably have met with a somewhat warmer reception. Yet the Health Committee preferred to stay in the mainstream of the British anti-tuberculosis movement, taking measures which were primarily aimed at eradicating unhealthy habits rather than controlling bacilli. In Britain, as in the United States, the fight against tuberculosis was conceived, first and foremost, as an educational campaign.[147] Promoting self-control and providing children and their parents with adequate information about healthy ways of life, it was argued, was not only the best way to build up children's resistance to tuberculosis and other diseases, but also to create good citizens. The BCG vaccine was a shortcut; it might save some children from tuberculosis, but it did not have the other important virtues of the educational approach. On the contrary, had the vaccine been introduced, people would no longer have been motivated to change their habits. Thus, while the Gothenburg authorities removed children from tuberculous homes or vaccinated them, the Birmingham authorities considered it preferable to send pre-tuberculous children to open-air schools to learn healthy ways of life and to breath fresh air. What both authorities ignored was that many pre-tuberculous children were actually malnourished and suffered from deficiency diseases such as rickets or anaemia. Neither the BCG vaccine nor the open-air school regime treated these conditions effectively.

Conclusion

Comparison of the Birmingham and Gothenburg anti-tuberculosis campaigns shows that scientific knowledge about tuberculosis allowed widely different definitions of the disease. In Gothenburg, where medical practitioners played a dominant role in the formulation of public health policies, tuberculosis was largely seen as a bacteriological and medical problem. Efforts to curb the ravages of the disease focused, firstly, on containing the spread of the bacillus: Infectious tubercular patients were isolated from the rest of society, and children born to high-risk families were boarded out in healthy foster-homes or, in the 1920s and 1930s, were vaccinated against the disease. Secondly, interventionist medicine, which required specialized skills and thus enhanced the professional status of tuberculosis physicians, took precedence over conservative methods in the actual treatment of tubercular patients. In other words, the campaign against tuberculosis was first and foremost a battle against the bacillus fought by experts – scientists, medical doctors and nurses – in laboratories, in hospitals and in the homes of tubercular patients. The efficiency of

---

[146] BCA PHC minutes 8 Apr. 1927, item 10392; 27 Jan. 1928, items 10921 and 10930; 17 Feb. 1928, item 11003; 23 Mar. 1928, items 11095 and 11103. See also F. Wilmot and P. Saul, *A Breath of Fresh Air: Birmingham's Open Air Schools 1911–1970* (Chichester 1998).

[147] Feldberg, *Disease and Class*.

the campaign was increased by instructing people in a healthy way of life, but the educational measures were subordinate to the medical and bacteriological strategies. The 'bacillocentric' approach adopted by the Gothenburg authorities justified control measures which might drastically encroach on the rights of individuals, but at the same time this approach assigned responsibility for disease prevention to experts and, to some extent, absolved individuals of blame for falling ill. The bacillocentric view served to make tuberculosis impersonal.

In Birmingham, where medical practitioners were less influential in shaping health policies, unhealthy habits rather than the bacillus were seen as the 'primary' cause of tuberculosis. In particular, the blame for the disease was placed on alcoholism, poor diet, lack of fresh air and the low standard of personal and domestic hygiene, which were all believed to weaken the body's own defence mechanism. In consequence, the Birmingham anti-tuberculosis campaign focused on instilling in people a sense of responsibility and on instructing them in healthy habits. Interventionist medicine in the treatment of tubercular patients did not gain widespread popularity in Birmingham until the 1930s, and the BCG vaccine was rejected as 'unsafe'. The educational approach was chosen for a variety of reasons. Firstly, educational measures were broadly in line with the British public health traditions, and secondly, the career of the tuberculosis officer was not particularly prestigious in Britain, so many of the officers concentrated their efforts on finding another job rather than on experimenting and introducing new therapies. Thirdly, the BCG vaccine, the isolation of advanced cases, and interventionist medical treatment were seen as measures which might nurture a false sense of security. Solving the problem of tuberculosis demanded nothing less than personal behaviour change. Control measures did not figure prominently in Birmingham, but since the anti-tuberculosis campaign concentrated on unhealthy habits, it inevitably blamed tubercular patients for their disease. The educational approach served to make tuberculosis personal.

Although there were great differences between the Birmingham and Gothenburg anti-tuberculosis campaigns, policy makers in both cities had based their campaigns on 'apolitical' facts. Scientific knowledge about tuberculosis could be reconstructed to justify both the educational approach and the medical approach. Furthermore, the death rate from tuberculosis declined sharply in Gothenburg and Birmingham during the period reviewed here, thus the health authorities in both cities were able to proclaim the success of their approaches (Figure 5.8).

These two anti-tuberculosis campaigns, both of which could be defended as scientific, rational and successful, clearly reflected the interests of the medical profession, but they also furthered other important political aims. Firstly, they served to maintain social order in cities by justifying official *intervention* in 'problem homes' and health promotion that involved constant record-taking, measuring and screening. Secondly, the anti-tuberculosis campaigns served to regulate the local economy by legitimizing both *intervention* and *non-intervention* in the housing market. In some situations, and especially when justifying municipal housing projects that provided homes for lower-middle-class and upper-working-class people, the health authorities emphasized how crucial decent housing was for the health of the population. In other cases, they were determined to show that health could be secured without major changes in the housing market. Justifying non-intervention was politically

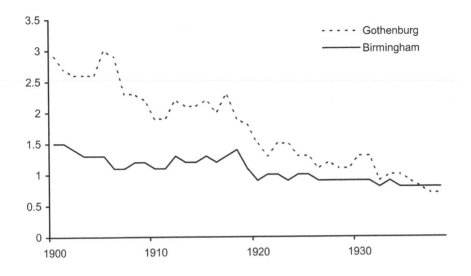

Figure 5.8   Tuberculosis mortality per 1,000 population in Gothenburg and Birmingham, 1900–1938.
Source: Annual Reports of the MOH for Birmingham, 1900–38; Göteborgs hälsovårdnämnds årsberättelser, 1900–38.

important. Colin G. Pooley, who has researched various housing strategies pursued in European countries in the early twentieth century, argues that 'while all main strategies provided good quality housing for more affluent working-class households, they failed to provide a solution to the problem of housing provision for those on genuinely low incomes'.[148]

This was clearly the case in both Birmingham and Gothenburg. In Birmingham, the poorest section of the population, among whom tuberculosis mortality was high, still lived in insanitary back-to-back houses in the late 1930s. The health authorities justified their non-interventionist policy by arguing that unhealthy habits, not defective housing, were the main problem in these unhealthy areas. In Gothenburg, the poorest of the poor lived in overcrowded, small flats throughout the period reviewed here. Public health officials acknowledged that small houses and tuberculosis were a dangerous combination, but they 'solved' the problem by removing infectious patients to hospitals, not by improving housing conditions. When tubercular patients were removed from their homes into a hospital, they became 'cases' and the circumstances in which they had lived and worked were no longer of interest. The problem of slum housing had been shelved in both Birmingham

---

[148]   See C.G. Pooley, 'Working-class housing in European cities since 1850', in Lawton, *The Rise and Fall of Great Cities*, 125–43.

and Gothenburg, and the way in which the problem of tuberculosis was defined legitimized the decision.

When it came to the question of tuberculosis and the family, the Birmingham and Gothenburg health authorities chose different paths. The Birmingham anti-tuberculosis campaign clearly reinforced the rights and responsibilities of biological parents, exhorting them to look after their children. In Gothenburg, by contrast, the mechanistic medicine and wide-ranging welfare calculations encroached on the rights of biological parents and, in many cases, overrode the wishes of tubercular patients and their families. For example, mothers suffering from tuberculosis were sometimes separated from their children. The main aim was that children would live in 'healthy' homes and in a healthy environment. Whether they were taken care of by their biological parents was of secondary importance.

CHAPTER 6

Contesting and Negotiating Public Health Policies

As the case studies in the preceding chapters illustrate, public health campaigns were, to an extent, political answers to political problems. The ways in which the authorities defined health problems and chose responses to them usually served to legitimize and maintain the existing political and socio-economic order in the cities. However, the definitions of health and disease could also challenge existing arrangements and become a vehicle for change. Much was at stake, and yet feelings rarely ran high. At the level of day-to-day policy making, in the meetings of Public Health Committees and City Councils, the political potential of health measures was dimly, if at all, perceived. In analysing urban health problems and in operating infant welfare centres and tuberculosis sanatoria, few health officials – elected or administrative – consciously viewed their activities as means of justifying the existing political and social arrangements.[1] They saw their responsibilities in much more practical terms: they investigated problems and sorted out solutions which were within the budget, could be incorporated into the existing services and were in line with the latest medical knowledge. Health officials may have been conscious of some political and social assumptions on which they based these solutions, but certainly not of all of them.

Health reforms did not arouse much political fervour on the opposing side either. Those who seriously questioned the existing political and economic order usually chose to voice their discontent in other fields than that of public health, even though there were exceptions to the rule. David Barnes, one of the few historians to analyse the extent to which radical groups contested the central tenets of the mainstream medicine, argues that revolutionary syndicalists in *belle époque* France rejected the dominant aetiology of tuberculosis. They claimed that the existing efforts to fight tuberculosis were ineffectual, since they were directed at the superficial manifestations of the disease. If the campaign was to succeed, efforts should be concentrated on tackling poverty and overwork and – in the long term – on overthrowing the capitalist system. In addition to leftist groups, some women's organizations fundamentally questioned the motives of health policies. Lynn Karlsson shows that in Sweden, female members of the Social Democratic Party and trade unions joined forces with middle-class feminists to campaign against a ban on night work that applied to women only. They argued that the ban, which was introduced to 'protect' the health

---

[1]   For the unintentionality of social control, see for example H. Waitzkin, 'A critical theory of medical discourse: ideology, social control, and the processing of social context in medical encounters', *Journal of Health and Social Behaviour* **30** (1989), 220–39.

of women and children, would only buttress the dual, gender-based labour market and therefore add to the hardships many women already suffered.[2]

However, raging debates about the political implications of health measures were usually limited to small circles of radical feminists and left-wing socialists. More moderate working-class and women's organizations, though sometimes seeing municipal and state welfare as a mixed blessing, rarely went so far as to question the dominant aetiology of diseases. Indeed, many people perceived health policies not as part of a wider political drama, but as measures which either alleviated or aggravated their immediate problems. For example, reforms improving access to medical treatment were welcomed by most working-class and middle-class people despite the ideological messages that doctors conveyed in their encounters with them. At the same time, routine medical inspections, which many people considered unnecessary, and health visiting, which entailed 'intrusion' into homes, were less popular, at least in the beginning.[3]

What insulated public health policies from political contention and conflict? The most effective shield against criticism, as the preceding chapters show, was the authority of science. The view that the basic tenets of health campaigns were apolitical and value-free was widely shared by both policy makers and the public.[4] Another factor that often saved health authorities the trouble of justifying their decisions was that health campaigns were not alone in promoting new attitudes to looking after one's body. During the period reviewed here, from the 1890s to the 1930s, stimuli and pressures for adopting a modern, rational and healthy way of life also came from below, from working-class organizations, women's groups and popular movements. Jonas Frykman, who has studied the transformation of 'peasants into Swedes', claims that if the process of discipline and 'civilization' is only examined as a process initiated from above and accepted down below, the rapid modernization of Sweden remains partly unexplained: 'Being on the fringe of Europe, they received new ideas from the Continent and England rather late. Still people were more thoroughly disciplined – in Foucault's sense of the word – than any comparable nation in Europe.'[5]

---

[2]   D.S. Barnes, *The Making of a Social Disease: Tuberculosis in Nineteenth-century France* (Berkeley, CA 1995), 215–46; L. Karlsson, 'The beginning of a "masculine renaissance": the debate on the 1909 prohibition against women's night work in Sweden', in U. Wikander, A. Kessler-Harris and J. Lewis (eds), *Protecting Women: Labor Legislation in Europe, the United States, and Australia, 1880–1920* (Urbana, IL 1995), 235–66.

[3]   P. Thane, 'The working class and state "welfare" in Britain, 1880–1914', *The Historical Journal* 27 (4) (1984), 877–900; L. Marks, *Metropolitan Maternity: Maternal and Infant Welfare Services in Early Twentieth Century London* (Amsterdam 1996), 263–89; R. Klein, *The New Politics of the National Health Service* (London 1995), 70.

[4]   Although people may have been sceptical about some research findings, they usually retained confidence in the ideal of science as a value-free means of resolving problems. For discussion, see R.D. Apple, *Vitamania: Vitamins in American Culture* (New Brunswick, NJ 1996); C. Hamlin, *A Science of Impurity: Water Analysis in Nineteenth-century Britain* (Bristol 1990), 1–15, 299–305.

[5]   J. Frykman, 'In motion: body and modernity in Sweden between the World Wars', *Ethnologia Scandinavica* 22 (1992), 36–51.

A third factor that helped persuade the public and win their approval for health measures was the ambiguity of health policies. No matter how coherent and internally organized policies appeared to be, they were always fissured by competing interests and aspirations. Owing to the contradictions, health policies were compatible with a variety of political perspectives. People subscribing to very different 'world views' – conservatism, socialism, militarism and feminism – could all feel that health policies reflected, at least to some extent, their values and interests. In examining the welfare reforms introduced in Britain between 1906 and 1914, David Vincent makes the same point, claiming that 'most Labour MPs saw [these reforms] as a stepping-stone towards something much better, and many Liberals regarded them as a bulwark against something much worse'.[6]

The ambiguity of health policies served to confine conflicts in another way, too. The contradictions in policies and the differences of opinion among health officials opened up opportunities for 'ordinary' city-dwellers to articulate their demands and to participate in the negotiation of policies. This chapter explores the ways in which health policies were contested and negotiated in Birmingham and Gothenburg, focusing in particular the layers of consensus and conflict in the debates concerning infant mortality and tuberculosis. The discussion begins with women activists and their perceptions about infant and maternal health care, and ends with working-class activists and their views of anti-tuberculosis work.

Women's Reform Activities

The burgeoning literature on women's voluntary efforts and the rise of the welfare states has shown that middle-class women, despite being at the margin of or entirely excluded from the official political process, had an important role in shaping health campaigns. They exerted influence on the campaigns, sometimes by openly protesting against the official policies, but more often by creating new innovative services which, in their opinion, answered the needs of women and children better than the existing services.[7] Among the most influential contributions to this debate have been Seth Koven's and Sonya Michel's articles on maternalist politics and the origins of the welfare states, in which they use the concept of 'maternalism' to describe ideologies that 'exalted women's capacity to mother and extended to society as a whole the values of care, nurturance, and morality'. As a prime example of maternalist activism in which women entered into political arena on the basis of

---

[6]   D. Vincent, *Poor Citizens: The State and the Poor in Twentieth-century Britain* (London 1991), 38.

[7]   See, for example, S. Koven and S. Michel, 'Womanly duties: maternalist politics and the origins of welfare states in France, Germany, Great Britain, and the United States, 1880–1920', *American Historical Review* **95** (4) (1990), 1,076–108; S. Koven and S. Michel (eds), *Mothers of a New World: Maternalist Politics and the Origin of Welfare States* (New York 1993); G. Bock and P. Thane (eds), *Maternity and Gender Policies: Women and the Rise of European Welfare States 1880s–1950s* (London 1994); B. Jordansson and T. Vammen (eds), *Charitable Women: Philanthropic Welfare 1780–1930: A Nordic and Interdisciplinary Anthology* (Odense 1998).

their 'difference' from men, and especially on the basis of their motherly qualities, Koven and Michel cite early twentieth-century maternal and child welfare campaigns. They also examine the extent to which women, individually and through voluntary organizations, were able to shape maternal and child welfare schemes in different countries. Their conclusion is that 'weak states' such as the United States and Britain, where women's organizations flourished, allowed women more political space in which to develop the welfare schemes than did 'strong states' such as Germany and France.[8]

The maternalism paradigm sheds light on important aspects of the emergence of state welfare structures, and in particular on the interaction between private and public welfare contributors. However, Koven's and Michel's approach also has its limitations. In emphasizing maternalism as the defining core of many women's vision of themselves and of politics, Koven and Michel virtually ignore other possible contexts of self-definition. Moreover, they have been criticized for presuming that motherhood as a common female instinct, if not experience, united women across racial, ethnic and class lines and enabled white middle-class women altruistically to identify with women less privileged than they.[9] Finally, as to the differences between weak and strong states, Nordic feminists especially have regarded the model as too restrictive, and have distanced themselves from the hostile attitude towards the state which Koven and Michel, among many other American feminists, have taken.[10] The following case study builds on these discussions and examines how women activists in Birmingham and Gothenburg contested policies pursued by male-dominated municipal departments and committees. Moreover, the aim is to explore the impact of local government structures on strategies available to women. Were women in Gothenburg, where policy making structures were centralized, less influential in shaping maternal and infant welfare schemes than women in Birmingham? The main attention in the section focuses on middle-class women, but there is some discussion about working-class women as well.

Birmingham

While middle-class women gave their time and money generously to many charitable activities in late nineteenth-century Birmingham, for some reason health

---

[8]   Koven and Michel, 'Womanly duties'; S. Koven and S. Michel, 'Introduction: "mother worlds"', in Koven and Michel, *Mothers of a New World*, 1–42.

[9]   For discussion see E. Boris and S.J. Kleinberg, 'Mothers and other workers: (re)conceiving labor, maternalism, and the state', *Journal of Women's History* **15** (3) (2003), 90–117; K.K. Sklar, A. Schuler and S. Strasser (eds), *Social Justice Feminists in the United States and Germany: A Dialogue in Documents, 1885–1933* (Ithaca, NY 1998).

[10]   For discussion about Koven and Michel's hypothesis, see for example C. Carlsson Wetterberg, 'Kvinnorörelse och välfärdsstat – Sverige/Schweiz: några tankar kring en komparativ studie', in B. Gullikstad and K. Heitmann (eds), *Kjønn, makt, samfunn i Norden i et historisk perspektiv*, vol. 1 (Dragvoll 1997), 155–81; A. Anttonen, 'Hyvinvointivaltion naisystävälliset kasvot', in A. Anttonen, L. Henriksson and R. Nätkin (eds), *Naisten Hyvinvointivaltio* (Tampere 1994), 203–26. See also J. Lewis, *Women in Britain since 1945: Women, Family, Work and the State in the Post-war Years* (Oxford 1992), 120–21.

education attracted relatively little philanthropic support. From the 1870s, the MOH tried in vain to encourage local 'philanthropic ladies' to follow the example set by the Ladies' Branch of the Manchester Sanitary Association and introduce a health visiting service. By 1899, no voluntary society had taken it upon itself to organize the service, and the Birmingham Health Committee saw no other option but to appoint municipal visitors.[11] The attempt to persuade middle-class women to establish a milk depot was not successful either.[12] However, the turn of the century witnessed a major change of heart among the women activists. Many women who had been thinking that alleviating urban health problems was not within the scope of their charitable activities became convinced that their contribution to maternity and child welfare was indispensable. The change in attitudes was soon reflected in the work of many old and newly established voluntary organizations. In 1916, voluntary agencies ran seven infant welfare centres, arranged sewing and cooking classes, supplied meals for nursing mothers, organized training courses for midwives and provided hospital beds for maternity cases.[13]

One of the most influential Birmingham societies working with mothers and infants was the Birmingham Infants' Health Society (BIHS) established in 1907. While the BIHS was largely run by women activists, it was not an exclusively female organization. To strengthen its role and authority, the Society formed strong ties with the local medical and public health establishment, a thoroughly male-dominated world. It included male medical practitioners and health officials on its Board, dutifully borrowed the MOH's words in its reports, and co-operated with the Public Health Department in its everyday work. The co-operation ran smoothly, since the services offered by the BIHS in St. Bartholomew's Ward had much in common with those provided by the Health Department in other slum areas.[14] However, there were also differences between the approaches.

Negotiating with the Authorities   Rather than accepting the 'official' definition of the infant mortality problem for the basis of their work, medical women and men working for the BIHS launched their own studies. As with the Health Department, their point of departure was the finding that breast-fed babies had a better chance of survival than their bottle-fed peers. However, while the MOH and the Health Committee

---

[11]   *Annual Report of the Medical Officer of Health for Birmingham* (hereafter *Annual Report*) *1877*, 10; *1880*, 22; *1899*, 34–9; Birmingham City Archives (BCA) Birmingham Health Committee (HC) minutes 24 Jan. 1899, item 5534; 14 Feb. 1899, item 5559; 28 Mar. 1899, items 5666–7.

[12]   BCA HC minutes 30 May 1899, item 5773; 26 Sept. 1899, item 5908.

[13]   BCA Birmingham Public Health and Housing Committee (PH&HC) minutes 22 Dec. 1911, item 78; 12 Jan. 1917, item 4167. *Report of the MOH on Child Welfare in 1913* (Public Health and Housing Department, Birmingham 1914), 13–16; 'Report of the MOH on maternity and child welfare during 1916', in *Annual Report 1916*, appendix, 13–14; J.E. Jones, *A History of the Hospitals and Other Charities of Birmingham* (Birmingham 1909), 55–8.

[14]   *Reports of the Birmingham Infants' Health Society* (hereafter *BIHS*) *1908–22*. From 1918, the name of the Society was The Floodgate Street Maternity and Infant Welfare Centre.

ended up emphasizing maternal ignorance and married women's employment as the major culprits responsible for the prevalence of bottle-feeding and therefore the high infant mortality, the BIHS doctors gave considerable weight to the role of poverty in influencing infant feeding. They pointed out that half-starved mothers, some of whom lived only on tea and toast, were unable to produce sufficient quantities of good quality breast-milk, and in consequence their babies, even if breast-fed, 'were considerably below the standard scale'. If the campaign was to succeed in desperately poor areas such as St Bartholomew's Ward, nursing mothers living below the poverty line should be provided with free meals, and infants who had to be bottle-fed should be provided with sterilized milk. The BIHS did not establish a milk depot, but it started supplying meals for nursing mothers in 1908, and expanded the service in 1913. Moreover, in the times of extreme hardships these efforts were intensified. For example, during the coal strike in 1912, the BIHS provided almost 2,000 lunches 'consisting of cocoa and meat or cheese sandwiches'.[15]

The problem of poverty figured more prominently in the reports of the BIHS than those of the Public Health Department, the difference being especially pronounced in the early 1910s, when the Department placed strong emphasis on individual responsibility.[16] The difference in approaches can be partly explained by the limited resources the BIHS had. No one expected a voluntary society with a budget of £100–200 a year to solve the problem of poverty, so the BIHS was able to address the issue. The Birmingham Corporation, by contrast, had means to alleviate poverty, but the majority of policy makers were ready to deal with it only if it was defined as a behavioural and not a structural problem.

In addition to meal provision, the BIHS developed other new services. In 1910, when the Health Department still concentrated exclusively on infants and their mothers, the BIHS introduced 'toddler consultations', where pre-school children were examined and their mothers were advised on child care. The BIHS doctors pointed out that there was a real need for this type of service in poor districts, where mothers often treated children 'more like grown-up people; they have the same food as their parents, and have a bath only occasionally'.[17] Apart from toddlers, the Society also sought to reach expectant mothers, who were offered general advice as to their health and, if necessary, were encouraged to seek medical attention.[18]

The BIHS programme was by no means a radical departure from the municipal policies. Indeed, more radical views were expressed within the Health Department, for example by an assistant MOH, Jessie Duncan. As a rule, the BIHS introduced services which the MOH, John Robertson, and other reform-minded health officials approved, but which they were unable or unwilling to push through in the sphere of municipal policy making. The BIHS did not contest any central tenets of the municipal campaign, least of all the links between infant welfare, the male-

---

[15]   *Report of the BIHS 1908*, 8–11; *1909*, 7–10; *1910*, 27; *1912*, 22–23; *1913*, 14, 25. See also V. Fildes, 'Breast-feeding in London, 1905–1919', *Journal of Biosocial Science* (1992), 53–70.

[16]   *Reports of the BIHS 1913–1915*; *Report of the MOH on Child Welfare in 1913*.

[17]   *Report of the BIHS 1910*, 15; *1911*, 20–22.

[18]   *Report of the BIHS 1910*, 18–19.

breadwinner family model and the ideal of self-supporting families. However, while the BIHS and the Health Department shared the same objectives, they diverged in the means by which to achieve them. The Department based the campaign rather strictly on normative patterns of familial dependence and maintenance. For example, they stuck to the principle that the father was responsible for maintaining the family and that the provision of free meals or any other measure undermining his sense of responsibility would be harmful, whatever the circumstances. The BIHS approach was more in line with the Minority Report of the Royal Commission on the Poor Laws (1909), which recommended that the treatment of poverty be 'adapted to the needs of individuals'.[19] The BIHS adapted its programme, to an extent, to the actual patterns of family maintenance, providing meals for the poorest mothers, many of whom were 'wives of either thriftless wastrels or men who were suffering from some long illness such as consumption'.[20] Some support at the right time and in the right place, the BIHS seemed to conclude, would save babies, but could also help families become self-supporting and (re-)establish the 'normal' gender roles.

Women's voluntary organizations clearly made an important contribution to the infant welfare campaign by addressing issues that the male-dominated municipal committees dismissed as controversial or relegated as unimportant. In Birmingham, the male-dominated committees and women-run voluntary organizations together managed to achieve something which neither side could have managed alone. The results of the interaction were manifest in specific plans and concrete measures in the years 1914–20, when the Birmingham authorities were reappraising their policies. For example, the Committee established a number of new infant welfare centres and extended the scope of their work by introducing medical check-ups for preschool children and ante-natal consultations for pregnant women, services that had been pioneered by the BIHS.[21] In 1916, the Committee finally decided to provide subsidized meals for the poorest mothers, a service that the BIHS had run for eight years.[22]

Paradoxically, the decision of the City Council to commit itself to defraying 80 per cent of voluntary infant welfare centres' expenses was the beginning of the end for voluntary centres. The decision, taken in 1919, meant that the municipal authorities together with the Ministry of Health shaped the course and goals of the campaign, and women activists running voluntary centres were pushed further and further from the centre of decision-making.[23] One after another, voluntary societies informed the Health Committee that they were unable to continue running centres because of difficulty in raising money and in finding voluntary workers. During the

---

[19] J. Harris, *Private Lives, Public Spirit: Britain 1870–1914* (London 1994), 239–41.

[20] BCA Birmingham Maternity and Child Welfare Sub-Committee (M&CWSC) minutes 4 Feb. 1916, item 36. See also *Annual Report 1914*, 20–21.

[21] 'Report of the MOH on maternity and child welfare during 1916'; *Report of the BIHS 1910*, 15, 18–19; *1911*, 20–25; *1914–15*, 20; *1915–16*, 15.

[22] BCA M&CWSC minutes 7 Jan. 1916, items 19–20; 4 Feb. 1916, items 36 and 36a; 3 Mar. 1916, item 62; 2 Mar. 1917, item 236; 4 May 1917, items 281–2; 5 Oct. 1921, item 992 and document 2. See also *Annual Report 1932*, 110–11.

[23] BCA M&CWSC minutes 7 Feb. 1919, item 563; Ministry of Health, *Maternity and Child Welfare: Circulars and Memoranda No 12, 1919* (London 1919).

period 1916–26, the number of voluntary centres in Birmingham declined from 7 to 1, while the number of municipal centres grew from 8 to 21.[24] Very few of the volunteer BISH activists managed to create new roles for themselves in municipal policy making. One member, Mrs Rosa Walker, who was involved in establishing the Society, was appointed as a co-opted member of the Maternity and Child Welfare Sub-Committee in 1915.[25] As a rule, however, organizations working exclusively among mothers and children were not stepping-stones to municipal committees. By looking at the affiliations of the nine women who were members of the Birmingham Public Health Committee and the Maternity and Child Welfare Committee during the period 1918–39, two paths to the committees may be discerned. For middle-class women, the best training grounds were the boards of guardians, other official bodies like the National Health Insurance committees, or voluntary societies dealing with wider social problems such as poverty and housing. The working-class women appointed to the Committees had acquired political expertise in trade unions, in the co-operative movement or in the Labour Party.[26] In the 1920s and 1930s, the content of child welfare services was determined by appointed and elected officials, men and women who had either professional qualifications or 'wider' political expertise, not by volunteer activists who focused their claims to develop welfare programmes exclusively on the traditional female sphere of competence.

Working-class women warmly welcomed the municipalization of maternity and infant services despite the fact that voluntary societies had usually been faster to react to their wishes than the municipal authorities.[27] The great appreciation of municipal services is manifest, for example, in the minute books of the Duddeston Branch of the Birmingham Women's Co-operative Guild. In the 1920s, the branch often invited officials from the Birmingham Health Department and the City Council to give talks about municipal services and arranged for its members to visit municipal hospitals and other institutions.[28]

Contesting the Authorities' Views   While the BIHS and other similar organizations working in close co-operation with the Birmingham Health Department shaped health policies in subtle ways, some other women's groups challenged the authorities' views more vigorously. They joined forces against some policy decisions where demographic or moral objectives were blatantly pursued at the expense of women's

---

[24]   'Report of the MOH on maternity and child welfare during 1916', 13–14; *Annual Report 1925*, 92–4; BCA Birmingham Maternity and Child Welfare Committee (M&CWC) minutes 10 Dec. 1920, item 691; 11 Mar. 1921, items 720 and 725; M&CWSC, minutes 2 Mar. 1921, item 886; 29 Jun. 1921, item 985; 24 Mar. 1926, item 1819. See also F. Woodcock, 'The voluntary worker in our welfare centre', *City of Birmingham Maternity and Child Welfare Magazine* (1934), June, 18.

[25]   BCA M&CWSC minutes 12 Nov. 1915, item 1; *Report of the BIHS 1908–17*.

[26]   *Cornish's Birmingham Year Books 1918–39*. See also P. Hollis, *Ladies Elect: Women in English Local Government 1865–1914* (Oxford 1987), ch. 9–10.

[27]   See, for example, BCA HC minutes 14 Jun. 1904, items 8710 and 8714; 14 Feb. 1905, item 9123; 11 Jul. 1905, item 9411; 22 Dec. 1911, item 78; 10 Jan. 1913, item 1063.

[28]   BCA Women's Co-operative Guild, Duddeston Branch minutes 12 Jul. 1926, 11 Jul. 1927; 5 Sept. 1927; 19 Mar. 1928; 16 Jul. 1928; 15 Oct. 1928.

health or where professional women were denied the opportunity to combine paid work with family life. The study of these protests does not lend support to Koven's and Michel's argument that women activists working with mothers and children entered into the political arena on the basis of their 'difference' from men, not their 'equality'. Rather, it substantiates Ann Taylor Allen's view that women activists did not find 'difference' and 'equality' mutually exclusive.[29]

A prime example of a policy decision where demographic and moral objectives were given priority over women's health was the Birmingham Health Committee's decision in 1931 not to provide family planning advice. As discussed in Chapter 4, the debate about birth control intensified in 1930, when the Ministry of Health gave local authorities permission to give birth control advice in 'cases where pregnancy would be detrimental to health'. Encouraged by the Ministry's memorandum, the Birmingham Women's Welfare Centre, the Birmingham Women's Co-operative Guild and the Women's Advisory Council of the Birmingham Labour Party urged the Maternity and Child Welfare Committee to establish a birth control clinic.[30] These requests found little favour with the Committee and the MOH, H.P. Newsholme, who warned that the mechanical methods of contraception were 'likely to lead to far graver evils that [they] purport to remedy'. He especially emphasized the damage caused to the marriage relationship by women who would apply the methods 'without the knowledge of the husband', and the harm done to children who would not have siblings. For the sake of their marriage and children, women should be ready to 'risk some degree of stress during the childbearing period'. Moreover, in cases where a future pregnancy posed a serious risk to the mother's life, abstinence would be a better choice than unreliable mechanical methods.[31]

The women campaigning for birth control advice, from both the middle and working class, were not easily defeated. A deputation consisting of female medical practitioners and representatives of working-class women's organizations drew the Committee's attention to the serious problems caused by too frequent pregnancies. Lack of access to advice on birth control was, so it was argued, 'responsible for much unhappiness and ill-health and [was] calculated to drive overburdened mothers to ignorant advisors and to agencies associated with dubious types of commerce'. In defending their case, the women sometimes used arguments based on the notion of 'equality' and the idea of women's individual rights, and sometimes arguments stemming from the notion of 'difference' and the idea of women's and men's complementary roles. While the MOH stated that mother's needs should be balanced against the needs of their children and their marriage, women activists argued that mothers whose health was at risk had a 'right' to birth control advice. However, at the same time women activists also used a maternalist argument, pointing out that the

---

[29] A. Taylor Allen, *Feminism and Motherhood in Germany 1800–1914* (New Brunswick, NJ 1991), 57–8.

[30] BCA M&CWC minutes 12 Dec. 1930, item 464; M&CWSC minutes 17 Dec. 1930, item 350.

[31] BCA M&CWSC minutes 14 Jan. 1931, item 369 and document 22. See also M&CWC 23 Jan 1931, items 519–20; 'Birth control problems: no instruction to be given in Birmingham' and 'Two maternity problems', *Birmingham Post*, 24 Jan. 1931.

establishment of a municipal birth control clinic would 'result in happier children'. Within a few years, the campaigners achieved their aim. In 1935, the Birmingham City Council decided by 58 votes to 55 to establish a clinic, where advice was given to married women suffering, for example, from tuberculosis or heart disease.[32]

Similarly, women activists stressed both women's individual rights and their complementary role, when the Health Committee decided in 1930 that female medical practitioners working for the infant welfare centres had to give up their positions upon marriage. The Birmingham Branch of the National Council of Women and the Birmingham District Medical Women's Association sent a deputation to impress upon the Committee that women doctors should be allowed to continue working after getting married. While some members of the deputation argued that an 'individual should have the right to take up such work as he or she was qualified to perform', some others used a maternalist argument, pointing out that it was in the interest of the authorities to employ married female doctors who were 'fully developed women' 'with an enthusiasm for marriage and children and a personal experience of the parent-craft which they were to teach'. The Committee assented to the request.[33] In the campaigns launched to improve the rights and welfare of women and children, the arguments based on 'equality' and those based on 'difference' coexisted. The women's campaigns to change the conventional gender contract, like the health authorities' campaigns to buttress it, were fraught with ambiguities.

Gothenburg

In nineteenth-century Gothenburg, *Sällskapet för uppmuntran av öm och sedlig modersvård* (The Society for Encouraging Tender and Moral Motherly Care) was the most important of the voluntary societies 'protecting' motherhood among the poorest of the poor. The Society offered either casual work such as sewing and weaving or direct financial assistance to women who had difficulty maintaining their children. By setting strict conditions for such assistance, the Society sought to ensure that in alleviating poverty, they also instilled a sense of responsibility in mothers. All unmarried mothers and mothers who sent their children out to beg were without exception deemed unworthy of philanthropic support.[34]

---

[32] BCA M&CWSC minutes 14 Jan. 1931 item 369; M&CWC minutes 23 Jan. 1931 item 519; 11 Mar. 1932 item 912; 8 Apr. 1932 item 919. See also 'Birth control problems', *Birmingham Post* 24 Jan. 1931; 'Birth control advice – Birmingham to have a clinic', *Birmingham Post*, 9 Jan. 1935; *Annual Report 1935*, 148.

[33] BCA M&CWC minutes 9 Jan. 1931 item 499; 23 Jan. 1931 item 514; 'Ban on marriage removed', *Birmingham Post*, 24 Jan. 1931.

[34] Göteborgs universitetsbibliotek (GUB) Kvinnohistorisk arkiv (KA) Sällskapet för uppmuntran af öm och sedlig modersvård, Handlingar 1877–1965: *Några anteckningar om Sällskapet för uppmuntran af öm och sedlig modersvård* (Göteborg 1914); *80-års berättelse, 1849–1929* (Göteborg 1930). See also B. Jordansson, 'Women and philanthropy in a liberal context: the case of Gothenburg', in Jordansson and Vammen, *Charitable Women*, 65–88.

Although 'the gospel of cleanliness, godliness, and needlework' which the Sällskapet för uppmuntran af öm och sedlig modersvård brought to working-class homes shared some goals with the early twentieth-century infant welfare campaign, there was no direct line of continuity between the campaigns. None of the ladies sitting on the Board of the Society was active in developing the infant welfare schemes in the early twentieth century.[35] While the old networks of philanthropic activity failed to become an innovative force, some new societies forged an important role for themselves. The most influential was *Föreningen Mjölkdroppen*, established in 1903, which operated milk depots. Within a few years the Society opened six outlets, which meant that Gothenburg was better provided with sterilized milk for its infants than Stockholm, where the same number of depots catered for a much larger potential clientele. An important contribution to the Gothenburg child welfare campaign was also made by *Föreningen Barnavärn* and other societies which provided nurseries for infants and toddlers, helping mothers reconcile work with childrearing.[36]

Negotiating with the Authorities   The dominance of the medical approach in the Gothenburg campaign was profoundly reflected in the work of Föreningen Mjölkdroppen. Unlike the BIHS and other similar Birmingham organizations, where volunteer lady activists played an important role, Föreningen Mjölkdroppen was firmly in the hands of medical practitioners. According to the rules of the Society, at least two of the eight Board members were to be medical practitioners, but it was standard practice that they had half of the seats. What further consolidated the power of medical experts was that the president of the Society was usually a medical practitioner holding a strong position in the community. For example, during the first five years, 1903–8, the Society was led by the First City Physician, Karl Gezelius. The central role of medical practitioners meant that the Society was fairly male-dominated. Unlike the exclusively male Health Committee, the Society provided women with an opportunity to participate in policy making from the early years of the twentieth century, and the women who were appointed as Board members, such as Dr Gärda Lidforss-af Geijerstam and foster care inspector Hilda Enander, certainly left their mark on the work of the Society. Yet the dominant position of men was always assured. From the establishment of the Society in 1903 to the 1940s, the majority of the Board members as well as medical practitioners working for the milk depots and infant welfare centres were men.[37]

---

35   GUB KA Sällskapet för uppmuntran af öm och sedlig modersvård, Handlingar 1877–1965: *Några anteckningar*; *80-års berättelse*. The quote is from F.K. Prochaska, *Women and Philanthropy in Nineteenth-century England* (Oxford 1980), 145.

36   *Göteborgs Stadsfullmäktiges Handlingar* (hereafter *GSH*) *1909:6*; *1909:252* and minutes 7 Jan. 1910, item 6; *1910:59*; *1911:27* and minutes 16 Feb. 1911, item 26; *1911:264*. See also F. Carlberg, 'Frivilligt arbete för späda barn i Göteborg', *Social Tidskrift* (1908), 537–8; I.-L. Lundén, 'Från mjölkdroppe till barnavårdscentral – historik och utveckling', *Tidskrift för Sveriges sjuksköterskor* **37** (1970), 198–201.

37   *GSH 1909:252*, 25–6; *1910:59*; *1911:27*; *Föreningen Mjölkdroppens barnavårdscentraler i Göteborg, Årsberättelser för 1930, 1935, 1938*; P. Karlberg, 'Barnhälsovården', in G. Carlson et al., *Sjukvården i Göteborg 200 år* (Göteborg 1982), 194–8.

Given the close contacts and the overlap of people between Föreningen Mjölkdroppen and the Health Department, differences in the aims were not likely to be significant. The work of the Society, like that of the Department, was based on the conception that infant mortality was largely a medical problem to be defined and resolved by experts. Infants whose mothers, according to a doctor's judgement, were unable to breast-feed successfully were provided with cow's milk modified under a doctor's direction to suit the nutritional needs of the infant. The infants were also examined fortnightly, and if necessary, offered medical treatment. Finally, home visiting nurses followed them to ensure that they were well taken care of and that the doctor's orders were carried out.[38] Both the Society and the authorities were pleased with the results. The mortality rate for the depot babies was lower than the overall infant mortality rate for the city, even though the vast majority of the depot babies were from deprived homes and some of them had been in very poor health when first brought to see a doctor.[39]

While emphasizing the medical approach, both Föreningen Mjölkdroppen and the Health Department recognized that part of the infant mortality problem stemmed from social causes, and in particular from the difficulties faced by unmarried and other poor mothers in maintaining and caring for their children. On the question of how to deal with the social causes, the approach of the Society diverged somewhat from that of the Health Department. The Gothenburg authorities, like their Birmingham counterparts, were reluctant to address the poverty problem directly because of the fear of opening the floodgates to innumerable claims on the public purse. The Gothenburg authorities stressed that a poor unmarried or married mother had two options: she should either bear the responsibility for maintaining her child, together with the father or by herself, or failing that, place her child in a foster home. What the authorities were ready to do was to offer expert advice to help the mother to obtain financial support from the father or to find a good foster home. Föreningen Mjölkdroppen offered more concrete help. For example, the Society provided some working mothers with financial assistance, enabling them to be away from work for child care for a few months. Without this assistance, many mothers would have had to resume factory work immediately after childbirth. In other words, the Society gave the poorest mothers the support they needed to get over the most difficult period immediately after the confinement, and therefore allowed them more time to consider the options available to them.[40]

The initial reason why Föreningen Mjölkdroppen started to support breast-feeding mothers seemed to be to silence the critics who argued that milk depots promoted artificial feeding.[41] Indeed, a sense of tokenism was palpable in the Society's report

---

[38]   *GSH 1909:252*, 25–6; *1911:27*. See also A. Höjer, 'Mjölkdroppar och barnavårdscentraler', in *Statens Offentliga Utredningar (SOU) 1929:28* (Stockholm 1929), 44–9; C.G. Sundell, 'Effektivare spädbarnsvård och spädbarnskontroll', *Social-Medicinsk Tidskrift* **6** (1929), 232–40; G. Weiner, 'De "olydiga" mödrarna: konflikter om spädbarnsvård på en Mjölkdroppe', *Historisk Tidskrift* **112** (4) (1992), 488–501.

[39]   *GSH 1911:27*, 5; *1912:120A*, 7.

[40]   *GSH 1909:252*, 3–5, 25–6; *1910:59*; *1911:27*; *1911:264*.

[41]   *GSH 1909:252*, 15–21; *1911:27*; *1926:192*; I. Jundell, 'Moderskydd', *Social Tidskrift* (1908), 51–62; H. Isberg, 'De oäkta barnen och fattigvård', *Social Tidskrift* (1906), 302–4;

of 1911, in which the special attention given to the new service almost hid the fact that direct financial assistance was offered to only eight mothers and that the amount of money used was minuscule compared to the sum spent on sterilized milk.[42] However, the situation was to change. In the late 1910s and early 1920s, the focus of the work was clearly twofold: firstly, to provide bottle-fed infants and nursing mothers with ready-to-use clean and bottled milk, and secondly, to help breast-feeding mothers financially so that they were able to stay at home and look after their newborn babies. The Society assisted 120–190 working mothers annually by giving them 15–40 crowns per month. The percentage of mothers receiving financial assistance was relatively small – approximately 3–5 per cent of all new mothers – but the service made a difference for many of those who received assistance.[43] Like the BIHS in Birmingham, Föreningen Mjölkdroppen took the stance that financial assistance at the right time would contribute to making families economically self-reliant in the long run.

Voluntary societies running nurseries for infants, toddlers and schoolchildren took up where the milk depots left off. They helped mothers returning to work after 'maternity leave' to combine child care and employment. Moreover, they catered for infants and small children whose mothers were undergoing hospital treatment and accommodated homeless mothers and their newborn babies. These societies also opened an opportunity for a wider range of women to become involved in the infant and child welfare work. While Föreningen Mjölkdroppen involved female medical practitioners, nurses and foster care inspectors – or in other words, women who had a formal training – the societies running nurseries relied on the efforts of both professional women and volunteer women activists.[44]

The Gothenburg societies, like the BIHS and other similar organizations in Birmingham, provided services which the leading health officials were unable or unwilling to offer within the system of municipal health care, but of which they often wholeheartedly approved. A clear indication that the milk depots and nurseries had the blessing of the health officials in Gothenburg was the increasing financial support these societies received from the City Council. For example, in the 1910s, when the milk depot activity was at its height, the proportion of municipal funding in the total income of Föreningen Mjölkdroppen rose from 25 per cent in 1911 to 60 per cent in 1919.[45] Although the voluntary societies attracted wide support among health officials and city councillors and among women activists, it does not mean that everyone supported them for the same reasons. On the contrary, nurseries were a good example of measures that were compatible with many political objectives. Male health officials and policy makers tended to emphasize that nurseries opened

---

H. Isberg, 'Barnavård', in G.H. von Koch (ed.), *Social Handbok* (Stockholm 1908), 67–8; K. Ohrlander, *I barnens och nationens intresse: Socialliberal reformpolitik 1903–1930* (Stockholm 1992), 73–8.

    [42] *GSH 1911:27; 1911:118A*, 11–15.

    [43] *GSH 1918:78; 1918:93; 1919:73* and minutes 27 Feb. 1919, item 28; *1919:174A*, 120–22; *1920:176B*, 19–21; *1920:308*; *1924:110* and minutes 27 Mar. 1924, item 24; *1925:145*, 2–3; *1926:406*, 12–13.

    [44] *GSH 1909:6; 1920:130* and minutes 26 Mar. 1920, item 18.

    [45] *GSH 1912:120A*, 4–5; *1919:174A*, 120–21.

up opportunities for poor mothers to work outside the home.[46] Women activists, by contrast, often put forward a more 'maternalistic' argument: nurseries made it possible for poor mothers to keep their children. For example, foster care inspectors Hilda Enander and Elin Hultén pointed out that children placed in foster homes, and especially those who lived outside Gothenburg, often lost contact with their mothers. Nurseries, by contrast, enabled unmarried mothers to combine work and motherhood, and at best strengthened the mother–child bond.[47] Hilda Enander based her views on her experience as a foster care inspector and on her work in Föreningen Barnavärn, which in the first decade of the twentieth century established three nurseries for infants.[48]

Contesting the Authorities' Views   In Gothenburg, as in Birmingham, more open protests against the official health policies usually came from the most reform-minded professional women and from women's organizations not working in close co-operation with the Health Department. As shown above, many professional women in Gothenburg participated actively in the campaigns to improve the situation of unmarried mothers. While middle-class women often considered unmarried mothers partly responsible for their own predicament, some of them also criticized the authorities harshly, accusing them not only of ignoring, but actually of exacerbating the plight of unmarried mothers. Frigga Carlberg, a writer and prominent campaigner for women's rights, pointed out that fathers who refused to support their children, together with (male) policy makers who allowed these fathers to evade their responsibilities, created a 'proletariat of women and children'. Women's voluntary organizations alleviated the problem, but the enthusiasm of some women activists was not enough to bring about fundamental improvements. Carlberg was convinced that a change in gender relations was needed to genuinely improve the situation of unmarried and other poor mothers.[49]

Social Democratic women's groups went a step further in their criticism. In their view, reform activities based on the assumption that single mothers were morally culpable for their plight missed the target. Municipal authorities and voluntary organizations would achieve little if they confined themselves to disciplining unmarried mothers, since men, the government and the capitalist economy were largely responsible for the hardships of unmarried mothers and their children.[50] In demanding changes in both class and gender structures, the Social Democratic women's groups challenged not only the views of health authorities and middle-class women activists, but also the official line of their own party.[51] In Malmö and

---

[46]   *GSH 1909:252*, 11 and minutes 7 Jan. 1910, item 6; *1926:192* and minutes 12 May 1926, item 24.

[47]   See, for example, *GSH 1917:284*, 2–4.

[48]   *GSH 1909:252*.

[49]   Carlberg, 'Frivilligt arbete'; H. Levin, *Kvinnorna på barrikaden: Sexualpolitik och sociala frågor 1923–36* (Stockholm 1997), 221.

[50]   'Kvinnokongressen i Stockholm', *Ny Tid*, 7 and 8 Aug. 1908.

[51]   Working-class organizations and parties in Sweden, like their counterparts in Britain, largely engaged in male-oriented politics and were not particularly receptive to women's proposals. C. Carlsson, *Kvinnosyn och kvinnopolitik: En studie av svensk socialdemokrati*

Norrköping in particular, the women's groups adopted a strident posture on the issue, comparing non-supporting fathers to strike-breakers and attacking them as traitors. Other Social Democratic women's groups, including those of Gothenburg and Stockholm, disassociated themselves from the rhetoric used by the Norrköping and Malmö groups, but they too demanded that the problems of unmarried mothers be placed in a wider context.[52]

While finding a common ground on the issue of unmarried motherhood was often difficult for middle-class and working-class women, creating a sense of shared interests in the question of birth control seemed easier. The Contraceptives Act of 1911 (Lex Hinke), which was in force until 1938, prohibited the dissemination of information on contraceptive methods in Sweden. The law was much criticized, as it prevented medical practitioners advising their clients, but failed to prevent newspapers publishing advertisements selling contraceptives under various pseudonyms. The protests against the law proliferated in the 1920s, and among the protestors there were both middle- and working-class women. In arguing for birth control, they used similar arguments to those used in Birmingham: all mothers should have a 'right' to birth control advice, and women would be 'better mothers' if they had access to family planning services.[53] One of the first practical steps to contest the law was taken by the Gothenburg Social Democratic women's group, which, together with Dr Gärda Lidforss-af Geijerstam, established a family planning clinic in 1924. The clinic, which gave advice to both married and unmarried mothers, was taken over by the municipality in 1930, at the instigation of a Health Committee member, Nathalia Ahlström.[54]

The Working Class and Tuberculosis

Tuberculosis was never the centre of attention in Gothenburg or Birmingham working-class politics, yet the question was often discussed in left-wing newspapers

1880–1910 (Lund 1986); L. Gordon, 'Introduction', in M. Llewelyn Davies (ed.), *Maternity: Letters from Working Women: Collected by the Women's Co-operative Guild* (New York 1978), v–xii.

    52   'Kvinnokongressen i Stockholm', *Ny Tid*, 7 and 8 Aug. 1908; Y. Hirdman, *Den socialistiska hemmafrun och andra kvinnohistorier* (Stockholm 1992), 59–63; Ohlander, 'The invisible child', 64–6; Carlsson, *Kvinnosyn*, 266–9.

    53   G. Byrman, 'From marital precautions to love power: gender construction in Swedish contraceptive brochures', *Nordic Journal of Women's Studies* 9 (2) (2001), 89–97; E. Elgán, *Genus och politik: En jämförelse mellan svensk och fransk abort- och preventivmedelspolitik från sekelskiftet till andra världskriget* (Uppsala 1994), 71–80; Levin, *Kvinnorna på barrikaden*, 187–218.

    54   T. Gårdlund, 'Förefintliga rådfrågningsbyråer för sexualupplysning i Sverige', in *SOU 1936:59* (Stockholm 1938), Appendix 12, 338–9; Göteborgs stadsarkiv (hereafter GSA) Göteborgs Hälsovårdsnämnd, II avdelningen (HVN II) minutes 5 Jan. 1928, item 16; 13 Jun. 1928, item 154; 10 Oct. 1930, item 446; 21 Jan. 1931, item 19; 27 Feb. 1931; Levin, *Kvinnorna på barrikaden*, 131, 204–17. Gärda Lidforss-af Geijerstam was a school medical officer and one of the pioneers of sexual health education in Sweden.

and pamphlets in the early twentieth century.[55] While left-wing writers, politicians and other activists rarely questioned the entire anti-tuberculosis campaigns or the scientific findings on which the campaigns were based, they lodged strong and strident protests against some individual anti-tuberculosis measures or certain aspects of the campaign. In addition to left-wing activists, 'ordinary' city-dwellers from lower social strata occasionally organized themselves in protest against anti-tuberculosis measures. The following section discusses some strategies which working-class activists and 'ordinary' city-dwellers adopted to change tuberculosis policies.

Gothenburg

In early twentieth-century Gothenburg, the Social Democratic newspaper *Ny Tid* actively campaigned for the provision of sanatorium and hospital treatment for poor tubercular patients. The newspaper followed international developments in both tuberculosis research and practical anti-tuberculosis work, and used this information to support their demands. For example, in 1903 the newspaper reported that the determined efforts of the German health insurance agencies and Danish voluntary organizations to provide tubercular patients with sanatorium treatment were beginning to show promising results. Referring to these examples, *Ny Tid* argued that in Sweden a large number of working-class people died of tuberculosis, since the treatment available to German and Danish workers was not offered to them. The newspaper wished that the Gothenburg City Council would, for once, be 'both practical and humane and not to make the same excuses' they always made when asked to take measures that would benefit the poorest of the poor.[56]

In addition to foreign examples, the newspaper also used other strategies to persuade policy makers to invest in hospitals and sanatoria. The writers contributing to *Ny Tid,* like middle-class women activists, were clearly aware of the differences of opinion between the leading health officers and the majority of the city councillors on some questions concerning health and welfare, and they used the situation to further their goals. For example, when the debate about providing new purpose-built hospital facilities to tubercular patients was at its height in the early years of the twentieth century, the newspaper sought to influence the decision-making process by backing up the First City Physician, Karl Gezelius, who actively campaigned for the new hospital. The newspaper argued that the suggested types of reforms would bring the Swedish campaign up to the standard which many other countries had already reached, and that Swedish society could well afford the cost of such reforms. In order to prove the point, one writer a few years later juxtaposed the millions that

---

[55]   On working-class views of public health, see D. Silbey, 'Bodies and cultures collide: enlistment, the medical exam, and the British working class, 1914–1916', *Social History of Medicine* **17** (1) (2004), 61–76; M. Sigsworth and M. Worboys, 'The public's view of public health in mid-Victorian Britain', *Urban History* **21** (2) (1994), 237–50; L. Bryder, *Below the Magic Mountain: A Social History of Tuberculosis in Twentieth-century Britain* (Oxford 1988), 199–226.

[56]   'Kampen mot tuberkulosen: förslaget om sanatorium för Göteborg', *Ny Tid,* 4 Sept. 1903; 'Tuberkulosen', *Ny Tid,* 12 Oct. 1903.

were spent on armaments to defend Sweden against its 'outside enemies' with the small amount of money available to fight 'the most formidable enemy' within the country: tuberculosis.[57]

Left-wing politicians and working-class organizations in Gothenburg remained generally favourable to sanatorium and hospital treatment of tuberculosis even in the 1920s and 1930s, when it became evident that the available therapies did not come up to expectations. Acceptance of the institutionalization of tubercular patients manifested itself, for example, in the motion which Councillors Ragnar Andersson and Einar Adamson, both Communists, put forward in 1930. They suggested that the Gothenburg Health Committee follow the example set by the Soviet authorities and establish yet another institution, a night sanatorium, for tubercular patients who were able to work but required some regular treatment.[58] Unlike Swedish and other Western health authorities, who preferred to remove tubercular patients from the city and expose them to beneficial influence of nature, the Soviet authorities thought it better to treat people where they lived. They were convinced that patients could be 'supervised medically more closely in factories than in agricultural enterprises'. Councillors Andersson and Adamson failed, however, in their effort to import this idea to Gothenburg.[59]

While left-wing activists and the general public agreed with the health officers that the generous provision of hospital beds served both the collective and individual good, the consensus might break down as soon as the question turned, for example, to a possible location of a new hospital. When the Gothenburg City Council in the early years of the twentieth century considered a plan to convert a former general hospital into a tuberculosis hospital, people living in the neighbourhood protested against the plan. In their letter to the City Council, they chose a line of reasoning which was very similar to that pursued by the First City Physician and the Health Committee. For example, the residents invoked the ideas of 'soil' and 'seed'. Firstly, they pointed out that people's resistance to infection would be weakened by the fear they would inevitably feel living near the 'death house'. Secondly, the risk of infection and continuous re-infection, already high in the overcrowded neighbourhood, would increase considerably if the authorities accommodated infectious tubercular patients in the area.[60] Such overt protests, together with the discrimination which many tubercular patients experienced, compelled the Health Committee time and again to revise its anti-tuberculosis schemes. The authorities in both Gothenburg and Birmingham depended to a certain extent on public fears to solicit funds, but at the same time public fears could also paralyse the campaign.

---

[57] 'Kampen mot tuberkulosen: förslaget om sanatorium för Göteborg', *Ny Tid*, 4 Sept. 1903; 'Sanatoriafrågan vinner gehör', *Ny Tid*, 10 Sept. 1903; 'Renströmska fonden', *Ny Tid*, 11 Sept. 1903; 'Renströmska fonden', *Ny Tid*, 12 Oct. 1903; 'Stadsfullmäktige i går', *Ny Tid*, 4 Dec. 1903. The quote is from 'Lungsoten: den fattiges öde', *Ny Tid*, 27 Jul. 1908.

[58] GSA Göteborgs Hälsovårdsnämnd, I avdelningen (HVN I) minutes 3 Dec. 1930, item 213; 13 May 1931, item 117; *GSH 1930:147*; *1931:86* and minutes 19 Mar. 1931, item 32.

[59] H.E. Sigerist, *Socialised Medicine in the Soviet Union* (London 1937), 236–41. See also *GSH 1925:3* and discussion 15 Jan. 1925, item 32, 10.

[60] *GSH 1902:90*, 6–8; GSA HVN I minutes 2 Apr. 1930, item 62 and documents K, L.

Finally, some left-wing politicians and writers in Gothenburg criticized the authorities for concentrating excessively on medical care. They pointed out that the improvements in patients' health brought about by sanatorium treatment were usually short-lived, since the authorities did very little to help patients readjust to 'normal' life after discharge from a sanatorium.[61] The municipal anti-tuberculosis campaign would succeed, so it was argued, only if the medical services were supplemented with measures that alleviated poverty and improved people's living and working conditions. In particular, in the 1910s and 1920s, when the housing problem was extremely severe in Gothenburg, the health authorities were criticized for ignoring social and environmental problems that made people susceptible to tuberculosis and other diseases. Instead of settling for half-measures, the health authorities should have ensured that tubercular patients had both medical care and healthy homes.[62]

Birmingham

While in Gothenburg the working class, or at least the most active politicians and writers, took the stance that the provision of institutional treatment for both early and advanced cases of tuberculosis was in the interests of the whole community, in Birmingham sanatorium treatment did not attract similar support. Michael Worboys argues that in Britain there is little evidence of any demand for sanatorium treatment directly by potential working-class patients. In his view, the demand was largely created by local authorities, general practitioners and voluntary organizations.[63] The Birmingham case seems to support his conclusion. For example, in 1905, when the Health Committee and the MOH set about investigating the possibility of establishing a sanatorium, working-class organizations showed relatively little interest. Friendly societies, however, were an exception. Sickness benefits that the friendly societies paid to the members suffering from tuberculosis were a major drain on their resources, and in consequence the societies were more than willing to share the burden with the municipal authorities. For example, Councillor S.G. Middleton, who was a member of the Ancient Order of Foresters, a friendly society that had traditionally opposed state welfare, campaigned actively for a municipal sanatorium in Birmingham.[64]

By the time the first sanatorium was opened in Birmingham in 1909, local authorities, general practitioners and voluntary organizations had managed to assure hundreds of tubercular patients that sanatorium treatment was their best hope for regaining their health. In consequence, only a proportion of the people who sought

---

[61]   'Lungsoten: den fattiges öde', *Ny Tid*, 27 Jul. 1908; 'Livet på sanatorierna behöver reformeras', *Ny Tid*, 9 May 1910. Left-wing politicians also critized living conditions in old sanatoria and hospitals. See *GSH 1923:328* and minutes and discussion 13 Sept. 1923, item 16.

[62]   'Kampen mot tuberkulosen', *Ny Tid*, 27 Aug. 1903; GSA HVN I minutes 1 Aug. 1928, item 115 and document C; 2 Apr. 1930, item 62 and document K.

[63]   M. Worboys, 'The sanatorium treatment for consumption in Britain, 1890–1914', in J.V. Pickstone (ed.), *Medical Innovations in Historical Perspective* (London 1992), 61.

[64]   BCA HC minutes 11 Apr. 1905, item 9233; 11 Jul. 1905, item 9395. See also Thane, 'The working class'; P. Thane, *The Foundations of the Welfare State* (London 1990), 28–30.

treatment in the years before the First World War could be admitted to sanatoria. However, the confidence that many patients might have had when they first entered these institutions soon ebbed. As discussed in Chapter 5, a considerable proportion of patients, sometimes more than 20 per cent, left the sanatorium before the end of the recommended treatment period.

While many left-wing politicians and writers in Birmingham accepted that unhealthy habits played a role in causing tuberculosis, they were rather sceptical about the educational approach that the Birmingham authorities had adopted. They pointed out that an unhealthy way of life might well be an important contributory factor to tuberculosis, but that unhealthy habits and behaviour, in turn, were largely due to defective housing. Poor living and working conditions, they argued, were having a demoralizing effect on the tenants. These writers castigated the health authorities for taking refuge behind the educational campaign and not tackling the 'real causes' of tuberculosis: defective housing and insanitary environment. As Councillor E.A. Wilson put it in 1913, the Public Health Committee had been 'amazingly active in creation of sanatoria, etc., but have allowed the housing question to be shelved'.[65]

Left-wing critics, like the health authorities, were convinced that scientifically sophisticated arguments were the key to persuading the public, or at least those townspeople 'who (were) concerned with the development and administration of local government'. Thus, in their analyses they often referred to experts on public health and medicine. J.A. Fallows, one of the first Labour councillors in Birmingham, often made use of material published by the Birmingham MOHs and other health experts, and used the differences of opinion between the leading officials and politicians to further his cause. He showed respect for the expertise of MOHs Alfred Hill and John Robertson, and at the same time he levelled fierce criticism against John Nettlefold, the chairman of the Housing Committee. Fallows argued that Nettlefold had set before the Housing Committee 'the impossible task of harmonising private greed and public benefit', and that he had spent public money in ways which 'can only benefit private speculators, whether in the form of compensation to property owners or of subsidies to builders'.[66]

Similarly, various working-class organizations rushed to back up the Medical Officer of Health, when he openly protested against the Public Works Committee's plans to build tenements for the poor to alleviate the housing shortage. The MOH argued that 'the general result of life in flats is that the young children suffer from ill-defined ailments and very definitely are much more prone to rickets'. Seventeen working-class organizations, many of them women's organizations or sections, wrote a letter supporting the MOH. For example, the Soho Ward Women's Labour Party protested against the proposal to erect flats, but also criticized plans to lower housing standards, and the Pineapple Women's Section stated that flats would be especially

---

[65]   J.A. Fallows, *The Housing of the Poor* (Birmingham 1899); J.A. Fallows and F. Hughes, *The Housing Question in Birmingham* (Birmingham 1905); C.E. Smith, *Memorandum on the Housing Question Submitted to the Housing Enquiry Committee of the Birmingham City Council on behalf of the Birmingham Socialist Centre, the Trades' Council and the Labour Representation Council* (Birmingham 1914).

[66]   Fallows and Hughes, *The Housing Question.*

'detrimental to the health of our women and children'. Despite the protests, the Public Works Committee built 180 flats in Garrison Lane, but the strong opposition contributed to making the Garrison Lane experiment a failure.[67]

Increasing awareness of the infectious nature of tuberculosis occasionally fuelled public panic, and in many cases the fear and anxiety found its expression in the discrimination and personal abuse of the sick. People did not necessarily make an open protest against the anti-tuberculosis campaign, but instead contested its principles in their everyday lives. In Birmingham, as in Gothenburg, employers, landlords, shop owners, neighbours and relatives often ignored the health authorities' recommendations by refusing to employ people suspected to suffer from tuberculosis, by evicting them from their homes, and by isolating them socially.[68]

Conclusion

In both Birmingham and Gothenburg, women and working-class activists challenged health policies and sought to change things to their advantage. The challenges took many forms, ranging from overt and obvious to covert and subtle, but what these groups had in common was that none of them had their own 'language' to discuss health issues or their own methods to examine them. Their success in shaping health policies depended on how they managed to draw upon the language and methods of the prevailing culture for their own ends, and how skilful they were in seizing on the inconsistencies in the existing policies and in capitalizing on the differences of opinion among health officials.

Middle-class women activists and their initiatives, commitments and visions profoundly influenced the maternal and infant welfare campaigns in both cities. While rarely questioning the main aims of the official campaigns, women activists explored alternative ways to achieve these aims. In so doing, they not only contributed to the welfare of women and children, but also participated in mediating gender and class conflicts in urban society. Sometimes their work was in line with the expectations of male health officers, sometimes they identified more with working-class women, emphasizing different aspects of scientific findings than male health officers did and reversing the order of priorities laid down by male councillors. The exact strategies available to women depended somewhat on local government structures. In Birmingham, where policy making structures were fragmented, women's organizations were influential in developing welfare schemes, and both 'philanthropic ladies' and professional women were involved in the work. In Gothenburg, where

---

[67]   BCA PHC minutes 23 Jan. 1925, item 8825; 25 Feb. 1925, item 8901; Women's Co-operative Guild, Duddeston Branch, minutes 12 Jul. 1926. See also A. Sutcliffe, 'A century of flats in Birmingham 1875–1973', in A. Sutcliffe (ed.), *Multi-storey Living: The British Working-class Experience* (London 1974), 190–92.

[68]   'Lungsoten: den fattiges öde', *Ny Tid*, 27 Jul. 1908; G.B. Dixon, 'The care of the consumptive in the home', reprint from the *Journal of the Royal Sanitary Institute* **25** (1904), 500; V. Berglund, 'Försäkring mot tuberkulos', *Social Tidskrift* (1908), 257–63. See also BCA HC minutes 22 Apr. 1902, items 7383–4; 'Renströmska fonden', *Ny Tid*, 12 Oct. 1903; GSA HVN I minutes 2 Apr. 1930, item 62 and documents K, L.

policy making structures were more centralized and experts had more important role in the formulation of policies, the choice of strategies for women was more limited. Women able to influence health policies were usually professional women who had managed to carve a niche for themselves in both municipal and voluntary health care systems. However, these differences should not be exaggerated. In both Birmingham and Gothenburg, women activists usually worked in or in close-co-operation with male-dominated institutions, and the maternal and infant welfare campaigns were constructed through the discourse and co-operation between men and women.

While women were often deprived of productive outlets for their concerns within the official political set-up, working-class (male) activists had a better opportunity to pursue their goals within it. The way in which working-class activists and – to some extent – 'ordinary' city-dwellers expressed their criticism about the tuberculosis campaigns reflected the health authorities' strategies to justify their policies. For example, in Gothenburg, where the health authorities often used foreign examples to legitimize their proposals, working-class organizations and groups used the same strategy to contest the authorities' views. In both Birmingham and Gothenburg, working-class activists protested against health policies by citing scientific findings that coincided their understanding of the problem, and by supporting health officials, whose views they shared.

CHAPTER 7

Conclusion

The cancer research establishment likes us to believe that a shortage of research funds is the primary problem. Ignorance, in this view, is the basic cause of cancer.

The key to cancer control is therefore knowledge – the great scientific breakthrough to wash away our stupor. But we already know a lot about cancer … We know … that cancer is the product of bad habits, bad government, bad business, and perhaps even bad science.

Robert N. Proctor, Cancer Wars (1995)[1]

Public health authorities campaigning against infant mortality and tuberculosis in the early twentieth century faced a problem very much analogous to that confronting the present-day cancer agencies. They knew a lot about the causes of infant mortality and tuberculosis, but were not always able or willing to use the knowledge they had. An important reason why many scientific findings were ignored or rejected was that the practical policies to which these findings seemed to lead were incompatible with the broader political and social goals of health campaigns. For example, studies linking infant mortality with poverty suggested that the well-being of infants could not be secured without a redistribution of economic resources between the well-to-do and the poor, between the childless and those with children, or between men and women. Most policy makers influential in the formulation of health policies were against profound structural changes or considered them to be beyond the scope of their rightful duties. Thus evidence of the link between economic deprivation and infant mortality was not taken to be knowledge, but was treated as a controversial research finding.

Similarly, studies linking tuberculosis with defective housing suggested that housing reform was an essential part of any successful attempt to control the disease. If the anti-tuberculosis campaign was to achieve its goals, municipalities or other non-speculative agencies should intensify their efforts to provide decent housing for those people who were most likely to fall ill: the poor. However, building healthy homes for those in the most acute housing need was extremely difficult as long as more important groups – upper-working-class and lower-middle-class people – also struggled to make decent homes for themselves and as long as the provision of municipal and co-operative housing was inextricably linked to free-market policies. Hence, health authorities had to choose their words carefully. On the one hand they argued that improving the standard of housing was an indispensable tool in the struggle against tuberculosis, and on the other they warned that studies concerning the

---

[1]   R.N. Proctor, *Cancer Wars: How Politics Shapes What We Know and Don't Know About Cancer* (New York 1995), 270.

housing–tuberculosis connection should not be taken too literally. This connection, so it was claimed, was extremely complicated, therefore it was only sensible to first try other possible means than housing reform to combat the disease. In discussing the housing–tuberculosis connection and the poverty–infant mortality connection, health authorities often ended up propagating ignorance to justify inaction. It was premature to draw conclusions, far too early to take measures.

While public health authorities were reluctant to translate some potentially important scientific findings into practical policy, they often lacked the kind of findings they would have liked to utilize. In other words, health officials had preconceptions about urban health problems and about responses to them, but they did not always have appropriate scientific evidence at hand to support their views. The comparison of the Swedish and British health campaigns reveals how creative health officials were in building scientific evidence to legitimize the ways in which they approached health issues and, more generally, the ways in which they managed the city. Furthermore, the comparison shows that health officials often convinced other policy makers and the public that if only they had more resources available and if only science advanced, the very approach they had chosen would yield even better results. The following sections discuss the ways in which health officials provided scientific legitimization for their policies, and the impact these scientific, 'value-free' policies had on urban development.

Unruly Urban Life and Neat Scientific Categories

The knowledge on which health policies were based was partly 'produced' by public health officials themselves. In both British and Swedish cities, health officers collected, collated and analysed information about the incidence of diseases among different sections of the population and about the links between particular ways of life and exposure to disease and death. Since the health officers used statistical techniques and other approved scientific methods, the maps, charts and tables they produced were usually taken to be value-free knowledge and the categories they used were seen as natural and obvious. However, by comparing the reports published in two different cities, it is easy to reveal some ways in which this information was structured by the questions the health officers asked and the answers they expected. Furthermore, it is possible to discuss what consequences this information and the apparently innocent categories that were used to organize it had on urban society.

The knowledge about urban health problems reflected the spatial and social arrangements in the city. In Birmingham, where the spatial separation of social classes had been an integral part of the city's economic and political development, the idea of socio-spatial segregation also informed the ways in which urban health problems were explored. The health authorities were interested in comparing mortality rates, environmental conditions and health habits in different city wards, and when analysing the results and proposing solutions, they sliced the city into three categories: 'unhealthy', 'less unhealthy' and 'healthy' areas. In the unhealthy areas, where both tuberculosis and infant mortality rates were highest, a large proportion of the inhabitants lived in old, ramshackle houses and their attitudes and behaviour

– their social contacts, their diet and the ways in which they looked after their own bodies, their children and their homes – were deemed irrational and unhealthy. The Birmingham health authorities were clearly drawn into a socio-spatial definition of how people did things, a definition which made a clear distinction between irrational and irresponsible people living in the 'unhealthy areas', and rational and responsible people living in the 'healthy' suburbs.

In Gothenburg, where socio-spatial segregation was less pronounced, the health authorities were not particularly interested in comparing different city wards. Instead, they devoted their time to comparing, for example, people living in different types of housing or infants born to different types of families. The Gothenburg health authorities, too, made a distinction between 'normal' and 'problem' families, but they did not associate these categories with any particular space in the city; rather, they built their campaigns on the assumption that problem families – people in low-quality housing, single mothers with their children, and tubercular patients with their families – lived scattered in the socially mixed city centre and in working-class areas.

The way in which the health officials categorized city-dwellers was not only an academic question, but had strong implications on urban form and the development of urban communities. In arranging unruly urban life into neat categories, the officials defined, for example, the frameworks of social action. In Birmingham, by defining the central wards as 'unhealthy areas', the authorities justified municipal intervention in all homes in these poor districts. Sanitary inspectors and health visitors were sent to inspect the houses and instruct the housewives in domestic hygiene. This system, whereby entire parts of the city were labelled and treated as problem areas, was self-reinforcing. As the unhealthy areas gained an increasingly residualized status, the incentive for 'respectable' working-class people to move out became greater and the patterns of residential segregation became more marked. In Gothenburg, by contrast, the authorities concentrated on people belonging to certain 'problem groups' largely irrespective of where these people lived in the city. The aim of the campaign – especially initially – was to track down the problem families and individuals, provide them with appropriate services, and keep them under close supervision. The Gothenburg authorities' approach, too, served to reinforce social-spatial segregation, but in a different, subtler way. Their health policies contributed to the fine-grained processes which created small pockets of poverty or ghettos apart in working-class and socially mixed areas. Inequality was expressed in the physical separation of one street from another, or even in the separation of upstairs and downstairs.

Spatial arrangements aside, categorizations had important implications for the other aspects of urban development, too. Many slum dwellers in Birmingham certainly led very unhealthy lives, and similarly, many people living in low-cost houses in Gothenburg were ignorant of important health matters. However, when, on the basis of specific unhealthy habits or of a specific disease, sweeping conclusions were drawn about the whole family or, as usually happened, about an entire category of people, health policies inevitably became a powerful means of pursuing politics. Defining the people living in poor neighbourhoods or people suffering from tuberculosis as 'problem groups' may have been important for the practical running of the health campaigns, but at the same time it meant that these people came to be seen as 'problem groups' in other contexts, too. For example, the Gothenburg authorities claimed that, more often than not, children living in tubercular families were neglected. In pondering why this was the case, the authorities jumped to the conclusion that tubercular families were generally more irresponsible than other families. Little thought was given to the possibility that, in some cases, these mothers and fathers may have appeared particularly bad parents mainly because their parenting was much more visible than that of other mothers and fathers. They were under scrutiny, therefore their faults and mistakes rarely went unnoticed.

Choosing the 'Right' Results

Public health officials, as a group, were able to influence which research questions were considered worth asking in society, and therefore what kind of research was being done by scientists. Furthermore, in utilizing the findings of medicine and the natural and social sciences, health officials were able to make choices. Scientists never spoke with a single voice on topical issues such as infant mortality and tuberculosis, therefore health officials could use scientific results that supported, at least to an extent, their own preconceptions of the problems. The family and mother ideals held up by the Birmingham and Gothenburg infant welfare campaigns and the scientific legitimization given to these ideals reveals the eclectic ways in which scientific findings were used.

In Birmingham, the ideal family consisted of the husband, who was a reliable breadwinner, and the wife, who was both a loving mother to the children and an efficient manager of the home. Scientific findings suggesting that this family model, and only this, promoted infant health and welfare were taken to be knowledge. The Birmingham authorities *knew* that work-shy and idle husbands who wasted their money on drink risked the welfare of their entire family. They *knew* that the full-time presence of the mother was indispensable to the development of young children, and that mothers who worked outside the home exposed their children to disease and death. Moreover, the Birmingham authorities *knew* that bottle-fed babies were susceptible to diseases, and therefore, in defiance of considerable public demand, they refused to establish milk depots. They also *knew* that in the 'unhealthy areas', children were at risk. Owing to the demoralizing effect of the slum life, families living in deprived areas were, or soon became, irresponsible and negligent. This knowledge was tailored to the opportunities and needs of a society in which married-couple families constituted the vast majority of families and where *per capita* income was relatively high, meaning that in most families there was a father who was, or was expected to be, capable of supporting the family. Moreover, this knowledge suited a society in which women's participation in the labour force was not deemed vital to the local economy.

In theory, the Gothenburg authorities probably embraced the same family ideal as their Birmingham counterparts, but in practice, they had to acknowledge that this ideal was too far removed from the working-class reality to be credible. The Gothenburg authorities simply could not afford to be concerned about such things as the appropriate roles of husbands and wives, since they had a much more urgent task ahead of them, namely to ensure that fathers and mothers fulfilled their parental responsibilities. In consequence, in the Gothenburg campaign, the ideal family consisted of parents who supported and protected their children, and scientific findings that served to legitimize this ideal were taken to be knowledge. The Gothenburg authorities *knew* that fathers and mothers neglecting their obligation to support their children were responsible for a large number of infant deaths. They *knew* that if the infant welfare campaign was to succeed, they had to make both fathers and mothers face up to their responsibilities, even if it meant forcing fathers to support their children and helping mothers to combine motherhood with paid work. Encouraging mothers to work was not particularly difficult for the Gothenburg authorities, since they *knew* that extra-familial child care – for example, nurseries – was not necessarily inimical to infant and child welfare. They also *knew* that, although breast-feeding was the best option, bottle-feeding could be safe, too. This knowledge was tailored to a society where the variety of family forms was relatively great, and in particular, where the number of single mothers was high. Furthermore, it suited a society where women were seen as a permanent part of the labour force and where local industries were keen to employ female workers.

Since the 'good mother' ideals were different in Birmingham and Gothenburg, the definitions of 'the problem mother' were likewise disparate. In Birmingham, the term 'problem mother' encompassed mothers living in slum areas, and in particular mothers working outside the home and bottle-feeding their babies. In Gothenburg, the 'problem mother' category consisted mainly of unmarried mothers, and especially mothers who handed over their children to bad foster-parents or who struggled without success to combine motherhood with economic survival. The Birmingham and Gothenburg campaigns stigmatized the problem mothers, but at the same time these mothers were given at least a slight opportunity to become good mothers. Slum mothers in Birmingham could become better mothers if they concentrated on motherhood and followed the experts' advice on child care – or ideally, if they moved to the new working-class suburbs with their families, which many of them did. To the great gratification of the Birmingham authorities, numerous families shook off the burdens and stresses of slum life and started 'from a clean slate' on a new council estate on the outskirts of Birmingham. Unmarried mothers in Gothenburg could become better mothers if they managed to support their children and protect their children's interests – or ideally, if they married the father of the child or someone else, which many of them did. For example, the illegitimate birth rate for Gothenburg decreased somewhat in the 1920s, and more rapidly in the 1930s.

While the problem mothers were given a chance to become better mothers, there were other groups of women in Birmingham and Gothenburg who were not given such a chance. In both cities, women with mental deficiencies were deemed unfit for motherhood, but there were other women, too, who shared their fate. In Birmingham, where the family ideal was given precedence over many other objectives, unmarried mothers were the ultimate 'bad' mothers, so much so that they were not only seen as harmful to their children, but they were also believed to have a contaminating effect on other mothers. Unmarried mothers were an alien element, a distinct 'other', in the British public health system and in British society in general. The Swedish authorities, by contrast, emphasized the rights of the child and the rights of society at the expense of the institution of family and family ties. Furthermore, they preferred to use medical rather than overtly moral criteria to define who was unfit for motherhood. Women who were believed to be at risk of transmitting serious hereditary defects or infectious diseases to their children were seen as an alien element that posed a grave threat to the health of the nation and to the Nordic stock. This threat was dealt with, for example, by sterilizing women suffering from mental deficiencies or epilepsy and by pressurizing mothers diagnosed with tuberculosis to place their children into foster care. The comparison between Birmingham and Gothenburg reveals sharply the elasticity of the 'problem mother' and 'bad mother' labels. In both Birmingham and Gothenburg, there were many mothers who neglected or even abused their children, there is no doubt of that. However, in both cities these labels were applied to far more women than to those whose actions really warranted it.[2]

Rival Interpretations

The comparison of the Birmingham and Gothenburg campaigns also shows how health authorities could draw different and yet equally logical conclusions from the same medical 'facts' and theories. What aspects of medical theories the health authorities emphasized depended on how far down in the chain of causation they looked when defining health problems. The Gothenburg authorities often stopped with micro-organisms or micro-events within the human body. They argued, or just assumed, that micro-organisms or micro-events were the 'real causes' of infant death and tuberculosis, and in consequence, medical doctors were to play the key role in the formulation and implementation of public health policies. The campaigns against tuberculosis or infant mortality were, to a large extent, scientific battles against disease-causing microbes. Infectious tubercular patients were isolated from the rest of society, and children born to high-risk tubercular families were either kept out of the way of tubercle bacilli by boarding them out in healthy foster-homes or were vaccinated against the disease. Similarly, in order to reduce death rates from infantile diarrhoea, the health authorities provided sterilized cow's milk for bottle-fed babies, and hospital beds for babies suffering from the disease. By attributing the cause of disease to micro-organisms or micro-events within the body, the health officials extended professional opportunities in medicine – a measure which was important in a country where doctors were dependent on central and local governments for their posts and pensions.

While for the Swedish authorities the interest was in information which could spin off in the direction of new therapies, the British authorities were more interested in information that might be useful for their educational health campaigns. Although the Birmingham authorities often utilized exactly the same medical theories as their Gothenburg counterparts, they usually emphasized that micro-organisms alone did not explain health problems such as tubercular diseases or infant mortality. Only a

---

[2]   See also M. Ladd-Taylor and L. Umansky, 'Introduction', in M. Ladd-Taylor and L. Umansky (eds), *'Bad' Mothers: The Politics of Blame in Twentieth-century America* (New York 1998), 1–28.

small proportion of people exposed to tubercular infection developed full-blown tuberculosis, and only some of the babies raised on cow's milk died of infantile diarrhoea. Seen from this perspective, the 'real causes' of tuberculosis and infant deaths seemed to be unhealthy habits which weakened bodily resistance and which facilitated the proliferation and transmission of disease-causing microbes in the homes. The campaigns against tuberculosis and infant mortality were educational projects aiming to instil in people a sense of responsibility and instruct them in a healthy way of life. These campaigns, while inspiring and empowering many city-dwellers to preserve their own health, did not take into account the unequal abilities of individuals to change their habits, and therefore often failed to address many problems, especially those confronting the poorest families.

By concentrating on disease-causing microbes or disease-causing unhealthy habits, the Gothenburg and Birmingham authorities took the stance that wider environmental or social factors were only secondary contributors to disease. This conclusion was 'politically' necessary, since the private, municipal and voluntary housing schemes all failed to provide decent housing for the poorest section of the population in both Birmingham and Gothenburg. In Birmingham, the poorest people, among whom both tuberculosis mortality and infant mortality were rampant, lived in ramshackle back-to-back houses throughout the period reviewed here. The health authorities justified the non-interventionist policy by arguing that unhealthy habits, not defective housing, were undermining people's health. In Gothenburg, the poorest of the poor, who had the highest risk of death and disease, still lived in small, overcrowded flats in the 1930s. The public health officials alleviated the problem by removing infectious patients to hospitals, not by improving housing conditions.

Science and Urban Society

The case studies of infant welfare and anti-tuberculosis campaigns show that public health officials, in spite of their ambitious rhetoric, sought solutions to urban health problems broadly within the existing gender and class structures. Hence, they often ended up reproducing the inequalities they professed to level out and perpetuating the problems they set out to solve. For example, measures aimed to improve women's health encouraged women to accept the inequalities in the family and on the labour market as a part of the natural order, thereby endorsing their second-class status, which, in turn, was the source of their many social and health problems. When profound socio-economic changes such as economic restructuring or demographic transition led to shifts in class and gender relations, health policies usually reflected and reinforced these shifts, but at the same time contributed to making them less dramatic. For example, health policies of the 1920s and 1930s reflected and reinforced the growing political significance of the lower middle class and upper working class. These groups were provided with new municipal services, which set them apart from the poor and brought them closer to the middle and upper middle classes, but which also sought to ensure that these groups were fully integrated into society and shared its core values.

Public health policies also had an important role in the redefinition of professional boundaries and statuses. As to the inter-professional boundaries, public health policies in both Britain and Sweden supported the efforts of the medical profession to establish and maintain its cultural domination over a wide range of issues. Medical practitioners were seen to have superior knowledge not only about diseases and injuries, but also about matters such as poverty, family life and the appropriate roles of women and men in society. When it came to the boundaries within the medical profession, the situation was different in Britain and Sweden. In Sweden, where the majority of medical practitioners worked in the public sector, the expansion of public health care rarely triggered serious boundary disputes within the profession. In Britain, where both the private and voluntary sectors had an important role in the field of health care, it was another story. The introduction of new publicly funded medical services threatened the boundaries between different groups – and especially between public health doctors and general practitioners – causing general practitioners fiercely to defend their territory. This meant that the health authorities had to devote much time and energy to mediate between the interests of different groups of the medical profession.

How influential were public health officials in regulating urban life? What complicated the matter was that public health officials themselves, though presenting a united front, often disagreed on how to tackle health problems and how to manage the city. The leading health officials – the MOH in Birmingham and the First City Physician in Gothenburg – were often ready to introduce more radical reforms than the majority of the Health Committee members or the city councillors, especially in the early twentieth century. The differences of opinion among the policy makers and the inconsistencies in the public policies opened up opportunities for city-dwellers – for example, middle-class women and working-class people – to influence policies and further causes they deemed important. The leading health officials, in turn, often utilized the support they attracted outside the municipal apparatus to push through reforms in council chambers or to get voluntary organizations to address certain health problems.

Finally, although the impact of health policies on social relations was profound, it was often unpredictable and unexpected. Changes were rarely unitary in their effects, and almost invariably involved trade-offs rather than unambiguous gains and losses. In other words, public health officials may have sought to reinforce existing economic and social arrangements, but they were never able to predict exactly how people would respond to their policies and what the consequences of their health measures would be. Measures designed to promote integration in urban society may have furthered segregation. Similarly, measures seeking to 'protect' a group of people, for example unmarried mothers and their children, could have subjected these people to demeaning supervision. This type of process was, as Jürgen Habermas has argued, an essential element of social modernization: the very (legal) means which secure freedom are often the means through which freedom is put in jeopardy.[3]

---

[3]   J. Habermas, *Der philosophische Diskurs der Moderne: Zwölf Vorlesungen* (Frankfurt am Main 1985), 336–43. See also J.R. Walkowitz, *City of Dreadful Delight: Narratives of Sexual Danger in Late-Victorian London* (Chicago, IL 1992), 81–120.

Bibliography

MANUSCRIPT SOURCES

Birmingham City Archives (BCA)

Birmingham Health Committee (HC), minutes 1898–1911.
Birmingham Maternity and Child Welfare Sub-Committee (M&CWSC), minutes 1915–33.
Birmingham Maternity and Child Welfare Committee (M&CWC), minutes 1920–33.
Birmingham Public Health and Housing Committee (PH&HC), minutes 1911–17.
Birmingham Public Health and Maternity and Child Welfare Committee (PH&MCWC), minutes 1933–39.
Birmingham Public Health Committee (PHC), minutes 1917–33.
Women's Co-operative Guild, Duddeston Branch (Birmingham), minutes 1926–28.

Göteborgs stadsarkiv (GSA) (Gothenburg City Archives)

Göteborgs Hälsovårdsnämnd (HVN), minutes 1900–1917.
Göteborgs Hälsovårdsnämnd, Samfälda nämnden (HVN SN), minutes 1917–33.
Göteborgs Hälsovårdsnämnd, I avdelningen (HVN I), minutes 1917–33.
Göteborgs Hälsovårdsnämnd, II avdelningen (HVN II), minutes 1917–33.

Göteborgs universitetsbibliotek (GUB) (Gothenburg University Library)

Kvinnohistorisk Arkiv (Women's History Archives).
Sällskapet för uppmuntran av öm och sedlig modersvård, Handlingar 1877–1965.

Public Record Office (PRO)

Ministry of Health 52/231, 'Birmingham County Borough Council, 1922–25 Maternity and Child Welfare and Tuberculosis Services, Investigation and Report of Borough Health Services'.

OFFICIAL PAPERS AND PRINTED REPORTS

Britain

British Parliamentary Papers

Royal Commission on the Poor Laws and Relief of Distress, 1909, Appendix, vol. IV.

Census of England and Wales

1911: vol. VIII: *Tenements in Administrative Counties and Urban and Rural Districts*; vol. X: *Occupations and Industries*; *Summary Tables: Area. Families or Separate Occupiers and Population.*
1931: *Occupation Tables.*
1951: *Industry Tables.*

City of Birmingham, Boundaries Committee

Report of the Boundaries Committee for Presentation at the Special Meeting of the Council on the 13th July, 1909 (1909).

City of Birmingham, Education Department

Birmingham Trades for Women and Girls (1914).

City of Birmingham, Health Department/Public Health and Housing Department

Annual Reports of the Medical Officer of Health for Birmingham for 1873–1940.
Duncan, Jessie (1911), *Report on Infant Mortality in St. George's and St. Stephen's Wards.*
Duncan, Jessie (1912), *Report on the Prevention of Infantile Mortality.*
Hill, Alfred (1877), *Report to the Health Committee on Infantile Mortality in the Borough of Birmingham.*
Quarterly Reports of the Medical Officer of Health for Birmingham for 1911.
Report of the Medical Officer of Health on Child Welfare in 1913 (1914).
'Report of the Medical Officer of Health on maternity and child welfare during 1916', in *Annual Report of the Medical Officer of Health for Birmingham for 1916*, Appendix.
Report of the Medical Officer of Health on the Unhealthy Conditions in the Floodgate Street Area and the Municipal Wards of St. Mary, St. Stephen, and St. Bartholomew (1904).
Report on the Spread of Tuberculosis by Indiscriminate Spitting (1909).
Robertson, John (1910), *Report on Industrial Employment of Married Women and Infantile Mortality.*

Robertson, John (1922), *The Milk Supply: Report on a Visit to American Cities in Regard to Milk Supply*.

Salterley Grange Sanatorium (1908).

Special Report by the Medical Officer of Health on Further Measures for the Prevention of Consumption in the City of Birmingham (1906).

Special Report of the Medical Officer of Health on Infant Mortality in the City of Birmingham (1904).

City of Birmingham, Public Works Department

MacMorran, James L. (1973), *Municipal Public Works and Planning in Birmingham: A Record of the Administration and Achievements of the Public Works Committee and Department of the Borough and City of Birmingham*, Birmingham: City of Birmingham.

Local Government Board

Newsholme, Arthur (1909–1910) 'Report on infant and child mortality', in *39th Annual Report of the Local Government Board*, London: HMSO, Supplement.

Ministry of Health

Interim Report of Departmental Committee on Maternal Mortality and Morbidity (1930), London: HMSO.

Maternity and Child Welfare: Circulars and Memoranda No. 12, 1919 (1919), London: HMSO.

Ministry of Labour

Local Unemployment Index, Unemployment Statistics, prepared by the Ministry of Labour, nos 48–91 (1929–34), London: HMSO.

Registrar General

Annual Reports of the Registrar General of Births, Deaths and Marriages in England and Wales, 1875–1920.

Statistical Reviews, 1910–1936.

Sweden

Bidrag till Sveriges Officiella Statistik, 1890–1910

A) Befolkningsstatistik.

D) Fabriker och Manufacturer.

Göteborgs stad

Göteborgs Stadsfullmäktiges Handlingar (GSH) för 1900–1940.
Statistiska årsböcker för Göteborg, 1900–1940.

Göteborgs stad, Hälsovårdsnämnden

Almquist, Ernst (1888), 'Dödorsakerna i Göteborg 1861–85', in *Göteborgs hälsovårdsnämnds årsberättelse för 1888*, Appendix, pp. 81–8.
Göteborgs hälsovårdsnämnds årsberättelser för 1888–1940.
'Sjukvårdsanstalten å Kålltorp: Göteborgs stads lungsotssjukhus: Historik', in *Göteborgs hälsovårdsnämnds årsberättelse för 1914*, Appendix.
Walter, Karl Axel (1900), 'Barnbördshuset i Göteborg verksamhet under tiden från 1 Oktober 1875 till 1 Juli 1900', in *Göteborgs hälsovårdsnämnds årsberättelse för 1900*, Appendix.
Westman, Abraham H. (1900), 'Barnbördsanstaltens historia', in *Göteborgs hälsovårdsnämnds årsberättelse för 1900*, Appendix.

Kommittébetänkanden

Betänkande angående åtgärder för spridande av kunskap om könssjukdomarnas natur och smittfarlighet m.m. avgivet av för ändamålet inom Kungl. Civildepartementet den 25 oktober 1918 tillkallade sakkunniga (1912), Stockholm.
Betänkande och förslag af den utaf Kungl. Maj:t den 20 oktober tillsatta kommitté för verkställande af utredning angående årgärder för människotuberkulosens bekämpande I (1907) and II (1908), Stockholm.
Dovertie G. (1907), 'Öfversikt öfver striden mot tuberkulos i Sverige och utlandet', in *Betänkande och förslag af den utaf Kungl. Maj:t den 20 oktober tillsatta kommitté för verkställande af utredning angående årgärder för människotuberkulosens bekämpande* I, Stockholm.

Statens Offentliga Utredningar (SOU)

Edin, K.A. (1929), 'Antalet barnaföderskor bland gifta industriarbeterskor', in *SOU 1929:28*, Stockholm, pp. 105–6.
Gårdlund, Torsten, 'Förefintliga rådfrågningsbyråer för sexualupplysning i Sverige', in *SOU 1936:59*, Stockholm, Appendix 12, pp. 331–49.
Höjer, A. (1929), 'Mjölkdroppar och barnavårdscentraler', in *SOU 1929:28*, Stockholm, pp. 44–55.
Jansson, Gunnar and Sterner, Richard (1935), 'Bostadssociala förhållanden inom vissa städer och stadsliknande samhällen', in *SOU 1935:2*, Stockholm, Bilaga 2.
Nyström, Bertil (1935), 'Åtgärder till förbättring av de mindre bemedlades bostadsförhållanden i vissa städer', in *SOU 1935:2*, Stockholm, Bilaga 1.
SOU 1929:28: Betänkande angående moderskapsskydd avgivet den 26 september 1929 av inom Kungl. Socialdepartementet tillkallade sakkunnige, Stockholm.

SOU 1935:2: Betänkande och förslag rörande lån och årliga bidrag av statsmedel för främjande av bostadsförsörjning för mindre bemedlade barnrika familjer jämte därtill hörande utredningar avgivet den 17 januari 1935 av Bostadssociala utredningen, Stockholm.

SOU 1936:59: Betänkande I sexualfrågan avgivet av Befolkningskommissionen, Stockholm.

Statistiska centralbyrån

Historisk statistik för Sverige. I: Befolkningen 1720–1950, Stockholm (1955).
Historisk statistik för Sverige. Del 1, Stockholm (1969).

NEWSPAPERS AND PERIODICALS

Birmingham Daily Mail.
Birmingham Daily Post.
Birmingham Post.
British Medical Journal.
Göteborgs Handels- och Sjöfartstidning.
Göteborgs Morgon-Posten.
Hygiea.
Lancet.
Maternity and Child Welfare.
Midland Medical Journal.
Ny Tid.
Public Health.

BOOKS AND ARTICLES PUBLISHED PRIOR TO 1940

Almquist, Ernst (1897), *Allmän hälsovårdslära med särskildt afseende på svenska förhållanden för läkare, medicine studerande, hälsovårdsmyndigheter, tekniker m. fl.*, Stockholm: P.A. Norstedt & Söners Förlag.

Almquist, Ernst (1902), *Hälsovårdslärans framsteg under senaste åren*, Stockholm: P.A. Norstedt & Söners Förlag.

Anderson, Hjalmar and Belfrage, Harald (1939), 'Ten years' experience of B.C.G.-vaccination at Gothenburg', *Acta Pædiatrica* **26**, pp. 1–11.

Annual Report of the Society for the Study of Heredity in Its Bearings on the Human Race, 1910–11 (1911), Birmingham.

Armstrong, Barbara N. (1939), *The Health Insurance Doctor: His Rôle in Great Britain, Denmark and France*, Princeton NJ: Princeton University Press.

Aronson, Anders (1924), 'Dispensärna och tuberkuloskampen', *Social-Medicinsk Tidskrift* **1**, pp. 210–13.

Bateman, A.G. (1904), 'Doctors in Parliament', *Midland Medical Journal* **3** (3), 38–9.

Berglund, Victor (1908), 'Försäkring mot tuberkulos', *Social Tidskrift*, pp. 257–63.

Black, Clementina (ed.) (1915/1983), *Married Women's Work: Being the Report of an Enquiry Undertaken by Women's Industrial Council*, London: Virago.

Body, W.S. (ed.) (1928), *Birmingham and Its Civic Managers: The Departmental Doings of the City Council*, Birmingham: The Corporation of the City of Birmingham – Stanford & Mann.

Brodin, Åke (1939), 'Spädbarnsdödligheten i Göteborg tiden 1908–1937', *Nordisk Medicin*, pp. 3,659–70.

Broomé, Emilia (1908), 'Kvinnofrågor och kvinnoarbete', in G.H. von Koch (ed.), *Social Handbok*, Stockholm: Aktiebolaget Ljus, pp. 184–207.

Buhre, B. (1906), 'Svenska Nationalföreningen mot tuberkulos, dess uppkomst, medel och mål', *Social Tidskrift*, pp. 12–17.

Buhre, B. (1908), 'Tuberkulosens bekämpande', in G.H. von Koch (ed.), *Social Handbok*, Stockholm: Aktiebolaget Ljus, pp. 325–32.

Carlberg, Frigga (1908), 'Frivilligt arbete för späda barn i Göteborg', *Social Tidskrift*, pp. 536–40.

Carver, A.E. (1913–14), *An Investigation into the Dietary of the Labouring Classes of Birmingham, With Special Reference to Its Bearing upon Tuberculosis*, Birmingham.

Chadwick, Edwin (1842/1965), *Report on the Sanitary Condition of the Labouring Population of Great Britain*, Edinburgh: Edinburgh University Press.

Cornish's Birmingham Year Books for 1918–39.

Dixon, Godfrey B. (*c.*1910), *Lectures on the Prevention of Consumption Delivered to the Birmingham and Derbyshire Tuberculosis Visitors*, Derby.

Dixon, Godfrey B. (1914), 'The care of the consumptive in the home', reprint from the *Journal of the Royal Sanitary Institute* **25**, Birmingham Central Library.

Dixon, Godfrey B. (*c.* 1921), 'The discharged soldier and sanatorium treatment', reprint from the *British Journal of Tuberculosis*, Birmingham Central Library.

Dixon, Godfrey B. (1928), 'Progress made in combatting tuberculosis', *Journal of the Royal Sanitary Institute* **48**, pp. 398–405.

Dixon, Godfrey B. (1931), 'Pulmonary tuberculosis in childhood', reprint from the *British Medical Journal*, 25 April, Birmingham Central Library.

Don, Alexander (1905), 'The sanatorium treatment of consumption: is it worthwhile?', *British Medical Journal*, 22 July, p. 214.

Drake, Barbara (1920/1984), *Women in Trade Unions*, London: Virago.

Elliot, A.O. (1930), *Minnen från det gamla Göteborg*, Stockholm: Wahlström & Widstrand.

Fallows, J.A. (1899), *The Housing of the Poor*, Birmingham: Birmingham Socialist Centre.

Fallows, J.A. and Hughes, Fred (1905), *The Housing Question in Birmingham*, Birmingham.

Föreningen Mjölkdroppens Barnavårdscentraler i Göteborg, *Årsberättelser för 1930, 1935, 1937, 1938*, Göteborg.

Gardiner, A.G. (1923), *Life of George Cadbury*, London: Cassell.

Gezelius, Karl Joh. (1923), 'Göteborgs stads hälso- och sjukvård', in Nils Wimarson (ed.), *Göteborg: En översikt vid trehundraårsjubileet 1923*, Göteborg: Göteborgs stad, pp. 338–85.

Glass, David Victor (1938), 'Population policies in Scandinavia', *Eugenics Review* **30** (2), pp. 89–100.

Göranson, Werner and Rosander, Gustaf (1936), 'Vad siffrorna säga om göteborgarens sätt att bo', in *Katalog för Göteborgs stads bostadsutställning 'Bo bättre', 1 Maj–1 Juni 1936*, Göteborg, pp. 25–41.

Göteborgare 1923: Biografisk uppslagsbok (1923), Göteborg: Hugo Brusewitz Aktiebolags Förlag.

Göthlin, Gösta (1917), 'Några bostadshygieniska reformkrav', in *Göteborgs Läkaresällskaps förhandlingar, Hygiea* **79** (21), pp. 1,151–69.

Gough, Alfred (1908), *Objections to the Housing and Town-Planning Bill of the Right Honourable John Burns; and to the Housing of the Working Classes Bill Introduced by Mr. Bowerman With Birmingham's Experience of the Housing Acts*, Birmingham: Birmingham and District Trades and Property Association.

Griffith, Ernest S. (1927), *The Modern Development of City Government in the United Kingdom and the United States*, vol. II, London: Oxford University Press.

Heyman, Elias (1879), 'Några statistiska uppgifter om sunda arberatebostäders inflytande på dödligheten', *Hygiea* **41**, pp. 73–85.

Heyman, Elias (1890), 'Bostadsfrågans betydelse ur sanitär synpunkt', *Hygiea* **52**, pp. 329–50.

Hill, Alfred (1888), 'The president's address', in Proceedings of the Society of Medical Officers of Health, *Public Health* **1**, pp. 2–10.

Hjärne, Urban (1930), 'Några drag ur engelsk barnavårdsverksamhet: från ett studieuppehåll i England sommaren 1929', *Nordisk Medicinsk Tidskrift* **2**, pp. 204–7.

Isberg, Hagb. (1906), 'De oäkta barnen och fattigvården', *Social Tidskrift*, pp. 302–4.

Isberg, Hagb. (1908), 'Barnavård', in G.H. von Koch (ed.), *Social Handbok*, Stockholm: Aktiebolaget Ljus, pp. 67–78.

Johansson, J.E. and Moosberg, R. (1908), *Lungsotsdödligheten i Sverige enligt prästerkapets anteckningar i dödböckerna 1901–1905*, Stockholm.

Johansson, Sven (1922), 'Göteborgs barnsjukhus' historia', *Hygiea* **84**, pp. 454–67.

Jones, J. Ernst (1909), *A History of the Hospitals and Other Charities of Birmingham*, Birmingham: Midland Educational Co.

Jundell, Isak (1908), 'Moderskydd', *Social Tidskrift*, pp. 51–62.

Kjellin, G. (1917), 'Bekämpandet av tuberkulosen bland barnen', in Alf Gullbring (ed.), Tuberkulosläkare-föreningens förhandlingar, *Hygiea* **79**, pp. 1,331–40.

Kjellin, G. (1929), 'Tuberkuloskampens organisation i större stadssamhällen', *Social-Medicinsk Tidskrift* **6**, pp. 224–31.

Lane-Claypon, Janet E. (1920), *The Child Welfare Movement*, London: G. Bell and Sons.

Linden, Gustav (1923), 'Town planning in Sweden after 1850', in Werner Hegemann (ed.), *International Cities and Town Planning Exhibition, Gothenburg, Sweden 1923: English Catalogue*, Gothenburg: Jubilee Exhibition Committee, pp. 250–61.

Lindman, Carl (1898), *Dödligheten i första lefnadsåret i Sveriges tjugo större städer 1876–95*, Stockholm: Nordin & Josephson.

Lindman, Carl (1911), *Sundhets- och befolkningsförhållanden i Sveriges städer 1851–1909*, vol. I: *Text* and vol. II: *Tabeller och diagram*, Helsingborg: Helsingborgs Litografiska Anstalt.

Lindsay, Dorothy E. (*c.* 1912), *Report upon a Study of the Diet of the Labouring Classes in the City of Glasgow Carried out During 1911–1912*, Glasgow: University of Glasgow.

Linroth, Klas (1890), 'Minnesteckning öfver Elias Heyman', *Hygiea* **52**, pp. 53–62.

Llewelyn Davies, Margaret (ed.) (1915/1978), *Maternity: Letters from Working-Women*, New York: W.W. Norton.

Macfie, Ronald (1905), 'The sanatorium treatment of consumption: is it worth while?', *British Medical Journal*, 29 July, p. 260.

MacGonigle, G.C.M. and Kirby, J. (1937), *Poverty and Public Health*, London: Gollancz.

McCleary, G.F. (1935), *The Maternity and Child Welfare Movement*, London: P.S. King & Son.

'Meddelanden från Göteborgs Läkaresällskaps förhandlingar 1910', *Hygiea* **73** (1911); '1914', *Hygiea* **77** (1915); '1915', *Hygiea* **78** (1916).

Neander, Gustaf (1926), 'Anti-tuberkulosarbetets financiering i Sverige. Återblick. Översikt. Önskemål', in *Det Fjärde Nordiska Tuberkulosläkarmötet i Stockholm, 25–27 augusti 1925*, Stockholm, pp. 104–13.

Nettlefold, J.S. (1908), *Practical Housing*, Letchworth: Garden City Press.

Newman, George (1906), *Infant Mortality: A Social Problem*, London: Methuen.

Newman, George (1907), *The Health of the State*, London: Headley Brothers.

Newsholme, Arthur (1905), 'Infantile mortality: a statistical study from the public health standpoint', *Practitioner*, pp. 489–500.

Newsholme, Arthur (1906a), 'An inquiry into the principal causes of the reduction in the death-rate from phthisis during the last forty years, with special reference to the segregation of phthisical patients in general institutions', *Journal of Hygiene* **6**, pp. 304–84.

Newsholme, Arthur (1906b), 'Domestic infection in relation to epidemic diarrhoea', *Journal of Hygiene* **6**, pp. 139–48.

Newsholme, H.P. (1930), *The Moral Health of the City*, Birmingham.

Petrén, Karl (1908), 'Tuberkuloskommitténs betänkande', *Social Tidskrift*, pp. 110–16.

Pooler, H.W. (1913), 'Infant mortality work in Berlin: a visit to the third international congress on infantile mortality', *Midland Medical Journal* **12** (1), pp. 1–7.

Ransome, Arthur, Armstrong, Henry E. and Sykes, John F.J. (1893–94), 'The training and qualification of medical officers of health', *Public Health*, pp. 242–8.

Reid, George (1892), 'Report of proceedings of public medicine section of annual general meeting of British Medical Association', *British Medical Journal*, pp. 275–8.

Reid, George (1906), 'Infant mortality and the employment of married women in factory labour before and after confinement', *Lancet* (Part II), pp. 423–4.

Reports of the Birmingham Infants' Health Society for 1908–1922, Birmingham.

Richert, J. Gust. (1929), *Minnesanteckningar*, Stockholm: P.A. Norstedt & Söner.

Robertson, John (1909), 'Prevention of tuberculosis among cattle', *Public Health* **22**, pp. 324–8.

Robertson, John (1919), *Housing and Public Health*, London: Cassell.

Robertson, John (1925), *The House of Health: What the Modern Dwelling Needs to Be*, London: Faber & Gisyer.

Robertson, John (1930–31), 'The slum problem', *Journal of the Royal Sanitary Institute* **51**, pp. 279–84.

Runborg, Carl and Sundbärg, Gustav (1905), 'Dödligheten af lungtuberkulos i Sveriges städer, åren 1861/1900', *Statistisk Tidskrift*, pp. 198–224.

Sigerist, Henry E. (1937), *Socialised Medicine in the Soviet Union*, London: Victor Gollancz.

Silbergleit (1895), 'Ueber den gegenwärtigen Stand der Kindersterblichkeit, ihre Erscheinungen und ihre Entwickelung in europäischen Großstädten', *Beilage zur Hygienischen Rundschau* 5, pp. 216–41.

Smith, C.E. (1914), *Memorandum on the Housing Question Submitted to the Housing Enquiry Committee of the Birmingham City Council*, Birmingham: Birmingham Socialist Centre.

Stéenhoff, G. (1917), 'Kampen mot tuberkulosen i England', in Tuberkulosläkareföreningens förhandlingar, *Hygiea* **79**, pp. 788–97.

Sundell, C.G. (1929), 'Effektivare spädbarnsvård och spädbarnskontroll', *Social-Medicinsk Tidskrift* **6**, pp. 232–40.

Sutherland, Halliday (1911), 'The extent of the disease and the sources of infection', in Halliday Sutherland (ed.), *The Control and Eradication of Tuberculosis: A Series of International Studies*, Edinburgh: William Green & Sons Medical Publishers, pp. 5–23.

Tennant, May (1908), 'Infantile mortality', in Gertrude M. Tuckwell et al., *Woman in Industry: From Seven Points of View*, London: Duckworth, pp. 85–119.

Thomas, Brinley (1936), *Monetary Policy and Crises: A Study of Swedish Experience*, London: George Routledge and Sons.

Thomson, Hyslop (1906), *Pulmonary Phthisis: Its Diagnosis, Prognosis and Treatment,* London: John Bale, Sons & Danielson.

Tuckwell, Gertrude, M. (1908), 'The regulation of women's work', in Gertrude M. Tuckwell et al., *Woman in Industry: From Seven Points of View,* London: Duckworth, pp. 1–23.

Vince, Charles Anthony (1902), *History of the Corporation of Birmingham, Volume III: 1885–1899*, Birmingham: Cornish Brothers.

von Koch, G.H. (1908), 'Bostadsfrågan', in G.H. von Koch (ed.), *Social Handbok*, Stockholm: Aktiebolaget Ljus, pp. 79–92.

Wallgren, Arvid (1927–28), 'Observations critiques sur la vaccination antituberculeuse de Calmette', *Acta Pædiatrica* **12**, pp. 120–37.

Wallgren, Arvid (1928), 'Intradermal vaccinations with BCG virus', *Journal of the American Medical Association* **91**, pp. 1,876–81.

Wallgren, Arvid (1930), Le rôle de la vaccination anti-tuberculeuse dans la lutte contre la tuberculose infantile', and discussion, *Acta Pædiatrica* **11**, *The Transactions of the Second International Pediatric Congress, Stockholm August 1930*, pp. 410–13.

Wallgren, Arvid (1934a), 'Barnavårdcentraler och deras förebyggande verksamhet i spädbarnsåldern: en betydelsefull social-medicinsk uppgift', *Social-Medicinsk Tidskrift* **11**, pp. 167–71.

Wallgren, Arvid (1934b), 'Value of Calmette vaccination in prevention of tuberculosis in childhood', *Journal of American Medical Association* **103**, pp. 1,341–5.

Wallgren, Arvid (1942), 'The neonatal mortality in Sweden, from a pediatric point of view', *Acta Pædiatrica* **29**, pp. 372–86.

Wallqvist, Hjalmar (1890), *Om arbetarebostäder*, Föredrag i Helsovårdsföreningen i Stockholm, 16. 12. 1889, Stockholm.

Wallqvist, Hjalmar (1891), *Bostadsförhållandena för de mindre bemedlade i Göteborg: Studie sommaren 1889*, Stockholm: Samson & Wallin.

Wellinder N.J. (1924), *Biografisk matrikel över svenska läkarkåren 1924*, Stockholm: A.B. Hasse W. Tullbergs Förlag.

Woodcock, Florence (1934), 'The voluntary worker in our welfare centre', *City of Birmingham Maternity and Child Welfare Magazine*, June, p. 18.

BOOKS AND ARTICLES PUBLISHED SINCE 1940

Åberg, Martin (1991), *En fråga om klass? Borgarklass och industriellt företagande i Göteborg, 1850–1914*, Göteborg: Göteborgs universitet.

Allen, Ann Taylor (1991), *Feminism and Motherhood in Germany 1800–1914*, New Brunswick, NJ: Rutgers University Press.

Andersson, Bertil (1996), *Göteborgs historia: Näringsliv och samhällsutveckling I: Från fästningsstad till handelsstad 1619–1820*, Stockholm: Nerenius & Santérus Förlag.

Anttonen, Anneli (1994), 'Hyvinvointivaltion naisystävälliset kasvot', in Anneli Anttonen, Lea Henriksson and Ritva Nätkin (eds), *Naisten Hyvinvointivaltio*, Tampere: Vastapaino, pp. 203–26.

Apple, Rima D. (1995), 'Constructing mothers: scientific motherhood in the nineteenth and twentieth centuries', *Social History of Medicine* **8** (1), April, pp. 161–78.

Apple, Rima D. (1996), *Vitamania: Vitamins in American Culture*, New Brunswick, NJ: Rutgers University Press, 1996.

Ariès, Philippe (1976/1994), *Western Attitudes Toward Death from the Middle Ages to the Present*, London: Marion Boyars.

Armstrong, David (1983), *Political Anatomy of the Body: Medical Knowledge in Britain in the Twentieth Century*, Cambridge: Cambridge University Press.

Arnold, David (1988), 'Introduction: disease, medicine and empire', in David Arnold (ed.), *Imperial Medicine and Indigenous Societies*, Manchester: Manchester University Press, pp. 1–26.

Arnold, David (1993), *Colonizing the Body: State Medicine and Epidemic Disease in Nineteenth-century India*, Berkeley, CA: University of California Press.

Arnot, Margaret L. (1994), 'Infant death, child care and the state: the baby-farming scandal and the first infant life protection legislation of 1872', *Continuity and Change* **9** (2), pp. 271–311.

Atkins, P.J. (1992), 'White poison? The social consequences of milk consumption, 1850–1930', *Social History of Medicine* **5** (2), August, pp. 207–27.

Atkins, Peter J. (2003), 'Mother's milk and infant death in Britain, circa 1900–1940', *Anthropology of Food*, 2, September.

Attman, Artur (1963), *Göteborgs Stadsfullmäktige 1863–1962*, vol. I.1: *Göteborg 1863–1913* and vol. I.2: *Göteborg 1913–1962*, Göteborg: Göteborgs stad.

Attman, Artur, Boberg, Stig and Wåhlstrand, Arne (1971), *Göteborgs Stadsfullmäktige 1863–1962*, vol. III: *Stadsfullmäktige, stadens styrelser och förvaltningar*, Göteborg: Göteborgs stad.

Baker, Jeffrey P. (1996), *The Machine in the Nursery: Incubator Technology and the Origins of Newborn Intensive Care*, Baltimore, MD: John Hopkins University Press.

Barnes, David S. (1995), *The Making of a Social Disease: Tuberculosis in Nineteenth-century France*, Berkeley, CA: University of California Press.

Barnsby, George J. (1989), *Birmingham Working People: A History of the Labour Movement in Birmingham 1650–1914*, Wolverhampton: Integrated Publishing Services.

Bergman, Helena (2001), '"En feministisk konspiration": kvinnors politiska aktivism för barnavårdsmannainstitutionens införande i 1910-talets Sverige', in Christina Florin and Lars Kvarnström (eds), *Kvinnor på gränsen till medborgarskap: Genus, politik och offentlighet 1800–1950*, Stockholm: Atlas Akademi, pp. 172–191.

Bergman, Rolf (1963), 'De epidemiska sjukdomarna och deras bekämpande', in Wolfram Kock (ed.), *Medicinalväsendet i Sverige 1813–1963*, Stockholm: AB Nordiska Bokhandelns Förlag, pp. 329–80.

Bergstrand, Hilding (1963), 'Läkarekåren och provinsialläkareväsendet', in Wolfram Kock (ed.), *Medicinalväsendet i Sverige 1813–1962*, Stockholm: AB Nordiska Bokhandelns Förlag, pp. 107–57.

Björkquist, Erik and Flygare, Ivar (1963), 'Den centrala medicinalförvaltningen', in Wolfram Kock (ed.), *Medicinalväsendet i Sverige 1813–1962*, Stockholm: AB Nordiska Bokhandelns Förlag, pp. 7–102.

Bland, Lucy (1995), *Banishing the Beast: English Feminism and Sexual Morality 1885–1914*, London: Penguin Books.

Bock, Gisela (1994), 'Anti-natalism, maternity and paternity in National Socialist racism', in Gisela Bock and Pat Thane (eds), *Maternity and Gender Policies: Women and the Rise of the European Welfare States, 1880s–1950s*, London: Routledge, pp. 233–55.

Bock, Gisela and Thane, Pat (eds) (1994), *Maternity and Gender Policies: Women and the Rise of the European Welfare States, 1880s–1950s*, London: Routledge.

Boris, Eileen and Kleinberg, S.J. (2003), 'Mothers and other workers: (re)conceiving labor, maternalism, and the state', *Journal of Women's History* **15** (3), pp. 90–117.

Bourdieu, Pierre (1998), *The State Nobility: Elite Schools in the Field of Power*, Cambridge: Polity Press.

Bourke, Joanna (1994), *Working-class Cultures in Britain 1890–1960: Gender, Class and Ethnicity*, London: Routledge.

Bramwell, Bill (1991), 'Public space and local communities: the example of Birmingham, 1840–80', in Gerry Kearns and Charles J. Withers (eds), *Urbanising Britain: Essays on Class and Community in the Nineteenth Century*, Cambridge: Cambridge University Press, pp. 31–54.

Brand, Jeanne L. (1965), *Doctors and the State: The British Medical Profession and Government Action in Public Health, 1870–1912*, Baltimore, MD: The John Hopkins Press.

Brändström, Anders (1988a), 'The impact of female labour conditions on infant mortality: a case study of the parishes of Nedertorneå and Jokkmokk, 1800–96', *Social History of Medicine* **1** (3), December, pp. 329–58.

Brändström, Anders (1988b), 'The silent sick: the life-histories of 19th century Swedish hospital patients', in Anders Brändström and Lars-Göran Tedebrand (eds), *Society, Health and Population During the Demographic Transition*, Stockholm: Almqvist and Wiksell International, pp. 343–68.

Brändström, Anders (1994), *'De kärlekslösa mödrarna': Spädbarnsdödligheten i Sverige under 1800-talet med särskild hänsyn till Nedertorneå*, Umeå: Umeå universitet.

Brändström, Anders, Edvinsson, Sören and Rogers, John (2002), 'Illegitimacy, infant feeding practices and infant survival in Sweden 1750–1950: a regional analysis', *Hygiea Internationalis* **3** (3), December, pp. 15–52.

Briggs, Asa (1952), *History of Birmingham, Volume II: Borough and City 1865–1938*, London: Oxford University Press.

Broberg, Gunnar and Tydén, Mattias (1996), 'Eugenics in Sweden: efficient care', in Gunnar Broberg and Nils Roll-Hansen (eds), *Eugenics and the Welfare State: Sterilization Policy in Denmark, Sweden, Norway, and Finland*, East Lansing, MI: Michigan State University Press, pp. 77–149.

Bryder, Linda (1988), *Below the Magic Mountain: A Social History of Tuberculosis in Twentieth-century Britain*, Oxford: Clarendon Press.

Bryder, Linda (1992), '"Wonderlands of buttercup, clover and daisies": tuberculosis and the open-air school movement in Britain, 1907–39', in Roger Cooter (ed.), *In the Name of the Child: Health and Welfare, 1880–1940*, London: Routledge, pp. 72–95.

Bryder, Linda (1996), '"Not always one and the same thing": the registration of tuberculosis deaths in Britain, 1900–1950', *Social History of Medicine* **9** (2), August, pp. 253–65.

Bryder, Linda (1999), '"We shall not find salvation in inoculation": B.C.G. vaccination is Scandinavia, Britain and the U.S.A, 1921–60', *Social Science and Medicine* **49** (1), pp. 157–67.

Bryder, Linda (2003), 'Two models of infant welfare in the first half of the twentieth century: New Zealand and the USA', *Women's History Review* **12** (4), pp. 547–58.

Burnett, John (1986), *A Social History of Housing 1815–1985*, London: Routledge.

Bynum, W.F. (1994), *Science and the Practice of Medicine in the Nineteenth Century*, Cambridge: Cambridge University Press.

Byrman, Gunilla (2001), 'From marital precautions to love power: gender construction in Swedish contraceptive brochures', *Nordic Journal of Women's Studies* **9** (2), pp. 89–97.

Cage, R.A. (1994), 'Infant mortality rates and housing: twentieth century Glasgow', *Scottish Economic and Social History* **14**, pp. 77–92.

Carlson, Gösta et al (1982), *Sjukvården i Göteborg 200 år*, Göteborg: Göteborgs Sjukvårdsstyrelse.

Carlsson, Christina (1986), *Kvinnosyn och kvinnopolitik: En studie av svensk socialdemokrati 1880–1910*, Lund: Arkiv.

Carlsson Wetterberg, Christina (1997), 'Kvinnorörelse och välfärdsstat – Sverige/ Schweiz: några tankar kring en komparativ studie', in B. Gullikstad and K. Heitmann (eds), *Kjønn, makt, samfunn i Norden i et historisk perspektiv*, vol. 1, Dragvoll: Norges teknisk-naturvitenskapelige universitet, pp. 155–81.

Castensson, Reinhold, Löwgren, Marianne and Sundin, Jan (1988), 'Urban water supply and improvement of health conditions', in Anders Brändström and Lars-Göran Tedebrand (eds), *Society, Health and Population During the Demographic Transition*, Stockholm: Almqvist and Wiksell International, pp. 273–98.

Cherry, Gordon E. (1994), *Birmingham: A Study in Geography, History and Planning*, Chichester: John Wiley & Sons.

Cherry, Steven (1996), *Medical Services and the Hospitals in Britain, 1860–1939*, Cambridge: Cambridge University Press.

Chinn, Carl (1988), *They Worked All Their Lives: Women of the Urban Poor in England, 1880–1939*, Manchester: Manchester University Press.

Chinn, Carl (1991), *Homes for People: 100 Years of Council Housing in Birmingham*, Exeter: Birmingham Books/Wheaton Publishers.

Condrau, Flurin (2001), '"Who is the captain of all these men of death?": the social structure of a tuberculosis sanatorium in postwar Germany', *Journal of Interdisciplinary History* **32** (2), Autumn, pp. 243–62.

Corbin, Alain (1988), *Pesthauch und Blütenduft: Eine Geschichte des Geruchs*, Frankfurt am Main: Fischer Taschenbuch Verlag.

Crowther, M.A. (1982), 'Family responsibility and state responsibility in Britain before the welfare state', *The Historical Journal* **25** (1), pp. 131–45.

Crowther, M.A. (1983), *The Workhouse System 1834–1929: The History of an English Institution*, London: Methuen.

Crowther, M. Anne (1988), *Social Policy in Britain 1914–1939*, London: Macmillan.

Daunton, M.J. (ed.) (2000), *The Cambridge Urban History of Britain, Volume III: 1840–1950*, Cambridge: Cambridge University Press.

Daunton, M.J. (2004), 'Taxation and representation in the Victorian city', in Robert Colls and Richard Rodger (eds), *Cities of Ideas: Civil Society and Urban Governance in Britain, 1800–2000*, Aldershot: Ashgate, pp. 21–45.

Davidoff, Leonore and Hall, Catherine (1992), *Family Fortunes: Men and Women of the English Middle Class 1780–1850*, London: Routledge.

Davies, Celia (1988), 'The health visitor as mother's friend: a woman's place in public health, 1900–14', *Social History of Medicine* **1** (1), April, pp. 39–59.

Dayus, Kathleen (1982), *Her People*, London: Virago.

Dierig, Sven, Lachmund, Jens and Mendelsohn, J. Andrew (2003), 'Introduction: toward an urban history of science', in Sven Dierig, Jens Lachmund and J. Andrew Mendelsohn (eds), *Science and the City/Osiris* **18**, pp. 1–19.

Digby, Anne (1994), *Making a Medical Living: Doctors and Patients in the English Market for Medicine, 1720–1911*, Cambridge: Cambridge University Press.

Digby, Anne and Bosanquet, Nick (1988), 'Doctors and patients in an era of national health insurance and private practice, 1913–1938', *Economic History Review* **41** (1), pp. 74–94.

Dingwall, R., Eekelaar, J. M. and Murray, T. (1984), 'Childhood as a social problem: a survey of the history of legal regulation', *Journal of Law and Society* **11** (2), pp. 207–32.

Dormandy, Thomas (2000), *The White Death: A History of Tuberculosis*, New York: New York University Press.

Doyle, Barry M. (2000), 'The changing functions of urban government: councillors, officials and pressure groups', in Martin Daunton (ed.), *The Cambridge Urban History of Britain, Volume III: 1840–1950*, Cambridge: Cambridge University Press, pp. 287–313.

Dowbiggin, Ian (1996), 'Back to the future: Valentin Magnan, French psychiatry, and the classification of mental diseases', *Social History of Medicine* **9** (3), December, pp. 383–408.

Dwork, Deborah (1987), *War is Good for Babies and Other Young Children: A History of the Infant and Child Welfare Movement in England 1890–1918*, London: Tavistock Publications.

Dyhouse, Carol (1981), 'Working-class mothers and infant mortality in England, 1895–1914', in Charles Webster (ed.), *Biology, Medicine and Society 1840–1940*, Cambridge: Cambridge University Press, pp. 73–98.

Dyhouse, Carol (1989), *Feminism and the Family in England 1880–1939*, Oxford: Basil Blackwell.

Dyos, H.J. and Reeder, D.A. (1973), 'Slums and suburbs', in H.J. Dyos and Michael Wolff (eds), *The Victorian City: Images and Realities*, vol. 1, London: Routledge and Kegan Paul, pp. 359–86.

Edvinsson, Sören (1992), *Den osunda staden: Sociala skillnader i dödlighet i 1800-talets Sundsvall*, Umeå: Umeå universitet.

Edvinsson, Sören and Rogers, John (2001), 'Hälsa och hälsoreformer i svenska städer kring sekelskiftet 1900', *Historisk tidskrift* **121** (4), pp. 541–64.

Elgán, Elizabeth (1990), 'Le législateur au secours de la mère célebataire: la solution de la responsabilité individuelle', in Marie C. Nelson and John Rogers (eds), *Mother, Father, and Child: Swedish Social Policy in the Early Twentieth Century*, Uppsala: Uppsala universitet, pp. 55–67.

Elgán, Elizabeth (1994), *Genus och politik: En jämförelse mellan svensk och fransk abort- och preventivmedelspolitik från sekelskiftet till andra världskriget*, Uppsala: Uppsala Universitet.

Elias, Norbert (1994), *The Civilizing Process: The History of Manners & State Formation and Civilization*, Oxford: Blackwell.

Elison, Ingela (1963), *Arbetarrörelse och samhälle i Göteborg 1910–1922*, Göteborg: Göteborgs universitet.

Enmark, Romulo (1984), 'Bo och leva i Annedal – kvarteret Ananasen', in *För hundra år sedan – skildringar från Göteborgs 1880-tal*, Göteborg: Göteborgs historiska museum, pp. 140–58.

Evans, Richard J. (1990), *Death in Hamburg: Society and Politics in the Cholera Years*, London: Penguin Books.

Fahl, Magnus (1963), *Göteborgs Stadsfullmäktige 1863–1962*, vol. II: *Biografisk matrikel*, Göteborg: Göteborgs stad.

Farganis, Sondra (1992), 'Feminism and the reconstruction of social science', in Alison M. Jaggar and Susan R. Bordo (eds), *Gender/Body/Knowledge: Feminist Reconstructions of Being and Knowing*, New Brunswick, NJ: Rutgers University Press, pp. 207–23.

Fausto-Sterling, Anne (1992), *Myths of Gender: Biological Theories about Women and Men*, New York: Basic Books.

Feldberg, Georgina D. (1995), *Disease and Class: Tuberculosis and the Shaping of Modern North American Society*, New Brunswick, NJ: Rutgers University Press.

Fildes, Valerie (1992), 'Breast-feeding in London, 1905–1919', *Journal of Biosocial Science* **24**, pp. 53–70.

Fildes, Valerie (1998), 'Infant feeding practices and infant mortality in England, 1900–1919,' *Continuity and Change* **13** (2), pp. 251–80.

Finer, S.E. (1952), *The Life and Times of Edwin Chadwick*, London: Methuen.

Flinn, M.W. (1976), 'Medical services under the New Poor Law', in Derek Fraser (ed.), *The New Poor Law in the Nineteenth Century*, London: Macmillan, pp. 45–66.

Foucault, Michel (1990), *The History of Sexuality, Volume 1: An Introduction*, London: Penguin Books.

Fox Keller, Evelyn (1992), *Secrets of Life. Secrets of Death: Essays on Language, Gender and Science*, New York: Routledge.

Fox Keller, Evelyn and Longino, Helen E. (1996), 'Introduction', in Evelyn Fox Keller and Helen E. Longino (eds), *Feminism and Science*, Oxford: Oxford University Press, pp. 1–14.

Fraser, Hamish (1993), 'Municipal socialism and social policy', in R.J. Morris and Richard Rodger (eds), *The Victorian City: A Reader in British Urban History 1820–1914*, London: Longman, pp. 258–80.

Fritz, Martin (1996), *Göteborgs historia. Näringsliv och samhällsutveckling II: Från handelsstad till industristad 1820–1920*, Stockholm: Nerenius & Santérus Förlag.

Frykman, Jonas (1992), 'In motion: body and modernity in Sweden between the World Wars', *Ethnologia Scandinavica* **22**, pp. 36–51.

Frykman, Jonas and Löfgren, Orvar (1979), *Den kultiverade människan*, Malmö: Gleerups.

Garside, Patricia (1988), '"Unhealthy areas": town planning, eugenics and the slums, 1890–1945', *Planning Perspectives* **3** (1), January, pp. 24–46.

Garside, Patricia (1997), 'Modelling the behaviour of non-profit housing agencies in Britain and France 1900–1939', in Clemens Zimmermann (ed.), *Europäische Wohnungspolitik in vergleichender Perspektive 1900–1939/European Housing*

Policy in Comparative Perpective 1900–1939, Stuttgart: Fraunhofer IRB Verlag, pp. 42–59.

Gilligan, Carol (1982), *In a Different Voice: Psychological Theory and Women's Development*, Cambridge, MA: Harvard University Press.

Good, Byron J. (1994), *Medicine, Rationality, and Experience: An Anthropological Perspective*, Cambridge: Cambridge University Press.

Gordon, Linda (1978), 'Introduction', in Margaret Llewelyn Davies (ed.), *Maternity: Letters from Working Women, Collected by the Women's Co-operative Guild*, New York: W.W. Norton, pp. v–xii.

Graham, David (1994), 'Female employment and infant mortality: some evidence from British towns, 1911, 1931 and 1951', *Continuity and Change* **9** (2), pp. 313–46.

Granshaw, Lindsay (1992a), 'The rise of the modern hospital in Britain', in Andrew Wear (ed.), *Medicine in Society: Historical Essays*, Cambridge: Cambridge University Press, pp. 197–218.

Granshaw, Lindsay (1992b), '"Upon this principle I have based a practice": the development and reception of antisepsis in Britain, 1867–90', in John V. Pickstone (ed.), *Medical Innovations in Historical Perspective*, London: Macmillan, pp. 17–46.

Green, David R. and Parton, Alan G. (1990), 'Slums and slum life in Victorian England: London and Birmingham at mid-century', in S. Martin Gaskell (ed.), *Slums*, Leicester: Leicester University Press, pp. 37–53.

Gröndahl, Jan (1990), 'Single mothers and poor relief in a Swedish industrial town (Gävle) at the beginning of the twentieth century', in Marie C. Nelson and John Rogers (eds), *Mother, Father, and Child: Swedish Social Policy in the Early Twentieth Century*, Uppsala: Uppsala universitet, pp. 31–53.

Guérin, Camille (1980), 'Early history', in Sol Roy Rosenthal (ed.), *BCG Vaccine: Tuberculosis – Cancer*, Littleton, MA: PSG Publishing Co., pp. 35–8.

Habermas, Jürgen (1985), *Der philosophische Diskurs der Moderne: Zwölf Vorlesungen*, Frankfurt am Main: Suhrkamp Verlag.

Hachten, Elizabeth A. (2002), 'In service to science and society: scientists and the public in late-nineteenth-century Russia', in Lynn K. Nyhart and Thomas Broman (eds), *Science and Civil Society/Osiris* **17**, pp. 171–209.

Hall, Catherine (1977), 'Married women at home in Birmingham in the 1920s and 1930s', *Oral History* **5** (2), pp. 62–83.

Hall, Thomas (1991a), 'Concluding remarks: is there a Nordic planning tradition?', in Thomas Hall (ed.), *Planning and Urban Growth in the Nordic Countries*, London: E. & F.N. Spon, pp. 247–59.

Hall, Thomas (1991b), 'Urban planning in Sweden', in Thomas Hall (ed.), *Planning and Urban Growth in the Nordic Countries*, London: E. & F.N. Spon, pp. 167–246.

Hall, Thomas (1994), 'Planning history: recent developments in the Nordic countries, with special reference to Sweden', *Planning Perspectives* **9** (2), April, pp. 153–79.

Hallström, Jonas (2002), *Constructing a Pipe-bound City: A History of Water Supply, Sewerage, and Excreta Removal in Norrköping and Linköping, Sweden, 1860–1910*, Linköping: Linköping University.

Hamlin, Christopher (1990), *A Science of Impurity: Water Analysis in Nineteenth-century Britain*, Bristol: Adam Hilger.

Hamlin, Christopher (1994a), 'Environmental sensibility in Edinburgh, 1839–1840: the fetid irrigation controversy', *Journal of Urban History* **20** (3), December, pp. 311–39.

Hamlin, Christopher (1994b), 'State medicine in Great Britain', in Dorothy Porter (ed.), *The History of Public Health and the Modern State*, Amsterdam: Editions Rodopi, pp. 132–64.

Haraway, Donna J. (1991), *Simians, Cyborgs, and Women: The Reinvention of Nature*, London: Free Association Books.

Harding, Sandra (1991), *Whose Science? Whose Knowledge? Thinking from Women's Lives*, Milton Keynes: Open University Press.

Hardy, Anne (1992), 'Rickets and the rest: child care, diet and the infectious children's diseases, 1850–1914', *Social History of Medicine* **5** (3), December, pp. 389–412.

Hardy, Anne (1994), '"Death is the cure of all diseases": using the General Register Office cause of death statistics for 1837–1920', *Social History of Medicine* **7** (3), December, pp. 473–92.

Hardy, Anne (2003), 'Reframing disease: changing perceptions of tuberculosis in England and Wales, 1938–70', *Historical Research* **76** (194), November, pp. 535–56.

Harris, Jose (1990), 'Economic knowledge and British social policy', in Mary O. Furner and Barry Supple (eds), *The State and Economic Knowledge: The American and British Experiences*, Cambridge: Cambridge University Press, pp. 379–400.

Harris, Jose (1994), *Private Lives, Public Spirit: Britain 1870–1914*, London: Penguin Books.

Harrison, Barbara (1995), 'Women and health', in June Purvis (ed.), *Women's History: Britain, 1850–1945: An Introduction*, London: UCL Press, pp. 157–92.

Harrison, Mark (1994), *Public Health in British India: Anglo-Indian Preventive Medicine 1859–1914*, Cambridge: Cambridge University Press.

Harrison, Michael (1995), 'Bournville 1919–1939', *Planning History* **17** (3), pp. 22–31.

Hellerström, Sven and Tottie, Malcolm (1963), 'De veneriska sjukdomarna', in Wolfram Kock (ed.), *Medicinalväsendet i Sverige 1813–1962*, Stockholm: AB Nordiska Bokhandelns Förlag, pp. 405–23.

Hendrick, Harry (1994), *Child Welfare: England 1872–1989*, London: Routledge.

Hendrick, Harry (1997), *Children, Childhood and English Society 1880–1990*, Cambridge: Cambridge University Press.

Hennock, E.P. (1973), *Fit and Proper Persons: Ideal and Reality in Nineteenth-century Urban Government*, London: Edward Arnold.

Hennock, E.P. (1998), 'Vaccination policy against smallpox, 1835–1914: a comparison of England with Prussia and Imperial Germany', *Social History of Medicine* **11** (1), April, pp. 49–71.

Hietala, Marjatta (1987), *Services and Urbanization at the Turn of the Century: The Diffusion of Innovations*, Helsinki: Finnish Historical Society.

Hirdman, Yvonne (1986), 'Särart – likhet: kvinnorörelsens scylla och karybdis? Reflektioner utifrån spröda empiriska iakttagelser rörande svensk kvinnorörelse historia under 1900-talet', in Inge Frederiksen and Hilda Rømer (eds), *Kvinder, mentalitet, arbejde: Kvindehistorisk forskning i Norden*, Århus: Aarhus Universitetsforlag, pp. 27–40.

Hirdman, Yvonne (1992), *Den socialistiska hemmafrun och andra kvinnohistorier*, Stockholm: Carlssons.

Hobson, Barbara (1993), 'Feminist strategies and gendered discourses in welfare states: married women's right to work in the United States and Sweden', in Seth Koven and Sonya Michel (eds), *Mothers of a New World: Maternalist Politics and the Origins of Welfare States*, New York: Routledge, pp. 396–429.

Hobson, Barbara and Takahashi, Meiko (1997), 'The parent–worker model: lone mothers in Sweden', in J. Lewis (ed.), *Lone Mothers in European Welfare Regimes: Shifting Policy Logics*, London: Jessica Kingsley, pp. 121–39.

Hollinger, David A. (1990), 'Free enterprise and free inquiry: the emergence of laissez-faire communitarianism in the ideology of science in the United States', *New Literary History* **21** (4), pp. 879–919.

Hollis, Patricia (1987), *Ladies Elect: Women in English Local Government 1865–1914*, Oxford: Clarendon Press.

Horrell, Sarah and Humphries, Jane (1997), 'The origins and expansion of the male breadwinner family: the case of nineteenth century Britain', in Angélique Janssens (ed.), *The Rise and Decline of the Male Breadwinner Family?/International Review of Social History* **42**, Supplement, pp. 25–64.

Howell, Joel D. (1989), 'Machines and medicine: technology transforms the American hospital', in Diana Elizabeth Long and Janet Golden (eds), *The American General Hospital: Communities and Social Contexts*, Ithaca, NY: Cornell University Press, pp. 109–34.

Humphries, Jane (1995), 'Women and paid work', in June Purvis (ed.), *Women's History: Britain, 1850–1945: An Introduction*, London: UCL Press, pp. 85–105.

Ito, Hirobumi (1980), 'Health insurance and medical services in Sweden and Denmark 1850–1950', in Arnold Heidenheimer and Nils Elvander (eds), *The Shaping of the Swedish Health System*, London: Croom Helm, pp. 44–67.

Johannisson, Karin (1988), 'Why cure the sick? Population policy and health programs within 18th-century Swedish mercantilism', in Anders Brändström and Lars-Göran Tedebrand (eds), *Society, Health and Population During the Demographic Transition*, Stockholm: Almqvist and Wiksell International, pp. 323–30.

Johannisson, Karin (1990), *Medicinens öga: Sjukdom, medicin och samhälle – historiska erfarenheter*, Stockholm: Norstedts.

Johannisson, Karin (1991), 'Folkhälsa: det svenska projektet från 1900 till 2:a världskriget', *Lychnos: Årsbok för idehistoria och vetenskapshistoria*, pp. 139–95.

Johannisson, Karin (1994), 'The people's health: public health policies in Sweden', in Dorothy Porter (ed.), *The History of Public Health and the Modern State*, Amsterdam: Editions Rodopi, pp. 165–82.

Johannisson, Karin (1995), *Den mörka kontinenten: Kvinnan, medicinen och fin-desiècle*, Stockholm: Norstedts.

Jones, Joseph (1940), *History of the Corporation of Birmingham*, vol. V, Parts I–II, Birmingham.

Jordanova, Ludmilla (1986a), 'Introduction', in Ludmilla Jordanova (ed.), *Languages of Nature: Critical Essays on Science and Literature*, London: Free Association Books, pp. 15–47.

Jordanova, Ludmilla (1986b), 'Naturalizing the family: literature and the bio-medical sciences in the late eighteenth century', in Ludmilla Jordanova (ed.), *Languages of Nature: Critical Essays on Science and Literature*, London: Free Association Books, pp. 86–116.

Jordanova, Ludmilla (1989), *Sexual Visions: Images of Gender in Science and Medicine between the Eighteenth and Twentieth Centuries*, New York: Harvester Wheatsheaf.

Jordanova, Ludmilla (1995), 'The social construction of medical knowledge', *Social History of Medicine* **8** (3), December, pp. 361–81.

Jordansson, Birgitta and Vammen, Tinne (eds) (1998), *Charitable Women: Philanthropic Welfare 1780–1930: A Nordic and Interdisciplinary Anthology*, Odense: Odense University Press.

Jordansson, Birgitta (1998), 'Women and philanthropy in a liberal context: the case of Gothenburg', in Birgitta Jordansson and Tinne Vammen (eds), *Charitable Women: Philanthropic Welfare 1780–1930: A Nordic and Interdisciplinary Anthology*, Odense: Odense University Press, pp. 65–88.

Kälvemark, Ann-Sofie (1977), 'Att vänta barn när man gifter sig: föräktenskapliga förbindelser och giftermålsmönster i 1800-talets Sverige', *Historisk Tidskrift* **97** (2), pp. 181–99.

Karlberg, Petter (1982), 'Barnhälsovården', in Gösta Carlson et al., *Sjukvården i Göteborg 200 år*, Göteborg: Göteborgs Sjukvårdsstyrelse, pp. 194–203.

Karlsson, Lynn (1995), 'The beginning of a "masculine renaissance": the debate on the 1909 prohibition against women's night work in Sweden', in Ulla Wikander, Alice Kessler-Harris and Jane Lewis (eds), *Protecting Women: Labor Legislation in Europe, the United States, and Australia, 1880–1920*, Urbana, IL: University of Illinois Press, pp. 235–66.

Kearns, Gerard (1988a), 'Private property and public health reform in England 1830–70', *Social Science and Medicine* **26** (1), pp. 187–99.

Kearns, Gerard (1988b), 'The urban penalty and the population history of England', in Anders Brändström and Lars-Göran Tedebrand (eds), *Society, Health and Population During the Demographic Transition*, Stockholm: Almqvist and Wiksell International, pp. 213–36.

Kearns, Gerard (1989), 'Zivilis or Hygaeia: urban public health and the epidemiologic transition', in Richard Lawton (ed.), *The Rise and Fall of Great Cities: Aspects of Urbanization in the Western World*, London: Belhaven Press, pp. 96–124.

Kearns, Gerard, Lee, W. Robert and Rogers, John (1989), 'The interaction of political and economic factors in the management of urban public health', in Marie C. Nelson and John Rogers (eds), *Urbanisation and the Epidemiologic Transition*, Uppsala: Uppsala universitet, pp. 9–81.

Kearns, Gerry (1995), 'Tuberculosis and the medicalisation of British Society, 1880–1920', in John Woodward and Robert Jütte (eds), *Coping with Sickness: Historical Aspects of Health Care in a European Perspective*, Sheffield: European Association for the History of Medicine and Health Publications, pp. 147–70.

Kessler-Harris, Alice, Lewis, Jane and Wikander, Ulla (1995), 'Introduction', in Ulla Wikander, Alice Kessler-Harris and Jane Lewis (eds), *Protecting Women: Labor Legislation in Europe, the Unites States, and Australia, 1880–1920*, Urbana, IL: University of Illinois Press, pp. 1–27.

King, Nicholas B. (2004), 'The scale politics of emerging diseases', in Gregg Mitman, Michelle Murphy and Christopher Sellers (eds), *Landscapes of Exposure: Knowledge and Illness in Modern Environments/Osiris* **19**, pp. 62–76.

Klein, Rudolf (1995), *The New Politics of the National Health Service*, London: Longman.

Kock, Wolfram (ed.) (1963), *Medicinalväsendet i Sverige 1813–1962*, Stockholm: AB Nordiska Bokhandelns Förlag.

Kock, Wolfram (1963), 'Lasaretten och den slutna kroppsjukvården', in Wolfram Kock (ed.), *Medicinalväsendet i Sverige 1813–1962*, Stockholm: AB Nordiska Bokhandelns Förlag, pp. 158–242.

Koven, Seth and Michel, Sonya (1990), 'Womanly duties: maternalist politics and the origins of welfare states in France, Germany, Great Britain, and the United States, 1880–1920', *American Historical Review* **95** (4), October, pp. 1,076–108.

Koven, Seth and Michel, Sonya (1993a), 'Introduction: "mother worlds"', in Seth Koven and Sonya Michel (eds), *Mothers of a New World: Maternalist Politics and the Origins of Welfare States,* New York: Routledge, pp. 1–42.

Koven, Seth and Michel, Sonya (eds) (1993b), *Mothers of a New World: Maternalist Politics and the Origins of Welfare States*, New York: Routledge.

Ladd-Taylor, Molly and Umansky, Lauri (1998), 'Introduction', in Molly Ladd-Taylor and Lauri Umansky (eds), *'Bad' Mothers: The Politics of Blame in Twentieth-century America*, New York: New York University Press, pp. 1–28.

Larkin, Gerald (1983), *Occupational Monopoly and Modern Medicine*, London: Tavistock Publications.

Latour, Bruno (1988), *The Pasteurization of France*, Cambridge MA: Harvard University Press.

Law, C.M. (1967), 'The growth of urban population in England and Wales, 1801–1911', *Transactions of the Institute of British Geographers* 41, pp. 125–43.

Lawrence, Christopher (1985), 'Incommunicable knowledge: science, technology and the clinical art in Britain 1850–1914', *Journal of Contemporary History* **20** (4), pp. 503–20.

Lawrence, Christopher (1994), *Medicine in the Making of Modern Britain, 1700–1920*, London: Routledge.

Lee, Roger (1988), 'Uneven zenith: towards a geography of the high period of municipal medicine in England and Wales', *Journal of Historical Geography* **14** (3), July, pp. 260–80.

Levin, Hjördis (1997), *Kvinnorna på barrikaden: Sexualpolitik och sociala frågor 1923–36,* Stockholm: Carlssons.

Lewis, Jane (1980), *The Politics of Motherhood: Child and Maternal Welfare in England, 1900–1939,* London: Croom Helm.

Lewis, Jane (1984), *Women in England 1870–1950: Sexual Divisions and Social Change,* London: Harvester Wheatsheaf.

Lewis, Jane (1986), *What Price Community Medicine? The Philosophy, Practice and the Politics of Public Health since 1919,* Brighton: Wheatsheaf Books.

Lewis, Jane (1992a), 'Gender and the development of welfare regimes', *Journal of European Social Policy* **2** (3), pp. 159–73.

Lewis, Jane (1992b), 'Providers, "consumers", the state and the delivery of health-care services in twentieth-century Britain', in Andrew Wear (ed.), *Medicine in Society: Historical Essays,* Cambridge: Cambridge University Press, pp. 317–45.

Lewis, Jane (1992c), *Women in Britain since 1945: Women, Family, Work and the State in the Post-war Years,* Oxford: Blackwell.

Lewis, Jane and Rose, Sonya O. (1995), '"Let England blush": protective labor legislation, 1820–1914', in Ulla Wikander, Alice Kessler-Harris and Jane Lewis (eds), *Protecting Women: Labor Legislation in Europe, the Unites States, and Australia, 1880–1920,* Urbana, IL: University of Illinois Press, pp. 91–124.

Lewis, Jane and Welshman, John (1997), 'The issue of never-married motherhood in Britain, 1920–70', *Social History of Medicine* **10** (3), December, pp. 401–18.

Løkke, Anne (1995), 'No difference without a cause: infant mortality rates as a world view generator', *Scandinavian Journal of History* **20** (2), pp. 75–96.

Lönnroth, Gudrun (1984), 'Stadsbilden – praktfulla palats och usla kåkar', in *För hundra år sedan – skildringar från Göteborgs 1880-tal,* Göteborg: Göteborgs historiska museum, pp. 26–62.

Loudon, Irvine (1992), *Death in Childbirth: An International Study of Maternal Care and Maternal Mortality 1800–1950,* Oxford: Clarendon Press.

Luckin, Bill (1990), *Questions of Power: Electricity and Environment in Inter-war Britain,* Manchester: Manchester University Press.

Lundberg, Anna (1999), *Care and Coercion: Medical Knowledge, Social Policy and Patients with Venereal Disease in Sweden 1785–1903,* Umeå: Umeå University.

Lundén, Inga-Lisa (1970), 'Från mjölkdroppe till barnavårdscentral – historik och utveckling', *Tidskrift för Sveriges sjuksköterskor* **37**, pp. 198–201.

Lundquist, John (1963), 'Tuberkulosen', in Wolfram Kock (ed.), *Medicinalväsendet i Sverige 1913–1962,* Stockholm: AB Nordiska Bokhandelns Förlag, pp. 381–404.

Lundquist, Tommie (1982), *Den disciplinerade dubbelmoralen: Studier i den reglementerade prostitutionens historia i Sverige 1859–1918,* Göteborg: Göteborgs universitet.

Lupton, Deborah (1995), *Medicine as Culture: Illness, Disease and the Body in Western Societies,* London: Sage Publications.

MacKenzie, Donald A. (1981), *Statistics in Britain, 1865–1930: The Social Construction of Scientific Knowledge*, Edinburgh: Edinburg University Press.

Marks, Lara V. (1994), *Model Mothers: Jewish Mothers and Maternity Provision in East London, 1870–1939*, Oxford: Clarendon Press.

Marks, Lara (1996), *Metropolitan Maternity: Maternal and Infant Welfare Services in Early Twentieth Century London*, Amsterdam: Editions Rodopi.

Marland, Hilary (1993), 'A pioneer in infant welfare: the Huddersfield scheme 1903–1920', *Social History of Medicine* **6** (1), April, pp. 25–50.

Marshall, R.J. (1993), 'Town planning in Sheffield', in Clyde Binfield et al. (eds), *The History of the City of Sheffield 1843–1993, Volume II: Society*, Sheffield: Sheffield Academic Press, pp. 17–32.

Maver, Irene (1996), 'Glasgow's civic government', in W. Hamish Fraser and Irene Maver (eds), *Glasgow, Volume II: 1830 to 1912*, Manchester: Manchester University Press, pp. 441–85.

Maver, Irene (2000), 'The role and influence of Glasgow's municipal managers, 1890s–1930s', in Robert J. Morris and Richard H. Trainor (eds), *Urban Governance: Britain and Beyond Since 1750*, Aldershot: Ashgate, pp. 69–85.

Mayne, Alan (1993), *The Imagined Slum: Newspaper Representation in Three Cities 1870–1914*, Leicester: Leicester University Press.

McEwen, William (1970), 'Working-class Politics in Gothenburg, Sweden 1919–1934: A Study of a Social Democratic Party Local in an Industrial and Urban Setting' (unpublished PhD thesis, Case Western Reserve University).

McFarlane, Neil (1989), 'Hospitals, housing, and tuberculosis in Glasgow, 1911–51', *Social History of Medicine* **2** (1), April, pp. 59–85.

McKeown, Thomas (1976), *The Modern Rise of Population*, London: Edward Arnold.

McKeown, Thomas (1979), *The Role of Medicine: Dream, Mirage or Nemesis?*, Oxford: Basil Blackwell.

McNay, Lois (1992), *Foucault and Feminism: Power, Gender and the Self*, Cambridge: Polity Press.

Megill, Allan (1991), 'Introduction: four senses of objectivity', *Annals of Scholarship* **8** (3), pp. 301–20.

Mein Smith, Philippa and Frost, Lionel (1994), 'Suburbia and infant death in late nineteenth- and early twentieth-century Adelaide', *Urban History* **21** (2), August, pp. 251–72.

Meller, Helen (2001), *European Cities 1890–1930s: History, Culture and the Built Environment*, Chichester: John Wiley & Sons.

Millward, Robert and Bell, Frances (2001), 'Infant mortality in Victorian Britain: the mother as medium', *Economic History Review* **54** (4), pp. 699–733.

Mitchell, B.R. (1990), *British Historical Statistics*, Cambridge: Cambridge University Press.

Mitchell, B.R. (1992), *International Historical Statistics: Europe 1750–1988*, New York: Stockton Press.

Morris, R.J. (1976), *Cholera 1832: The Social Response to an Epidemic*, New York: Holmes & Meier Publishers.

Morris, R.J. (1992), 'The state, the elite and the market: the "visible hand" in the British industrial city system', in Herman Diederiks, Paul Hohenberg and Michael Wagenaar (eds), *Economic Policy in Europe Since the Late Middle Ages: The Visible Hand and the Fortune of Cities*, Leicester: Leicester University Press, pp. 177–99.

Morris, R.J. (2000), 'Governance: two centuries of urban growth', in Robert J. Morris and Richard H. Trainor (eds), *Urban Governance: Britain and Beyond Since 1750*, Aldershot: Ashgate, pp. 1–14.

Moscucci, Ornella (1993), *The Science of Woman: Gynaecology and Gender in England, 1800–1929*, Cambridge: Cambridge University Press.

Nelson, Marie Clark and Rogers, John (1992), 'The right to die? Anti-vaccination activity and the 1874 smallpox epidemic in Stockholm', *Social History of Medicine* **5** (3), December, pp. 369–88.

Nelson, Marie Clark and Rogers, John (1994), 'Cleaning up the cities: application of the first comprehensive public health law in Sweden', *Scandinavian Journal of History* **19** (1), pp. 17–39.

Niemi, Marjaana (1999a), 'Challenging authorities' views: women and health in British and Swedish cities, 1900–1920', in Marjatta Hietala and Lars Nilsson (eds), *Women in Towns: The Social Position of European Urban Women in a Historical Context*, Stockholm: Stockholms universitet, pp. 125–42.

Niemi, Marjaana (1999b), 'In the public interest and for private gain: Finns' study trips abroad from the 16th to the 20th century', in Timo Tuomi et al. (eds), *En Route! Finnish architects' Studies Abroad*, Helsinki: Museum of Finnish Architecture, pp. 10–29.

Niemi, Marjaana (2000), 'Public health discourses in Birmingham and Gothenburg 1890–1920', in Sally Sheard and Helen Power (eds), *Body and City: A Cultural History of Urban Public Health*, Aldershot: Ashgate, pp. 123–42.

Niemi, Marjaana (2001), 'The "disappearance" of environmental problems: the refocusing of public health policies in British and Swedish cities, 1890–1920', in Christoph Bernhardt (ed.), *Environmental Problems in European Cities in the 19th and 20th Century*, Münster: Waxmann, pp. 121–41.

Nilsson, Hans (1994), *Mot bättre hälsa: Dödlighet och hälsoarbete i Linköping 1860–1894*, Linköping: Linköping Universitet.

Nilsson, Hans (1995), 'Hälsa och stadsrenhållning under 1800-talet', *Nordisk Arkitekturforskning* **8** (1), pp. 19–26.

Nilsson, Lars (1989), *Den urbana transitionen: Tätorterna i svensk samhällsomvandling 1800–1980*, Stockholm: Stadshistoriska institutet.

Norton, Bernhard (1981), 'Psychologists and class', in Charles Webster (ed.), *Biology, Medicine and Society 1840–1940*, Cambridge: Cambridge University Press, pp. 289–314.

Oakley, Ann (1997), *Man and Wife: Richard and Kay Titmuss: My Parents' Early Years*, London: Flamingo.

Öberg, Lars (1983), *Göteborgs Läkaresällskap: En historik*, Göteborg: Göteborgs läkaresällskap.

Ohlander, Ann-Sofie (1994), 'The invisible child? The struggle for a Social Democratic family policy in Sweden, 1900–1960s', in Gisela Bock and Pat Thane (eds), *Maternity and Gender Policies: Women and the Rise of the European Welfare States, 1880s–1950s*, London: Routledge, pp. 60–72.

Ohrlander, Kajsa (1992), *I barnens och nationens intresse: Socialliberal reformpolitik 1903–1930*, Stockholm: Stockholms universitet.

Olsson, Britt-Marie (1984), 'Stadens styrelse – ett upplyst fåvälde', in *För hundra år sedan – skildringar från Göteborgs 1880-tal*, Göteborg: Göteborgs historiska museum, pp. 227–40.

Olsson, Kent (1972), *Hushållsinkomst, inkomstfördelning och försörjningsbörda: En undersökning av vissa yrkesgrupper i Göteborg 1919–1960*, Göteborg: Göteborgs universitet.

Olsson, Kent (1996), *Göteborgs historia: Näringsliv och samhällsutveckling III: Från industristad till tjänstestad 1920–1995*, Stockholm: Nerenius & Santérus Förlag.

Olsson, Ulf (1970), *Lönepolitik och lönestruktur: Göteborgs verkstadsarbetare 1920–1949*, Göteborg: Göteborgs universitet.

Östberg, Kjell (1995), 'Män, kvinnor och kommunalpolitik under mellankrigstiden', in Marja Taussi Sjöberg and Tinne Vammen (eds), *På tröskeln till välfärden: Välgörenhetsformer och arenor i Norden 1800–1930*, Stockholm: Carlssons, pp. 202–26.

Pedersen, Susan (1995), *Family, Dependence, and the Origins of the Welfare State: Britain and France, 1914–1945*, Cambridge: Cambridge University Press.

Perkin, Harold (1990), *The Rise of Professional Society: England since 1880*, London: Routledge.

Pestre, Dominique (1997), 'Science, political power and the state', in John Krige and Dominique Pestre (eds), *Science in the Twentieth Century*, Amsterdam: Harwood Academic Publishers, pp. 61–75.

Peterson, M. Jeanne (1978), *The Medical Profession in Mid-Victorian London*, Berkeley, CA: University of California Press.

Pickstone, John V. (1985), *Medicine and Industrial Society: A History of Hospital Development in Manchester and Its Region 1752–1946*, Manchester: Manchester University Press.

Pickstone, John V. (1992a), 'Dearth, dirt and fever epidemics: rewriting the history of British "public health", 1780–1850', in Terence Ranger and Paul Slack (eds), *Epidemics and Ideas: Essays on the Historical Perception of Pestilence*, Cambridge: Cambridge University Press, pp. 125–48.

Pickstone, John V. (1992b), 'Introduction', in John V. Pickstone (ed.), *Medical Innovations in Historical Perpective*, London: Macmillan, pp. 1–16.

Pinker, Robert (1966), *English Hospital Statistics 1861–1938*, London: Heinemann.

Platt, Harold. L. (2004), '"Clever microbes": bacteriology and sanitary technology in Manchester and Chicago during the Progressive Age', in Gregg Mitman, Michelle Murphy and Christopher Sellers (eds), *Landscapes of Exposure: Knowledge and Illness in Modern Environments/Osiris* **19**, pp. 149–66.

Pomfret, David (2001), 'The city of evil and the great outdoors: the modern health movement and the urban young, 1918–40', *Urban History* **28** (3), December, pp. 405–27.

Pooler, H.W. (1948), *My Life in General Practice*, London: Christopher Johnson Publishers.

Pooley, Colin G. (1989), 'Working-class housing in European cities since 1850', in Richard Lawton (ed.), *The Rise and Fall of Great Cities: Aspects of Urbanization in the Western World*, London: Belhaven Press, pp. 125–43.

Pooley, Colin G. (1992), 'England and Wales', in Colin G. Pooley (ed.), *Housing Strategies in Europe, 1880–1930*, Leicester: Leicester University Press, pp. 73–104.

Poovey, Mary (1988), *Uneven Developments: The Ideological Work of Gender in Mid-Victorian England*, Chicago, IL: University of Chicago Press.

Poovey, Mary (1993), 'Curing the "social body" in 1832: James Phillips Kay and the Irish in Manchester', *Gender & History* **5** (2), Summer, pp. 196–211.

Porter, Dorothy (1991), 'Stratification and its discontents: professionalization and conflict in the British public health service', in Elizabeth Fee and Roy M. Acheson (eds), *A History of Education in Public Health: Health that Mocks the Doctors' Rules*, Oxford: Oxford University Press, pp. 83–113.

Porter, Dorothy and Porter, Roy (1988), 'The politics of prevention: anti-vaccinationism and public health in nineteenth-century England', *Medical History* **32**, pp. 231–52.

Porter, Theodore M. (1995), *Trust in Numbers: The Pursuit of Objectivity in Science and Public Life*, Princeton, NJ: Princeton University Press.

Porter, Theodore M. (1997), 'The management of society by numbers', in John Krige and Dominique Pestre (eds), *Science in the Twentieth Century*, Amsterdam: Harwood Academic Publishers, pp. 97–110.

Poulain, Michel and Tabutin, Dominique (1980), 'La mortalité aux jeunes âges en Europe et en Amérique du Nord du XIXe à nos jours', in Paul-Marie Boulanger and Dominique Tabutin (eds), *La mortalité des enfants dans le monde et dans l'histoire*, Liège: Ordina Editions, pp. 119–57.

Powell, Martin (1992), 'Hospital provision before the National Health Service: a geographical study of the 1945 hospital surveys', *Social History of Medicine* **5** (3), December, pp. 483–504.

Powell, Martin (1995), 'Did politics matter? Municipal public health expenditure in the 1930s', *Urban History* **22** (3), December, pp. 360–79.

Preston, Samuel H. and van de Walle, Etienne (1978), 'Urban French mortality in the nineteenth century', *Population Studies* **32** (2), pp. 275–97.

Prochaska, Frank K. (1980), *Women and Philanthropy in Nineteenth-century England*, Oxford: Clarendon Press.

Proctor, Robert N. (1991), *Value-free Science? Purity and Power in Modern Knowledge*, Cambridge, MA: Harvard University Press.

Proctor, Robert N. (1995), *Cancer Wars: How Politics Shapes What We Know and Don't Know About Cancer*, New York: Basic Books.

Puranen, Britt-Inger (1984), *Tuberkulos: En sjukdoms förekomst och dess orsaker: Sverige 1750–1980*, Umeå: Umeå universitet.

Purvis, June (1995), 'From "women worthies" to poststructuralism? Debate and controversy in women's history in Britain', in June Purvis (ed.), *Women's History: Britain, 1850–1945: An Introduction*, London: UCL Press, pp. 1–22.

Richardson, Ruth (1988), *Death, Dissection and the Destitute*, London: Penguin Books.

Riska, Elianne (1993), 'The medical profession in the Nordic countries', in Frederic W. Hafferty and John McKinlay (eds), *The Changing Medical Profession: An International Perspective*, New York: Oxford University Press, pp. 150–61.

Roberts, Elizabeth (1985), *A Woman's Place: An Oral History of Working-class Women 1890–1940*, Oxford: Blackwell.

Rodger, Richard (1989), *Housing in Urban Britain 1780–1914: Class, Capitalism and Construction*, London: Macmillan.

Rodger, Richard (1992), 'Managing the market – regulating the city: urban control in the nineteenth-century United Kingdom', in Herman Diederiks, Paul Hohenberg and Michael Wagenaar (eds), *Economic Policy in Europe since the Late Middle Ages: The Visible Hand and the Fortune of Cities*, Leicester: Leicester University Press, pp. 200–219.

Rodger, Richard (2000), 'Slums and suburbs: the persistence of residential apartheid', in Philip Waller (ed.), *The English Urban Landscape*, Oxford: Oxford University Press, pp. 233–68.

Rogers, John and Nelson, Marie Clark (1989), 'Controlling infectious diseases in ports: the importance of the military in central–local relations', in Marie C. Nelson and John Rogers (eds), *Urbanisation and the Epidemiological Transition*, Uppsala: Uppsala universitet, pp. 83–107.

Romlid, Christina (1998), *Makt, motstånd och förändring: Vårdens historia speglad genom det svenska barnmorskeväsendet 1663–1908*, Stockholm: Vårdförbundet.

Rosenberg, Charles E. (1989), 'Community and communities: the evolution of the American hospital', in Diana Elizabeth Long and Janet Golden (eds), *The American General Hospital: Communities and Social Contexts*, Ithaca, NY: Cornell University Press, pp. 3–17.

Rosenthal, Sol Roy (1980), 'The history of BCG in the United States as a tuberculosis vaccine', in Sol Roy Rosenthal (ed.), *BCG Vaccine: Tuberculosis – Cancer*, Littleton, MA: PSG Publishing.

Saegert, Susan (1980), 'Masculine cities and feminine suburbs: polarized ideas, contradictory realities', *Signs* **5** (3), Supplement, pp. 96–111.

Savage, Gail (1996), *The Social Construction of Expertise: The English Civil Service and Its Influence, 1919–1939*, Pittsburgh, PA: University of Pittsburgh Press.

Savage, Mike (1988), 'Trade unionism, sex segregation, and the state: women's employment in "new industries" in inter-war Britain', *Social History* **13** (2), pp. 209–30.

Savage, Mike and Warde, Alan (1993), *Urban Sociology, Capitalism and Modernity*, London: Macmillan.

Schiebinger, Londa (1994), *Nature's Body: Sexual Politics and the Making of Modern Science*, London: Pandora.

Schönbeck, Gun (1991), *Victor von Gegerfelt – arkitekt i Göteborg: En yrkesman och hans verksamhetsfält 1841–1896*, Göteborg: Göteborgs Universitet.

Scott, Joan Wallach (1988), *Gender and the Politics of History*, New York: Columbia University Press.

Scott, Joan Wallach (1996), *Only Paradoxes to Offer: French Feminist and the Rights of Man*, Cambridge, MA: Harvard University Press.

Searle, G.R. (1971), *The Quest for National Efficiency: A Study in British Politics and Political Thought, 1899–1914*, Oxford: Basil Blackwell.

Searle, G.R. (1981), 'Eugenics and class', in Charles Webster (ed.), *Biology, Medicine and Society 1840–1940*, Cambridge: Cambridge University Press, pp. 217–42.

Sears, Alan (1992), '"To teach them how to live": the politics of public health from tuberculosis to AIDS', *Journal of Historical Sociology* **5** (1), pp. 61–83.

Sellers, Christopher (2004), 'The artificial nature of fluoridated water: between nations, knowledge, and material flows', in Gregg Mitman, Michelle Murphy and Christopher Sellers (eds), *Landscapes of Exposure: Knowledge and Illness in Modern Environments/Osiris* **19**, pp. 182–200.

Shaw, Clifford (1993), 'Aspects of public health', in Clyde Binfield et al. (eds), *The History of the City of Sheffield, 1843–1993, Volume II: Society*, Sheffield: Sheffield Academic Press, pp. 100–117.

Shortt, S.E.D. (1983), 'Physicians, science, and status: issues in the professionalization of Anglo-American medicine in the nineteenth century', *Medical History* **27**, pp. 51–68.

Sigsworth, Michael and Worboys, Michael (1994), 'The public's view of public health in mid-Victorian Britain', *Urban History* **21** (2), August, pp. 237–50.

Silbey, David (2004), 'Bodies and cultures collide: enlistment, the medical exam, and the British working class, 1914–1916', *Social History of Medicine* **17** (1), April, pp. 61–76.

Skarin Frykman, Birgitta (1990), *Arbetarkultur – Göteborg 1890*, Göteborg: Etnologiska föreningen i Västsverige.

Sklar, Kathryn Kish, Schuler, Anja and Strasser, Susan (eds) (1998), *Social Justice Feminists in the United States and Germany: A Dialogue in Documents, 1885–1933*, Ithaca, NY: Cornell University Press.

Skocpol, Theda (1985), 'Bringing the state back in: strategies of analysis in current research', in Peter B. Evans, Dietrich Rueschemeyer and Theda Skocpol (eds), *Bringing the State Back In*, Cambridge: Cambridge University Press, pp. 3–37.

Skocpol, Theda (1992), *Protecting Soldiers and Mothers: The Political Origins of Social Policy in the United States*, Cambridge, MA: The Belknap Press of Harvard University Press.

Smart, Carol (1992), 'Disruptive bodies and unruly sex: the regulation of reproduction and sexuality in the nineteenth century', in Carol Smart (ed.), *Regulating Womanhood: Historical Essays on Marriage, Motherhood and Sexuality*, London: Routledge, pp. 7–32.

Smith, Barbara M.D. (1964), 'Industry and trade 1880–1960', in W.B. Stephens (ed.), *A History of the County of Warwick, Volume VII: The City of Birmingham*, London: Oxford University Press.

Smith, Bonnie (1981), *Ladies of the Leisure Class: The Bourgeoisie of Northern France in the Nineteenth Century*, Princeton, NJ: Princeton University Press.

Smith, Dennis (1982), *Conflict and Compromise: Class Formation in English Society 1830–1914: A Comparative Study of Birmingham and Sheffield*, London: Routledge & Kegan Paul.

Smith F.B. (1988), *The Retreat of Tuberculosis 1850–1950*, London: Croom Helm.

Smith F.B. (1990), *The People's Health 1830–1910*, London: Weidenfeld and Nicolson.

Smith, Roger (1992), *Inhibition: History and Meaning in the Sciences of Mind and Brain*, Berkeley, CA: University of California Press.

Sommestad, Lena (1997), 'Welfare state attitudes to the male breadwinning system: the United States and Sweden in comparative perspective', in Angélique Janssens (ed.), *The Rise and Decline of the Male Breadwinner Family?/International Review of Social History* **42**, Supplement, pp. 153–74.

Starr, Paul and Immergut, Ellen (1987), 'Health care and the boundaries of politics', in Charles S. Maier (ed.), *Changing Boundaries of the Political: Essays on the Evolving Balance Between the State and Society, Public and Private in Europe*, Cambridge: Cambridge University Press, pp. 221–54.

Stenhammar, Ann-Marie, Ohrlander, Kajsa, Stark, Ulf and Söderlind, Ingrid (2001), *Mjölkdroppen – Filantropi, förmynderi eller samhällsansvar?*, Stockholm: Carlssons.

Ström, Justus (1963), 'Den förebyggande barnavården', in Wolfram Kock (ed.), *Medicinalväsendet i Sverige 1813–1962*, Stockholm: AB Nordiska Bokhandelns Förlag, pp. 528–35.

Strömberg, Thord (1992), 'Sweden', in Colin G. Pooley (ed.), *Housing Strategies in Europe, 1880–1930*, Leicester: Leicester University Press, pp. 11–39.

Sturdy, Steve (1992), 'The political economy of scientific medicine: science, education and the transformation of medical practice in Sheffield, 1890–1922', *Medical History* **36**, pp. 125–59.

Sutcliffe, Anthony (1974a), 'A century of flats in Birmingham, 1875–1973', in Anthony Sutcliffe (ed.), *Multi-storey Living: The British Working-class Experience*, London: Croom Helm, pp. 181–206.

Sutcliffe, Anthony (1974b), 'Introduction', in Anthony Sutcliffe (ed.), *Multi-storey Living: The British Working-class Experience*, London: Croom Helm, pp. 1–18.

Sutcliffe, Anthony and Smith, Roger (1974), *History of Birmingham, Volume III: Birmingham 1939–1970*, Oxford: Oxford University Press.

Sutherland, Gillian (1981), 'Measuring intelligence: English local education authorities and mental testing 1919–1939', in Charles Webster (ed.), *Biology, Medicine and Society 1840–1940*, Cambridge: Cambridge University Press, pp. 315–35.

Szreter, Simon (1988), 'The importance of social intervention in Britain's mortality decline c. 1850–1914: a reinterpretation of the role of public health', *Social History of Medicine* **1** (1), April, pp. 1–37.

Szreter, Simon and Mooney, Graham (1998), 'Urbanization, mortality, and the standard of living debate: new estimates of the expectations of life at birth in nineteenth-century British cities', *Economic History Review* **51** (1), pp. 84–112.

Tesh, Sylvia (1981), 'Disease, causality and politics', *Journal of Health Politics, Policy and Law* **6** (3), pp. 369–90.

Tesh, Sylvia (1988), *Hidden Arguments: Political Ideology and Disease Prevention Policy*, New Brunswick, NJ: Rutgers University Press.

Thane, Pat (1984), 'The working class and state "welfare" in Britain, 1880–1914', *The Historical Journal* **27** (4), pp. 877–900.

Thane, Pat (1990), *The Foundations of the Welfare State*, London: Longman.

Thane, Pat (1994), 'Visions of gender in the making of the British welfare state: the case of women in the British Labour Party and social policy, 1906–1945', in Gisela Bock and Pat Thane (eds), *Maternity and Gender Policies: Women and the Rise of the European Welfare States 1880s–1950s*, London: Routledge, pp. 93–118.

Thane, Pat (2003), 'What difference did the vote make? Women in public and private life in Britain since 1918', *Historical research* **76** (192), May, pp. 268–85.

Thane, Patricia M. (1993), 'Women in the British Labour Party and the construction of state welfare, 1906–1939', in Seth Koven and Sonya Michel (eds), *Mothers of a New World: Maternalist Politics and the Origins of Welfare States*, New York: Routledge, pp. 343–77.

Therborn, Göran (1989), *Borgarklass och byråkrati i Sverige: Anteckningar om en solskenshistoria*, Lund: Arkiv Förlag.

Thomson, Mathew (1998), *The Problem of Mental Deficiency: Eugenics, Democracy, and Social Policy in Britain, c.1870–1959*, Oxford: Clarendon Press.

Tiles, Mary (1987), 'A science of Mars or of Venus?', *Philosophy* **62**, July, pp. 293–306.

Topalov, Christian (1993), 'The city as *terra incognita*: Charles Booth's poverty survey and the people of London, 1886–1891', *Planning Perspectives* **8** (4), pp. 394–425.

Torstendahl, Rolf (1992), 'Engineers in Sweden and Britain 1820–1914: professionalisation and bureaucratisation in a comparative perspective', in Werner Conze and Jürgen Kocka (eds), *Bildungsbürgertum im 19. Jahrhundert. Teil I: Bildungssystem und Professionalisierung in internationalen Vergleichen*, Stuttgart: Klett-Cotta, pp. 543–60.

Vallgårda, Signild (1996), 'Hospitalization of deliveries: the change of place of birth in Denmark and Sweden from the late nineteenth century to 1970', *Medical History* **40**, pp. 173–96.

Vincent, David (1991), *Poor Citizens: The State and the Poor in Twentieth-century Britain*, London: Longman.

Waddington, Ivan (1984), *The Medical Profession in the Industrial Revolution*, Dublin: Gill and Macmillan.

Waddington, Ivan (1992), 'Medicine, the market and professional autonomy: some aspects of the professionalization of medicine', in Werner Conze and Jürgen Kocka (eds), *Bildungsbürgertum im 19. Jahrhundert, Teil I: Bildungssystem und Professionalisierung in internationalen Vergleichen*, Stuttgart: Klett-Cotta, pp. 388–416.

Wåhlstrand, Arne (1971), *Göteborgs Stadsfullmäktige, 1863–1962*, vol. III: *Stadsfullmäktige, stadens styrelser och förvaltningar*, Göteborg: Göteborgs stad.

Waitzkin, Howard (1989), 'A critical theory of medical discourse: ideology, social control, and the processing of social context in medical encounters', *Journal of Health and Social Behaviour* **30**, June, pp. 220–39.

Walker, Janet (1991), 'Interventions in families', in David Clark (ed.), *Marriage, Domestic Life and Social Change*, London: Routledge, pp. 188–213.

Walkowitz, Judith R. (1980), *Prostitution and Victorian Society: Women, Class, and the State*, Cambridge: Cambridge University Press.

Walkowitz, Judith R. (1992), *City of Dreadful Delight: Narratives of Sexual Danger in Late-Victorian London*, Chicago, IL: Chicago University Press.

Wallentin, Hans (1978), *Arbetslöshet och levnadsförhållanden i Göteborg under 1920-talet,* Göteborg: Göteborgs universitet.

Walton, W.S. (1956), 'The history of the Society of Medical Officers of Health 1856–1956', *Public Health* **69** (8), May, pp. 160–226.

Waterhouse, Rachel (1962), *Children in Hospital: A Hundred Years of Child Care in Birmingham*, London: Hutchinson.

Watts, D.G. (1964), 'Public health', in W.B. Stephens (ed.), *A History of the County of Warwick, Volume VII: The City of Birmingham*, London: Oxford University Press, pp. 339–50.

Weiner, Gena (1992), 'De "olydiga" mödrarna: konflikter om spädbarnsvård på en Mjölkdroppe', *Historisk Tidskrift* **112** (4), pp. 488–501.

Weir, Margaret and Skocpol, Theda (1985), 'State structures and the possibilities for "Keynesian" responses to the Great Depression in Sweden, Britain, and the United States', in Peter B. Evans, Dietrich Rueschemeyer and Theda Skocpol (eds), *Bringing the State Back In*, Cambridge: Cambridge University Press, pp. 107–63.

Wetterberg, Ola and Axelsson, Gunilla (1995), *Smutsguld och dödligt hot: Renhållning och återvinning i Göteborg, 1864–1930*, Göteborg: Göteborgs Renhållningsverk.

Williams, Naomi and Mooney, Graham (1994), 'Infant mortality in an "Age of Great Cities": London and the English provincial cities compared, c.1840–1910', *Continuity and Change* **9** (2), pp. 185–212.

Wilmot, Frances and Saul, Pauline (1998), *A Breath of Fresh Air: Birmingham's Open Air Schools 1911–1970*, Chichester: Phillimore.

Wilson, Elizabeth (1991), *The Sphinx in the City: Urban Life, the Control of Disorder, and Women*, London: Virago.

Witz, Anne (1992), *Professions and Patriarchy*, London: Routledge.

Wohl, Anthony S. (1984), *Endangered Lives: Public Health in Victorian Britain*, London: Methuen.

Woods, Robert (1978), 'Mortality and sanitary conditions in the "Best governed city in the world" – Birmingham, 1870–1910', *Journal of Historical Geography* **4** (1), pp. 35–56.

Woods, Robert, Watterson, P.A. and Woodward, J.H. (1988–89), 'The causes of rapid infant mortality decline in England and Wales, 1861–1921, Part I', *Population Studies* **42** (3), pp. 343–66, and 'Part II', *Population Studies* **43** (1), pp. 113–32.

Worboys, Michael (1992), 'The sanatorium treatment for consumption in Britain, 1890–1914', in John V. Pickstone (ed.), *Medical Innovations in Historical Perspective*, London: Macmillan, pp. 47–71.

Zacke, Brita (1971), *Koleraepidemien i Stockholm, 1834: En socialhistorisk studie*, Stockholm: Nordstedt.

Index

age relations 6, 148–52, 158
Ahlström, Nathalia 173
alcoholism 123, 156, *see also* drinking
Almquist, Ernst 118, 121
ambiguity of health policies 6, 22–3, 65–7, 76, 79, 81, 84–6, 90, 108–10, 116–18, 120–21, 129–30, 144, 149–50, 156–61, 187–8
antenatal care 98–9, 165
Ariès, Philippe 131
Armstrong, David 56
Atkins, Peter 75

baby-farmers 62
back-to-back houses 35–6, 38, 124, 157, 187
bacteriological solutions 58, 74, 115–116, 121, 130, 155–6
bacteriologists 58, 61, 69, 115, 146
BCG vaccine 144–8, 151–2, 155–6, 186
Britain
    health officials 2, 4–13, 23, 16–19, 23, 47–8, 52–6, 58–9, 61–4, 70, 113–18, 139, 148–50, 156, 182, 185–6, 188
    hospital provision 47, 53, 59
    public health legacies 47–8, 52–6, 58–9, 62
    public health legislation 11–12, 43, 52–6, 58–9, 77, 62–3, 91, 98, 143
British Medical Journal 38, 139
Birmingham
    city council 23–5, 28, 58, 70, 73, 92, 98–9, 139, 143, 146, 165–6, 168, 188
    death rates 4, 30, 36, 54, 68, *see also* infant, maternal and tuberculosis mortality rates
    economic structure 25–6, 41–3
    housing 28–9, 35–8, 69, 72, 74–5, 94, 123–5, 127–9, 157, 177, 187

    Housing Committee/ Department 1, 27, 74, 85, 177
    image 25, 68
    Maternity and Child Welfare Committee 93, 95, 97–9, 166–7
    party politics 23–5, 166–7, 177
    population 27, 29–30, 97
    Public Health Committee/ Department 1, 43, 58, 68–70, 73–4, 77, 79, 85, 91–4, 99, 109, 127, 129, 139–40, 143–4, 152, 155, 163–8, 176–7, 188
    unemployment 41–2
Birmingham Branch of the National Council of Women 168
Birmingham District Medical Women's Association 168
Birmingham Infants' Health Society 163–6, 169, 171
Birmingham Women's Co-operative Guild 166–7
Birmingham Women's Welfare Centre 167
birth control 17, 92–3, 167–8, 173
Booth, Charles 74
bottle-feeding 61, 73, 75, 87–8, 92, 99, 109, 163–4, 170–71, 184–6
Bournville, garden village 38
Bradford 98, 100
breast-feeding 63, 72–3, 77, 88, 106, 163–4, 170–71, 185
bronchitis 61–2, 71, 77, 81–2, 84–5, 114
Budin, Pierre 64

Cadbury family 95, 153
Calmette, Albert 146–8, 152
Canada 146
capitalism 5, 21, 55, 159, 172
Carlberg, Frigga 172
Carnegie Infant Welfare Institute, Birmingham 95
Cassie, Ethel 95, 108

central government grants 38, 57, 59, 94, 98, 135, 140, 152
central-local government relations 5, 48–9, 52–9, 77–8, 100, 135, 145–6
Chadwick, Edwin 54–5, 76
Chamberlain, Joseph 25, 138
chemotherapy 141
child care advisers 106
child maintenance 87, 102–103, 170, 172–3, 185
children 3, 22, 41, 43, 56, 62, 65, 71, 76–8, 92, 94, 106, 164, 167–8, 171–2, 177–8, 181, 184–6, 188
    access to medical care 74, 82–4, 97, 100–102, 108–109, 164
    illegitimate 44–5, 86–88, 100–103, 110, 172
    and poverty 76, 88, 103, 105, 110, 152, 170, 172
    pre-tuberculous 150–5, *see also* tuberculosis
    socialization of 81, 152
Children's Hospital, Birmingham 74
Children's Hospital, Gothenburg 83– 4, 101–102, 106, 146
cholera 49, 52, 54–5, 115
city councils 1–2, 13–18, 159, *see also* Birmingham, Gothenburg
city physicians 48, 51, 56, *see also* Gezelius, Karl
city planning 3, 27–8, 31–2, 124
civil servants 5, 48
class
    background of health care providers 9–11, 63, 90–91
    conflict 2, 6, 10, 66, 137, 178
    hierarchies, legitimation of 14–15, 21–2, 187
    and urban space 28–32, 35, 67, 90, 110, 118, 124–6, 182–3
    see also middle classes, working classes
collapse therapy 134
Collegium Medicum 48–9
colonies, for children 151
Contagious Diseases Act (1864), the repeal of 56
Contraceptives Act (1911) (Lex Hinke) 173
Cropwood open-air school 153–4

death at home/in institution 122–3, 131
death rates, *see* Birmingham, Gothenburg, and infant, maternal and tuberculosis mortality rates
democracy 15, 18
Denmark 108, 146, 174
discrimination
    of tubercular patients 132, 144, 175, 178
    see also unmarried mothers
Dixon, Godfrey (Chief Tuberculosis Officer for Birmingham) 144, 146, 148–9, 152, 155
doctor-patient relationship 100, 144
domestic science teachers 105
drinking 75, 92, 127–8, 184
Duncan, Jessie 70, 72, 75, 78, 91–2, 164

educational approach 75, 90–2, 95–6, 98, 100, 105–106, 108, 117, 129–30, 138–9, 142–3, 145, 155–6, 177, 186–7, *see also* environmental approach, medical approach
emigration 29, 40
Enander, Hilda 169, 172
environmental approach 38, 48, 53–5, 72, 80–81, 90–91, 117, 121, 187, *see also* educational approach, medical approach
environmental problems 27, 50–51, 68–9, 75, 97, 127, 129, 176–7, 182
Epidemic Act (1857) (*Epidemistadgan*) 49–50
epidemic diseases 12, 48–9, 52–6, 115
ethnic tensions 2, 5–6, 162

Fallows, J.A. 177
family 3, 5–6, 22, 60–7, 117, 118, 152, 183, 188
    division of labour within 28, 41, 76, 92, 103–104, 109–110, 184–6
    ideal/real 44–5, 67, 75, 79, 92, 99, 109–110, 124, 158, 164–5, 184–6
    male bread-winner model 6, 40–41, 43–4, 66–7, 76, 79, 108–110, 164–5, 184–6
    middle-class 28, 35, 38, 44–5, 51, 68, 79, 124

self-supporting/self-reliant 66–7, 73, 79, 108–110, 164–5, 184–6
working-class 32, 35, 38, 40–41, 44–5, 124–5
with a tubercular patient 121–4, 128, 130, 132, 136–7, 141–4, 146, 151–2, 155, 158
family planning, *see* birth control
fathers
absent/non-supporting 86–7, 90, 102, 170, 172–3, 185
negligent 75–6, 86–7, 103, 184–5
see also men
feminists 16, 19–21, 44, 159–62
financial assistance to mothers 72, 79, 168, 170–71
First World War 38, 45, 75, 92, 94, 141
flats 31–5, 52, 118–119, 121–5, 130, 136–8, 151, 157, 177–8, 187
Föreningen Barnavärn 169, 172
Föreningen Mjölkdroppen 102, 105, 169–71
foster care inspectors 169, 171–2
foster homes 86–8, 104, 151, 152, 155, 170, 172, 185–6
blamed for the high infant mortality 86, 88
supervision of 63, 88, 102–3
Foucault, Michel 160
France 76, 83, 162
BCG vaccine 146–8, 151–2
infant mortality 63–4, 66
tuberculosis 117, 119–121, 159
friendly societies 53, 140, 176,
Frykman, Jonas 160

garden cities 27, 31, 38
gender
concept of 20
conflicts 2, 6, 62, 66, 172, 178
inequality 5, 14, 20
roles 22, 76, 79, 86, 90, 104, 165, 168, 187
segregation of the labour market 39, 43, 87, 160, 187
General Board of Health 54
Germany 38, 51, 162
hospitals 50, 83, 174
infant mortality 66

town planning 27
tuberculosis 117, 139, 146, 152, 174
Gezelius, Karl (First City Physician for Gothenburg) 57–8, 82, 88, 114, 119, 123, 131–2, 169, 174–5, 188
Glasgow 25
congenital anomalies 61, 71, 81–2, 84
Gothenburg
Child Welfare Committee 102
city council 23–4, 34–5, 56–8, 83–7, 101–102, 105–106, 120–21, 136–7, 145, 152, 171, 174–5, 188
death rates 4, 30, 84, 186, *see also* infant, maternal and tuberculosis mortality rates
economic structure 26, 39–41, 87, 185
housing 31–5, 86, 101, 118–23, 125–6, 130–31, 136–8, 157, 176, 187
Housing Committee/Department 120, 137
image 26–7
party politics 23–4, 27, 34–5, 137, 172–5
population 29–31
Public Health Committee/ Department 1, 56–8, 82, 84–5, 102–4, 106, 132, 169–70, 172–3, 175, 188
unemployment in 39
Gothenburg Social Democratic women's group 172–3
Göthlin, Gösta (Chief Tuberculosis Officer for Gothenburg) 119–20, 123, 136–7, 144, 146
government intervention
in homes 22, 62, 73, 149–50, 118, 123, 129–30, 136, 143, 149–150, 156, 183
in the housing market 3, 22, 34–5, 38, 118–120, 123, 129, 137, 156–7, 187
in the labour market 103, 110, 160
in the medical market 3, 11–12, 22, 48, 73, 81, 90, 100, 102, 108–9, 188
Guérin, Camille 146–7

Habermas, Jürgen 188
Hamlin, Christopher 52

health authorities, conflicting roles of 2–3,
    6, 22, 65–6, 108–10, 116–18, 122,
    156–8
health visitors 43, 77, 90–7, 110, 143–4,
    163, 183
Hemmet för lungsotssjuka 130
Heyman, Elias 51
Hill, Alfred 36, 55, 68–9, 123–4, 177
hospitals
    children's 74, 82–5, 98–102, 108–9,
        146, 186
    general 50, 53, 57, 175
    isolation 49, 53
    maternity 74, 82–5, 97–102, 109, 152,
        163
    municipal 50, 53, 57, 82–5, 101–102,
        146, 166
    poor law/ workhouse infirmaries 50,
        53, 97
    special 50
    voluntary 9, 47, 53, 97, 100–101, 118
    see also sanatoria, tuberculosis hospitals
hospitalization
    advantages of 84–6, 122–3, 130
    of deliveries 83–4, 97, 101
    of tubercular patients 122–3, 130–31,
        143, 151, 175
    see also hospitals, sanatoria,
        tuberculosis hospitals
household management 41, 76, 105, 108
housing
    co-operative 34–5, 119–20, 137
    council/municipal 34–5, 38, 69, 94, 119,
        137
    company 34
    defective 17, 28–9, 31–2, 35, 36–8,
        51–2, 54, 72, 74–5, 86, 101,
        117–124, 127–9, 137, 157, 177,
        187
    overcrowded 32, 35–6, 101, 118–121,
        123, 137–8
    and sanitary provision 35–6, 52, 54, 69,
        75, 123–4
    shortage of 34, 38, 137–8, 177
    speculative/private 34, 38, 119–20, 137
    see also flats, terraces houses
housing inspection 121, 123, 130, 136–8
housing market 3, 22, 32, 35, 118–120, 123,
    129, 137, 156

housing policies 17, 34–6, 38, 69, 74, 86,
    94, 119–20, 124, 127, 129, 137–8,
    157
Hull 97

illegitimacy 44–5, 86–88, 99, 100, 102–103,
    110, 185
Illegitimate Children Act (1917) (Lagen om
    barn utom äktenskap) 103
illegitimate birth rate 44–5, 185
infant consultations 90–91, 94, 97–8
Infant Life Protection Act (1872) 62
infant mortality
    and artificial feeding 72, 74–5, 77, 86–8,
        92, 99, 109, 163, 170–71, 184–7
    and defective housing 72, 74–5
    and environmental problems 68, 72,
        79–81, 90–91, 97
    and fathers negligence 75–6, 86–7, 103,
        184–5
    and foster care 86–8, 185
    and gender roles 76–9, 86, 90, 109–110,
        165
    and illegitimacy 86–7, 99–100, 103, 185
    and lack of medical care/ advice 74, 78,
        82–4, 93, 97, 100, 109, 167–8,
        170–71, 173
    and maternal ignorance 76–8, 86–7,
        90–91, 105–106, 108, 164,
        184–5
    and milk supply 73, 75, 88–9, 107
    neonatal 61, 83, 98–9 and poor hygiene
        72–3, 75, 84, 86
    post-neonatal 61
    and poverty 71–2, 78, 81, 88, 90, 103,
        164–5, 170, 172, 181
    and women's employment 76–9, 86–8,
        92, 99, 104, 109, 159–60, 164,
        184
infant mortality rates 63, 66, 69, 71–2
    in Birmingham 67–9, 77–9, 93–4, 100,
        109, 111
    in Gothenburg 67, 79–81, 88, 102,
        110–111, 170
infant welfare centres 159
    in Birmingham 93, 94–8, 108, 165, 168
    in Gothenburg 106, 108, 169
    voluntary centres in Birmingham 163,
        165–6

infantile diarrhoea 61, 63, 68–72, 75, 81–2, 84–5, 87, 98, 186–7
Infectious Disease (Notification) Act (1889) 52
innovations 144–6
institutionalization, *see* hospitalization
international anti-tuberculosis movement 144–6, 174
international contacts 4, 26, 116–117, 144–5
    see also study trips
international infant welfare movement 63–4, 81, 83
international rivalry 65, 85, 116
isolation of the sick, *see* segregation

Journal of the American Medical Association 147

Karlsson, Lynn 159
Kingstanding, Birmingham 96–7
Kirby J. 38
Koch, Robert 114–5
Koven, Seth 161–2, 167

labour market, *see* gender, government intervention
Lancet 139
landlords 55, 72, 121, 137–8, 178
Lane-Claypon, Janet 70
Lawrence, Christopher 9
Leicester 100
Lidforss-af-Geijerstam, Gärda 169, 173
lifestyle theory of disease causation 108
Lilienberg, Albert 31
Lindman, Carl 80
Liverpool 25, 42, 49, 54, 69, 92, 97, 98
local economy, regulation of 3, 117, 156, 184–5, *see also* government intervention
Local Government Board 1, 54, 70, 78, 97
local government structures 47, 162, 178–9
London 24, 26, 69, 97–8

MacCallum, Alexandra 70, 78, 93
MacGonigle, G.C.M. 38
Macirone, Clara 93
Malmö 26, 80, 103, 172–3
malnourishment 75, 105, 119, 128, 130, 149, 155–6
Manchester 42, 69, 97–8, 163

Manchester Sanitary Association, the Ladies Branch of 163
Marks, Lara 24
Marland, Hilary 59
marriage bar 40, 43–4
maternal mortality rates 63, 83, 99
maternalism, the concept of 161–2
Maternity and Child Welfare Act (1918) 59, 98
maternity care
    institutional 82–4, 87, 97–101, 163
    the quality of 61, 73, 82–4, 97–101
    see also midwives
maternity leave 77, 104, 171
meals for mothers 98, 163–5, 171
mediation of urban conflicts 6, 10, 22–3, 116–18, 122, 161, 178
Medical Act (1858) 11
medical approach 82–6, 90, 97–102, 104, 109, 117, 130–5, 155–6, 169–170, 176, *see also* educational approach, environmental approach
medical care, access to 50, 52–3, 74, 79, 82–5, 90, 97–102, 105, 108–10, 131–5, 140–41, 143, 148, 151, 160, 164–5, 167
medical market 3, 11–12, 22, 48
medical officers of health 10–12, 17–18, 54, 58, *see also* Hill, Alfred; Robertson, John; Newsholme, H.P., and assistant MOHs Duncan, Jessie, MacCallum, Alexandra; Cassie, Ethel
medical knowledge, *see* scientific knowledge
medical practitioners
    female 12, 167–8, 171, 91
    general practitioners 10–12, 47, 61, 67, 71, 73, 90, 97, 100, 102, 108–109, 118, 176, 188
    hospital consultants 10, 47, *see also* medical officers of health, public health officers, first city physicians and tubeculosis officers
medical profession
    authority of 8–9, 12–13, 17, 47, 62, 64, 131, 134, 143, 152, 155–6, 169, 186, 188
    hierarchies within 8–11, 13, 188

interests of 8–13, 22, 67, 81, 100, 102, 109, 118, 156, 186, 188
and the state bureaucracy 11–13
status 7, 11, 22, 84–5, 109, 118, 135, 142
medicine, *see* science
men
  as policy makers 14, 20–21, 23–4, 166, 169, 178–9
  role in the family 20–21, 41, 43, 75–6, 79, 108–110, 165, 172, 184–5
  wages 40–3, 109
  work 3, 39–40, 42
Michel, Sonya 161–2, 167
middle classes
  and child care 71
  and family life 28, 32, 44–5, 71, 79, 108, 124, 184–5
  and health care 50, 71, 94, 108, 110, 140, 160, 173
  and housing 32, 35, 38, 51, 124, 156, 181
  and political power 15, 28, 51, 161, 166, 178–9, 186, 188
  and suburban migration/suburbs 28, 30, 38, 68, 90
  and women's organizations 162–9, 172
  and work 40, 43–4, 159
midwives 11, 73, 87, 108
  regulation of 48, 63
  training of 63, 97–8, 163
  untrained in Birmingham 71, 97
milk (cow's) 72–5, 88–9, 106, 107, 110, 169, 170–1, 187
milk depots 58, 73, 88–90, 92, 98, 105–107, 163–4, 169–71, 184
milk inspectors 107
milk shops 73, 89
Ministry of Health, Britain 70, 92–3, 100, 134, 148, 150, 152, 165, 167
Mooney, Graham 68
mothers
  biological 62
  Catholic 93
  with epilepsy 104, 110, 186
  feeble-minded 99, 104–105
  foster 88, 185, *see also* foster homes
  full-time 41, 86–7, 92, 108, 184–5
  with mental illness/deficiencies 99, 104, 110, 185–6
  single *see* unmarried mothers
  with tuberculosis 104–105, 110, 152, 158, 186
  working 41, 76–9, 87–8, 92, 99, 104, 108–110, 170–71, 184–5
mothers' clubs 94
Municipal Maternity Hospital, Gothenburg 82–4, 101

National Board of Health, Sweden 49, 57
National Conference on Infant Mortality (1906) 77
national efficiency movement 65, 68, 86, 116
National Insurance Act (1911) 12, 59
nationalism 5, 38, 65–6, 99, 110, 116, 145, 186–7
Nettlefold, John 27–8, 177
networking, *see* international contacts, study visits
Newman, George 70, 76
Newsholme, Arthur 70, 78
Newsholme, H.P. 93, 98–9, 146, 167
Norrköping 26, 80, 173
Notification of Births Act (1907) 91
notification of tuberculosis 58–9, 144
nurseries 87, 90, 92, 98, 104, 110, 169, 171–2, 185
Ny Tid 41, 174

obstetrics 81, 85
open-air schools 153–5
open-air treatment 132–4, 139
outpatient services 136, 143
overcrowding, *see* housing, tuberculosis

paediatrics 81, 85
Pasteur Institute 146
Pedersen, Susan 24
pneumonia 61–2, 71, 81–2, 84, 114
police 49, 51, 62, 64
pollution 3, 28, 128–9
poor
  and family life 67, 75–6, 86–8, 90–2, 103, 108–9, 183–6

and health care 74, 82–3, 90–2, 97–9,
  100–102, 109, 121–3, 130–3,
  135, 167, 170, 173–6, 186, *see
  also* poor law medical care
and infant/child care 72–3, 75–9, 86–92,
  97–9, 106, 108–110, 164–5,
  183–6
irresponsibility of 72, 75–9, 86–8, 92–3,
  99, 104, 123–4, 127–30, 165,
  168, 184–6
and lack of political power 15
and living conditions 29, 31–2, 35, 38,
  68, 71–2, 74–5, 90–1, 100–102,
  118–20, 123–9, 136–8, 157–8,
  176–7, 182–3
and poor hygiene 72, 75, 86, 90–91,
  123, 128, 156, 182–3
supervision of 91–2, 99, 102–106, 109–
  110, 129–30, 136–40, 142–4,
  149–50, 152, 168, 185–6
and unhealthy habits 75–6, 120, 123,
  127–9, 156, 177, 182–3
Poor Law Amendment Act (1834) 52
poor law authorities
  Birmingham 97, 99, 101–102, 109, 134,
    140, 144
  Gothenburg 87, 102, 131–2
Poor Law Commission 52
poor law medical care 50, 52–3, 56, 97, 99,
  101–102, 109, 131–2, 134, 140, 144
Porter, Theodore M. 9
post-natal care 99, 101
poverty and health 38, 47, 50, 52–3, 67–8,
  71–4, 77–9, 86, 88–90, 106, 108,
  117–119, 121, 128, 136–7, 157–9,
  164–5, 170, 174, 176, 181–3, 188
Powell, Martin 24
prematurity 61, 71, 82, 99
press 43, 62, 69–70, 73
Privy Council 54
Proctor, Robert N. 181
prostitution, regulation of 49, 56
  opposition to the regulation 50, 56
protests against health policies 17, 55–6
  by general practitioners 67, 73, 90, 100,
    102, 108–9, 188
  by tubercular patients 141–2
  by women 161, 166–8, 172–3, 178–9

by working-class organizations 173–8,
  179
see also vaccination, prostitution
public health
  and interests of the medical profession
    8–13, 22, 67, 81, 84–5, 100,
    102, 109, 118, 156, 186, 188
  and political pressures 1–7, 13–17,
    22–4, 27, 64–7, 70, 82, 90, 94,
    110, 113–117, 121, 136–7, 140,
    145, 156–61, 171–2, 178–9,
    181–8
Public Health Act (1848) 53–4
Public Health Act (1874)
  (Hälsovårdsstadgan) 51–2
public health legacies, *see* Britain, Sweden
public health officers 3, 5, 7–13, 16–18, 47,
  57–8, 64–5, 115, 117–18, 135, 139,
  142, 145–6, 150, 152, 178, 182, *see
  also* individual officers
Public Health (Tuberculosis) Act (1921) 59
pubs 127–8

Rawlinson, Robert 54
recession 29, 39, 41–2, 98
rickets 98, 155, 177
Robertson, John (MOH for Birmingham)
  27–8, 36, 58, 69–76, 78, 91–3, 115,
  124, 127–9, 139–40, 142–4, 146,
  163–4, 176–7
Rowntree, Seebohm 74
Royal Commission on the Poor Laws 91
  Minority Report of 165

St Helens 58, 92
Sällskapet för uppmuntran av öm och sedlig
  modersvård 168–9
Salterley Grange Sanatorium 140–1
sanatoria 57, 59, 102, 122, 132–6, 138–44,
  150, 152
sanitary reform/engineering 50–5, 68–9, 72,
  79–81, 90–91, 124–7
science/medicine
  confidence in 18–19, 64, 160
  criticism against 19–22, 140, 148
  as a source of authority 7–11, 13, 18,
    22, 57–8, 85, 95, 122, 140, 143,
    148, 152, 159, 186

Soviet 21, 175
scientific/medical knowledge 4, 7, 9–11,
    18–21, 65, 115, 149, 181–8
    as a legitimizer 1–3, 5–7, 15, 17–22, 64,
        66, 140–5, 148, 156, 184–8
    production/deployment of 5–6, 19–20,
        65, 156, 182, see also statistical
        knowledge
scientific techniques 5, 9–11, 13–14, 18,
    56, 116, 182, see also statistical
    techniques
Scott, Joan 20
segregation
    of the healthy and the sick 49, 53,
        121–2, 127, 129, 130–31, 135,
        138, 151–2, 155–6, 186
    spatial/residential 28–31, 110, 124–6,
        182–3
    see also class, gender
sex 17, 44
sexual difference 20–1
Sheffield 58, 69
Sjukvårdsanstalten å Kålltorp 132–3
Skocpol, Theda 24, 47
slums 17, 21, 28–9, 35, 54, 70–72, 74–5,
    85–6, 93–4, 108–109, 124, 127,
    157–8, 163, 183–5
    slum clearance 35, 74
social order
    and health policies 2–3, 10, 85, 91–2,
        99, 117, 122, 138–9, 156, 159
Society of Medical Officers of Health 17
Sommestad, Lena 40
spatial expressions
    of health problems/ solutions 93–6, 110,
        124–6, 182–3
    of urban inequality 28–31, 67
spitting, prohibition of 141
state bureaucracies 8, 11–13, 135
Statistical Bureau (Tabelverket) 48, 63
statistical knowledge 3, 5, 15, 18, 48, 63, 74
    differing interpretations of 77–8, 92,
        139–40, 142 ,147–8
    as a legitimizer 15, 18,140
statistical techniques 5, 18, 182
sterilization, in Sweden 104–105, 186
Stockholm 26, 35, 40, 44, 48, 49, 51, 80, 89,
    118, 149, 152, 169, 173

study trips 4, 27, 57, 78, 97–8, 108,
    116–17, 139, 144–6, 152, see also
    international contacts
Sturdy, Steven 10
suburbanization 28–30, 38, 124, 138
suburbs 27–8, 38, 71, 90, 93–4, 96–7,
    108–109, 123–5, 129, 183, 185
Sundhetskollegium 49
sunlight 121, 123
Sutcliffe, Anthony 35
Sweden
    health officials 2, 4–9, 11–13, 16–19,
        23, 47–52, 56–7, 61–4, 81, 104,
        109, 113–119, 135, 147–50, 182,
        185–6, 188
    hospital provision 47–50, 57, 100
    local government reform (1862–63) 51
    public health legacies 47–52, 56–8, 63, 85
    public health legislation 49–52, 56–7,
        63, 103–4, 173
Taylor Allen, Ann 167
terraced houses 35
Thane, Pat 16
trade unions 40–1, 43, 79, 87, 159, 166
tubercle bacillus 113–15, 117, 120–21, 123,
    127–8, 130, 146, 148, 152, 155–6,
    186
tubercular infection 113, 117, 120–22,
    142–4, 146, 149, 175
    breaking the chain of 105, 121–3, 135,
        140, 150–2
    building resistance to 127–9, 138–9,
        142–3, 150–1, 155, 187
tuberculin
    skin tests 148–9
    treatment 139, 146
tuberculosis (non-pulmonary) 82, 84, 114
tuberculosis (pulmonary)
    and children 121, 123, 131–2, 135, 143,
        145–55, 158, 184, 186
    and defective housing 117–131, 136–7,
        151, 156–7, 176–8, 181–2, 187
    and drinking 123, 127–8, 156
    and environmental problems 117, 127,
        129, 176–7
    and ignorance 122–3, 143–4

and lack of medical care 131–2, 155–6, 174–6,
and malnourishment 119, 128, 130, 149, 155–6
and overcrowding 118–20, 123, 128–9, 136–8, 157, 175, 187
and overwork 119, 130, 159
and poor hygiene 123, 128, 156
and poverty 117, 119, 136, 159, 176
and tubercle bacillus 113, 117, 120–21, 123, 127, 130, 146, 152, 155, 186–7
and unhealthy habits 117, 120, 127–9, 155, 177, 187
and workshop conditions 127–9
Tuberculosis Committee, governmental (Sweden) 115, 118–119, 122, 134
tuberculosis hospitals 57, 59, 121–2, 130–136, 139, 141–3, 150, 152, 155–7, 174–5, *see also* sanatoria
tuberculosis inspection 136, 143
tuberculosis mortality rates 119, 122, 135, 145
    Birmingham 114-116, 123–5, 156–7
    Gothenburg 114–116, 119, 125–6, 137, 156–7
typhus 52, 115

unemployment 39, 41–2
unhealthy areas 74, 90, 93, 110, 124–7, 144, 157, 182–4
United States of America 29, 145–6, 152, 155, 162
unmarried mothers 3, 40–1, 44–5, 86–8, 90, 102–3, 109, 172–3, 183
    stigmatization/discrimination of 99, 105, 109, 168, 185
    supervision of 103–104, 110, 170, 172–3, 185, 188
urban space, *see* class and urban space
urbanization, of Sweden 12

vaccination 49, 52, 144–8, 151-5
    opposition to 50, 56
Vaccination Act (1898) 56
Variot, Gaston 64
venereal diseases 49
Vincent, David 161

voluntary societies 58, 64, 72–3, 81, 86, 88, 91, 93–4, 104–5, 109–10, 155, 161–74, 176, 178–9,187–8, *see also* hospitals (voluntary)

Wallgren, Arvid 106, 146–7
wasting diseases 71, 82, 98
water closets 69, 79
water supply 36, 51–2, 54, 79, 124
welfare states 76, 161
Weoley Castle, Birmingham 97
widows 44
Williams, Naomi 68
Willesden 100
women
    difference from/equality with men 14–16, 161–2, 167–8, 173
    and health 17, 71, 74–5, 82–4, 93, 97–102, 104–105, 108–110, 143, 163–73, 186–7
    as policy makers 1, 14–16, 20–21, 161–73, 178–9
    professional 12, 43, 108, 163, 166–8, 169, 171–3, 178–9
    role in the family 20–22, 28, 44–5, 76, 79, 86–7, 108–110, 165, 172–3, 184–8, 187
    wages 40, 42–3, 103
    work 3, 39–44, 76–9, 87–8, 92, 103, 108–110, 159–160, 164, 168, 172–1
    see also mothers, unmarried mothers, widows
Women's Advisory Council of the Birmingham Labour Party 167
women's organizations 93, 159–160, 162–173, 178–9
Worboys, Michael 176
work ethic 3, 22
working classes
    difference between upper and lower 15, 28–9, 32, 35, 38, 47, 50, 52–3, 90, 93–4, 99, 108–110, 144, 157, 187
    and family life 32, 44–5, 124, 128, 184–5

and health care 50, 71, 93–4, 99–100,
    105, 108, 110, 140, 160, 173–4,
    176
and housing 32–6, 38, 101, 124, 137,
    156–7, 181
and infant care 71–3, 75–9
and organizations 36, 160, 167, 175–7
and political power 15, 24, 166, 178–9,
    186, 188

and suburban migration/suburbs 28–9,
    38, 90, 124, 129, 138, 185
and women's organizations 166–7,
    172–3, 177–8
and work 39–44, 62, 76, 159, 169
see also poor

Yardley Road Sanatorium 141